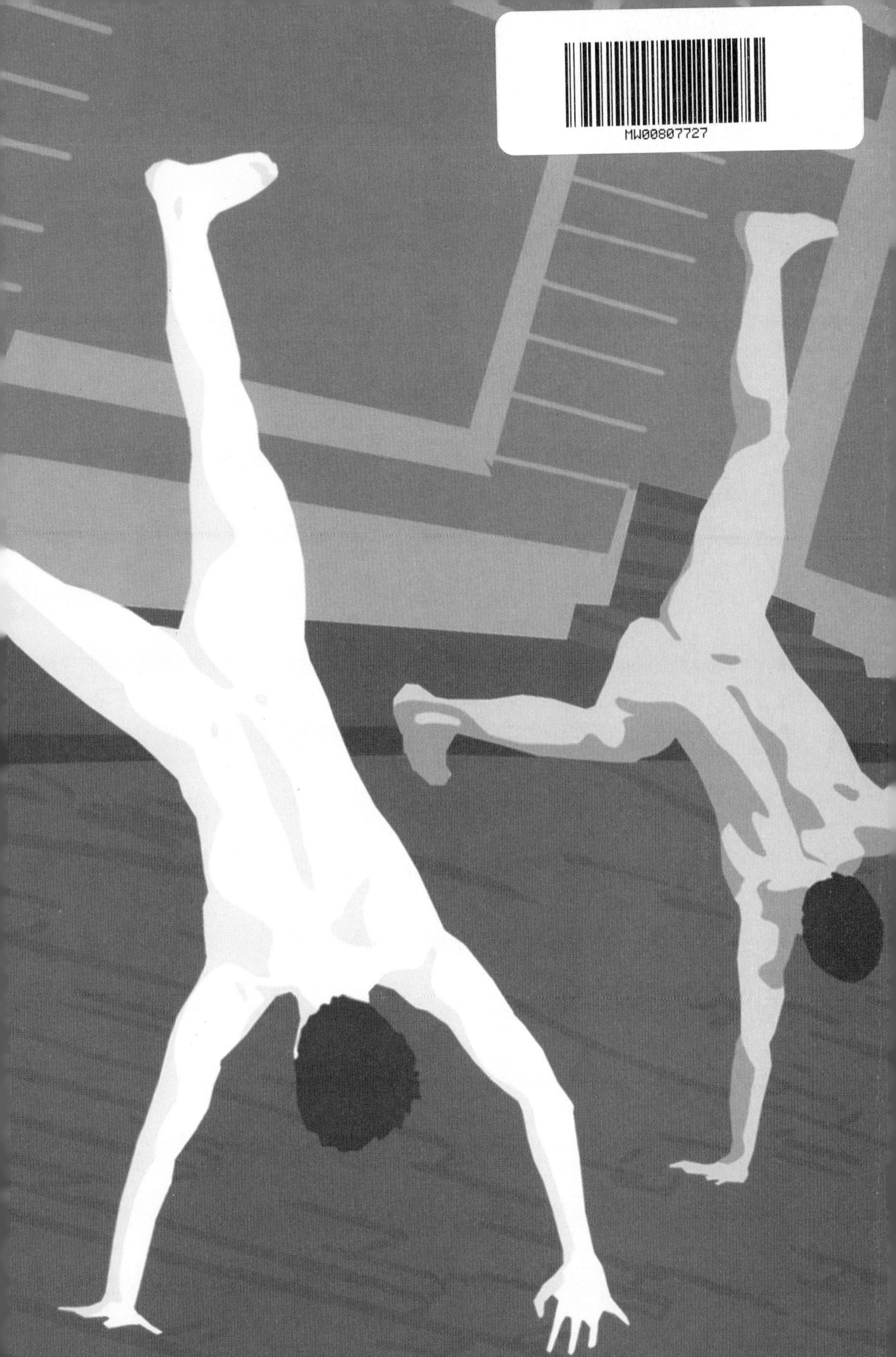

produced by man of action entertainment, los angeles, ca / new york, ny
published by image comics, portland, or

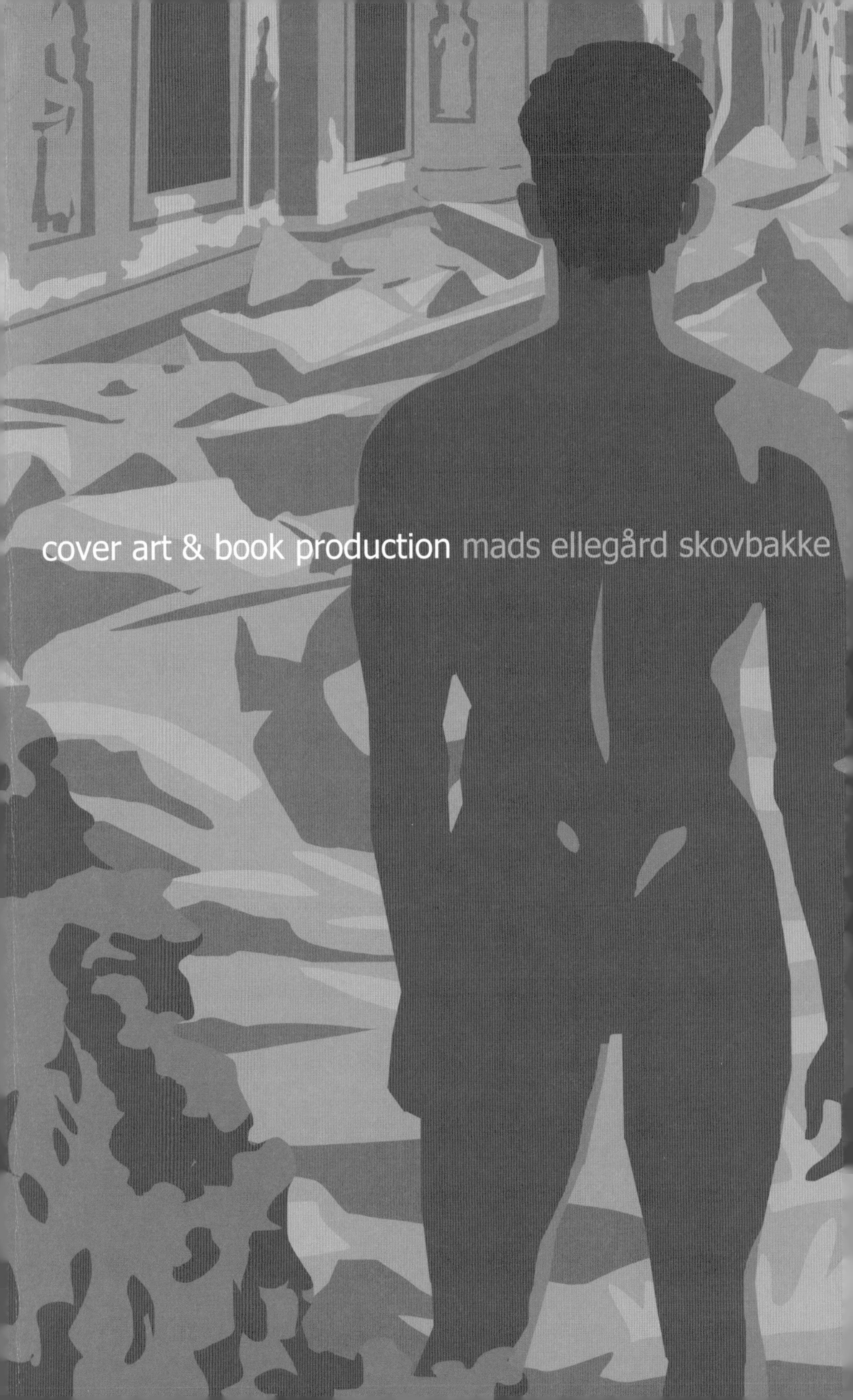
cover art & book production mads ellegård skovbakke

travel posters & design images

emei olivia burell

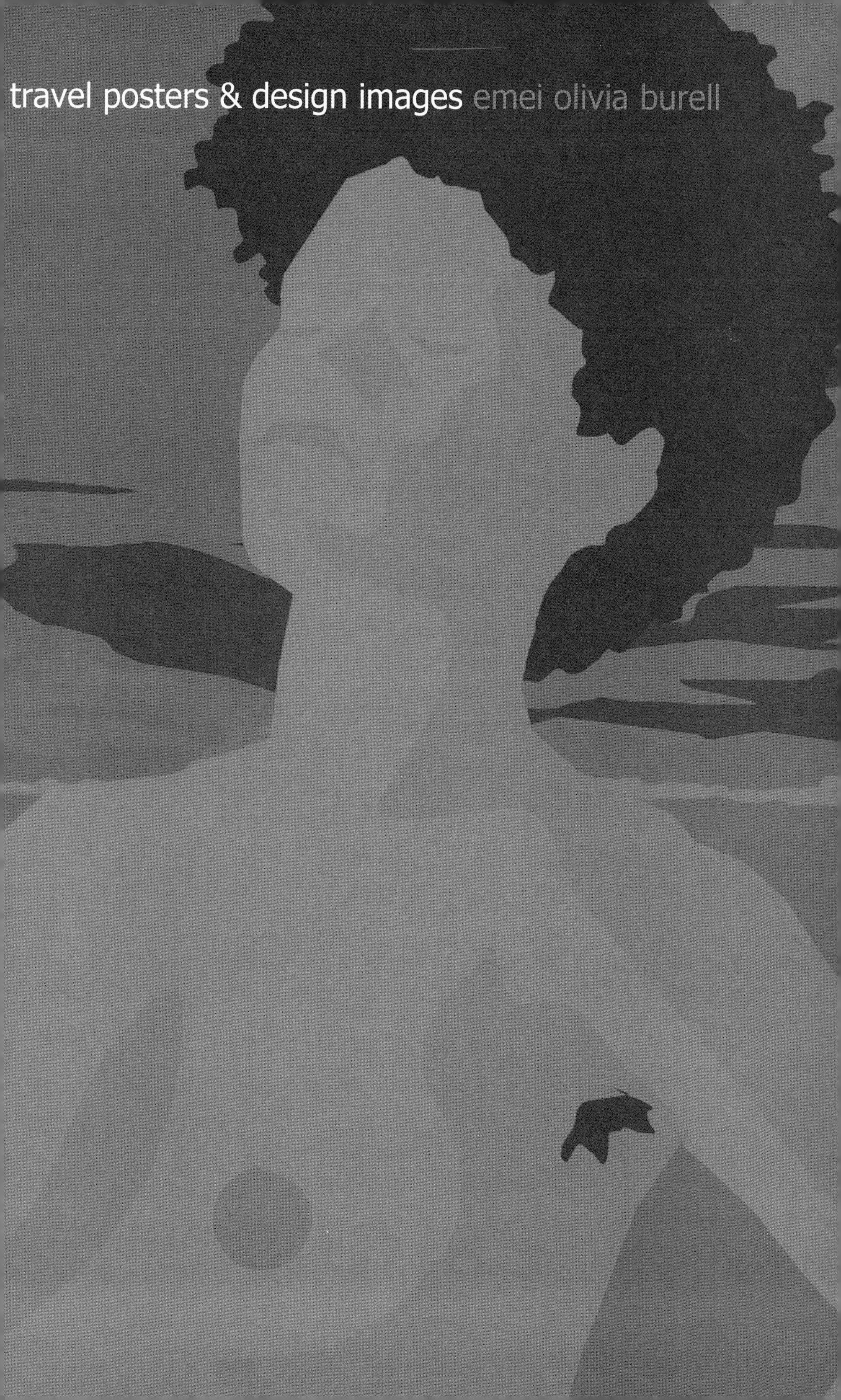

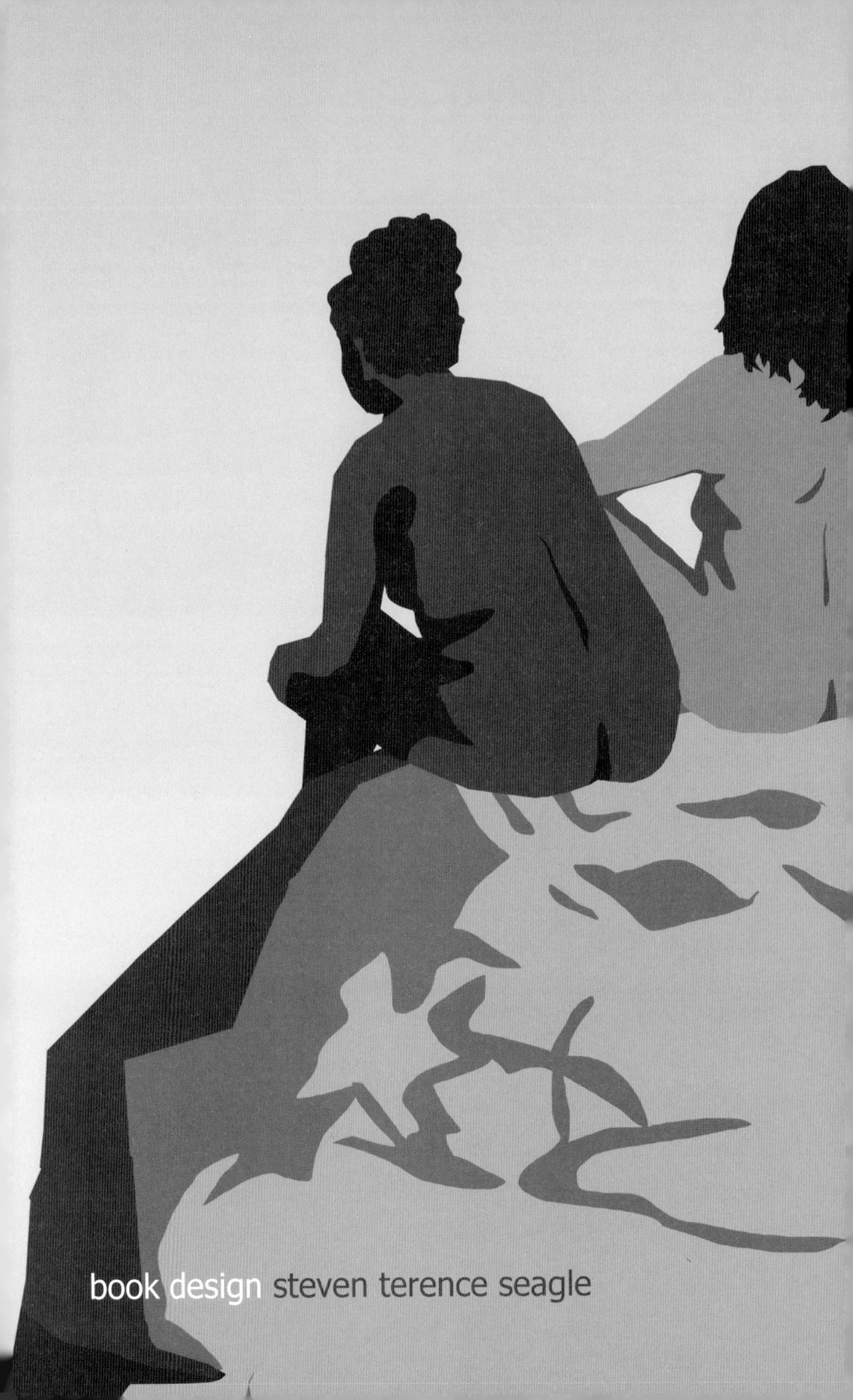
book design steven terence seagle

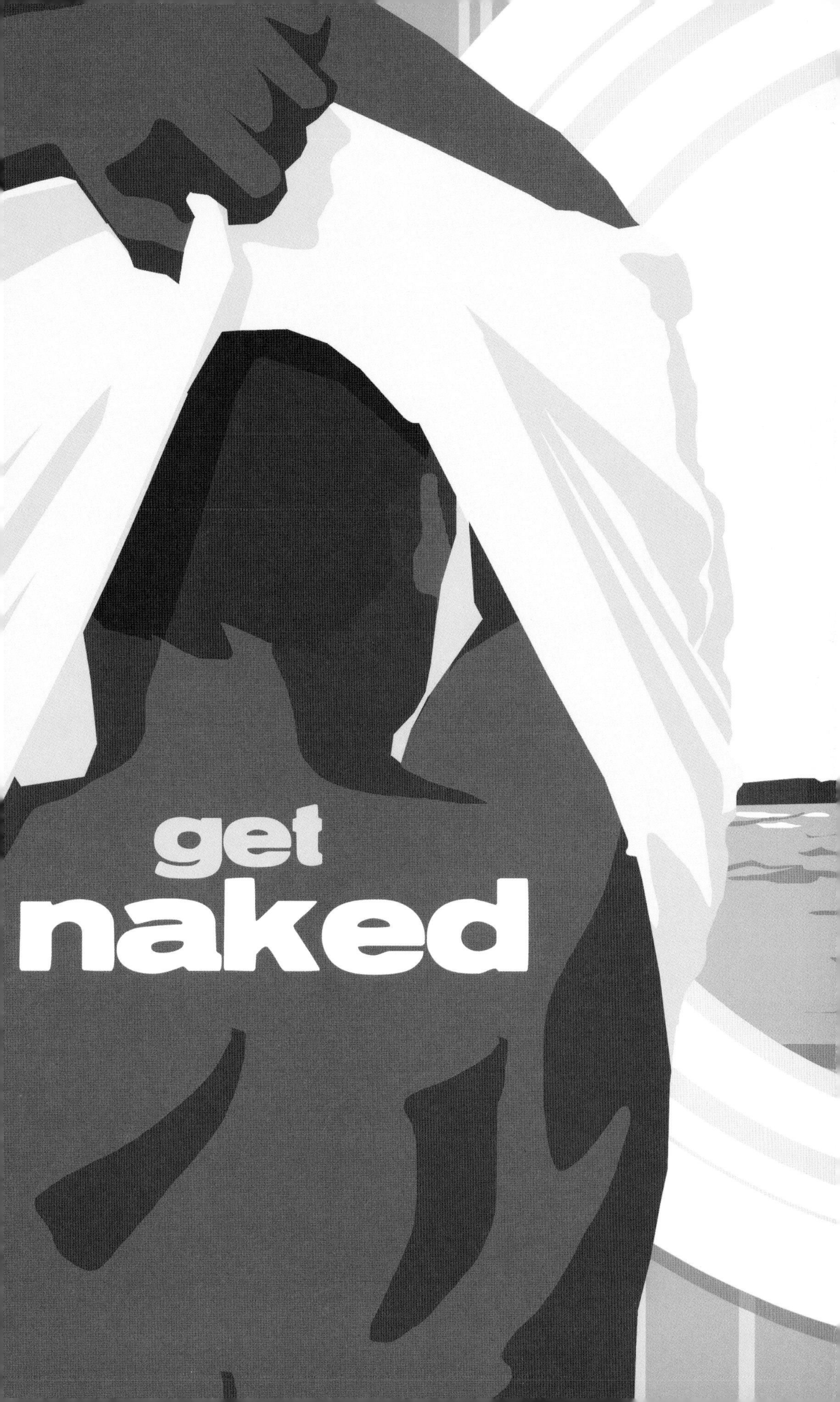
get
naked

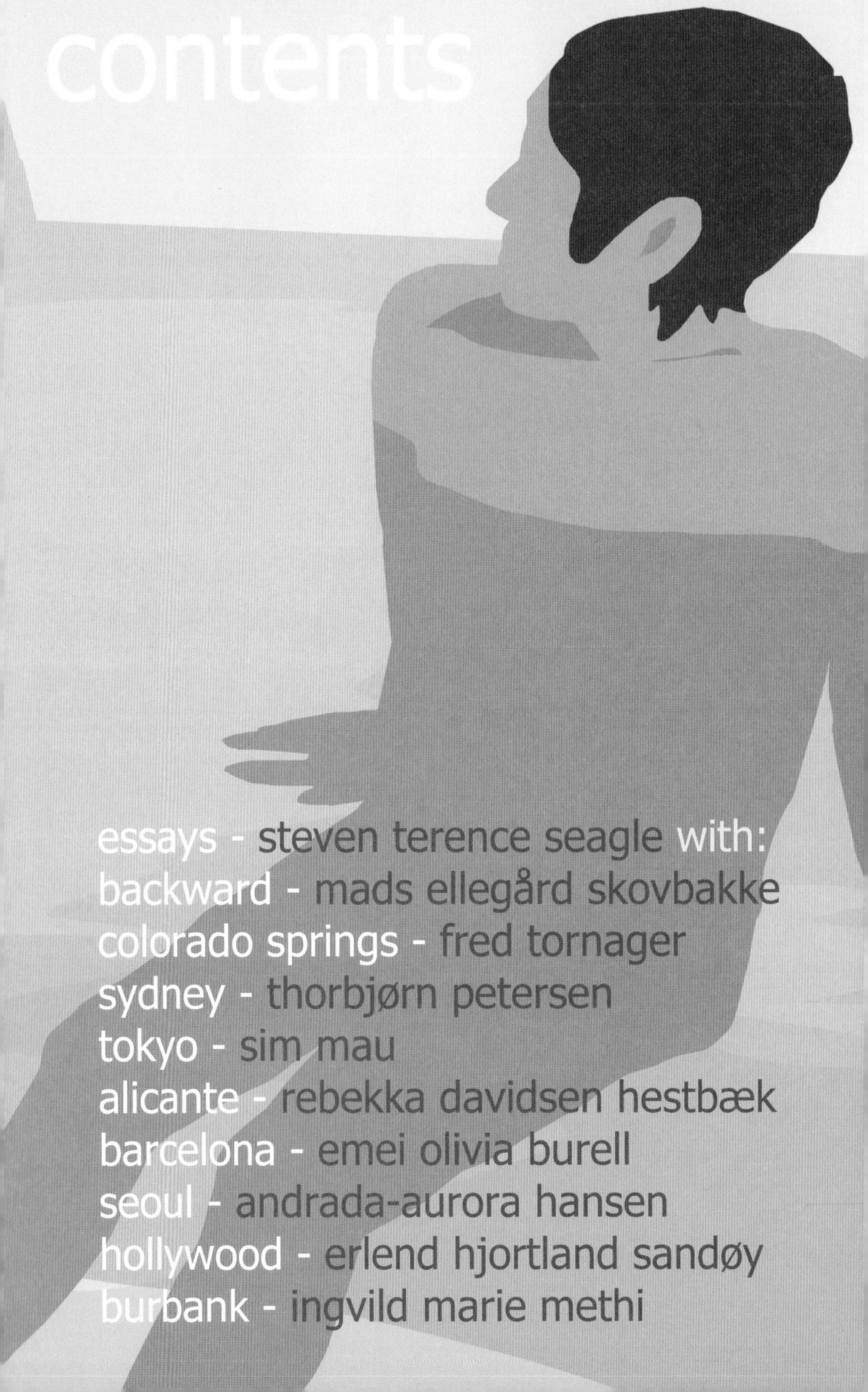

contents

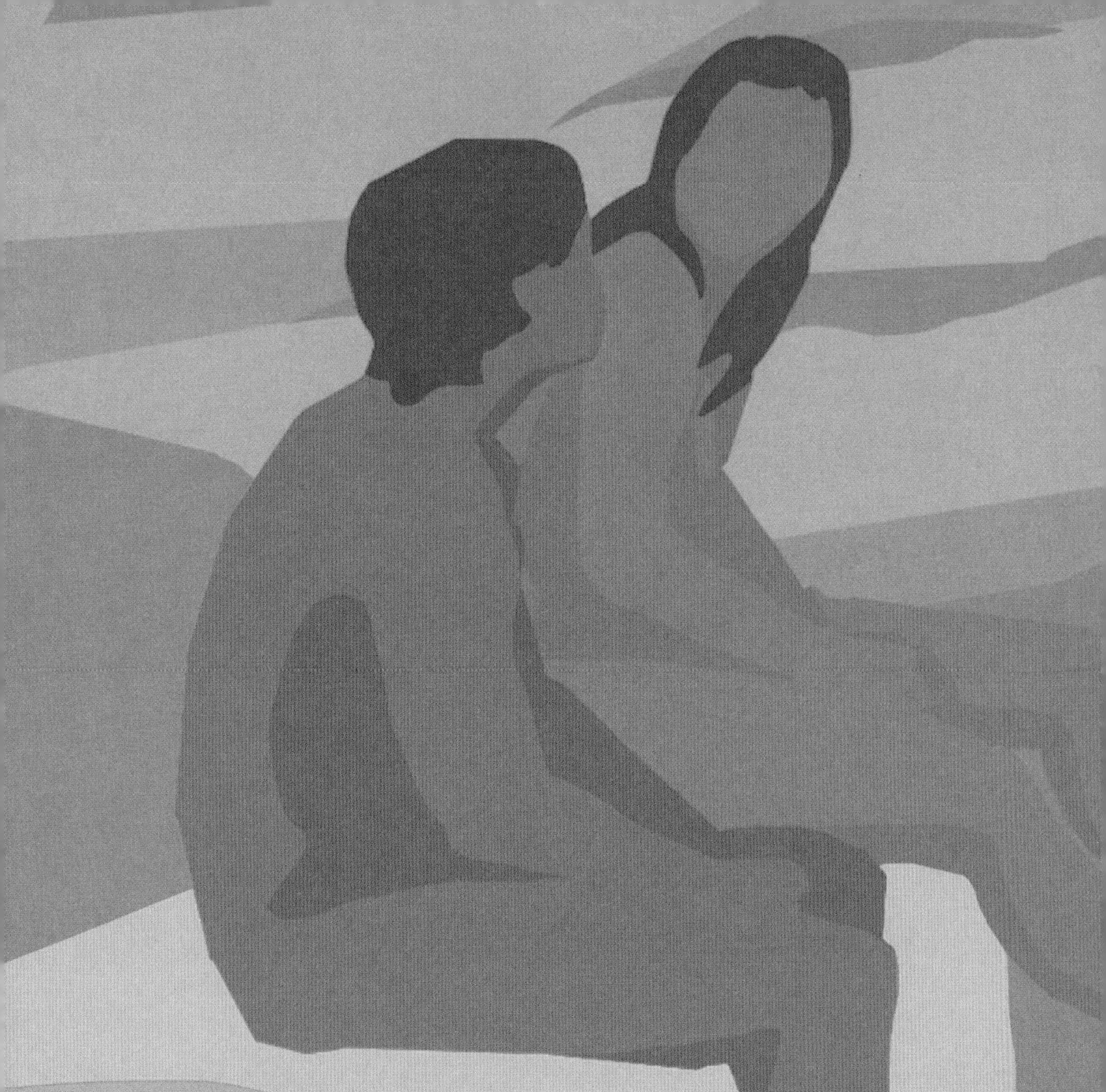

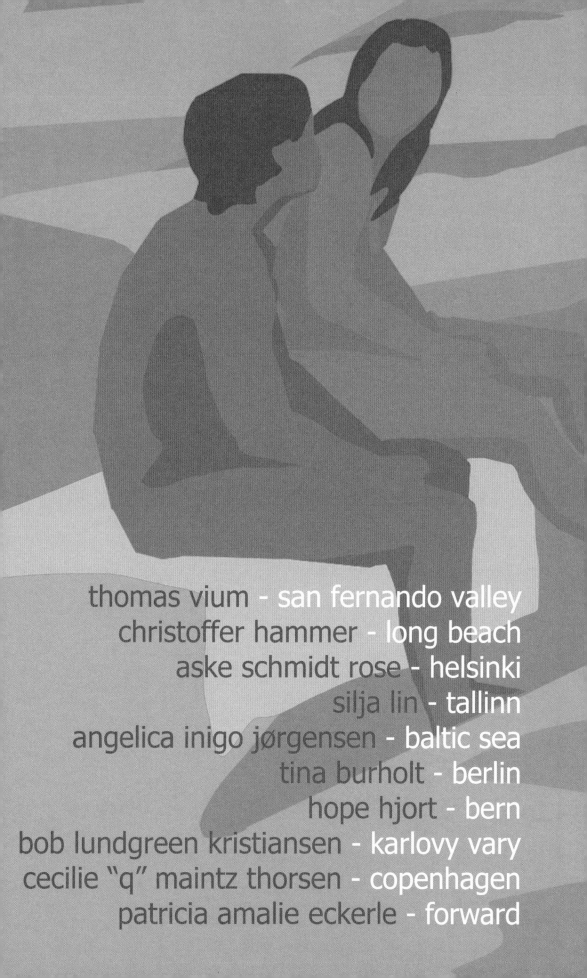

thomas vium - san fernando valley
christoffer hammer - long beach
aske schmidt rose - helsinki
silja lin - tallinn
angelica inigo jørgensen - baltic sea
tina burholt - berlin
hope hjort - bern
bob lundgreen kristiansen - karlovy vary
cecilie "q" maintz thorsen - copenhagen
patricia amalie eckerle - forward

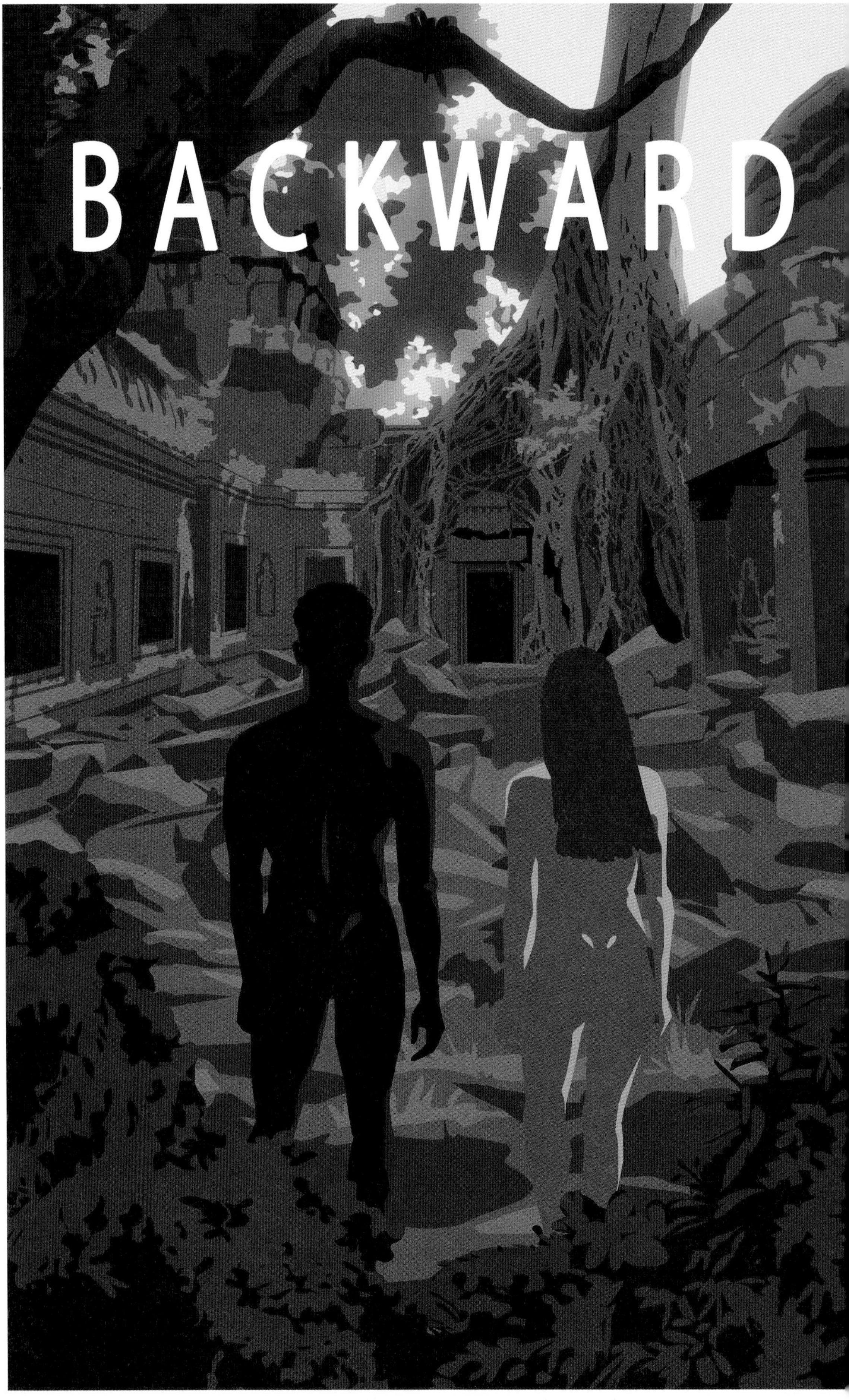
BACKWARD

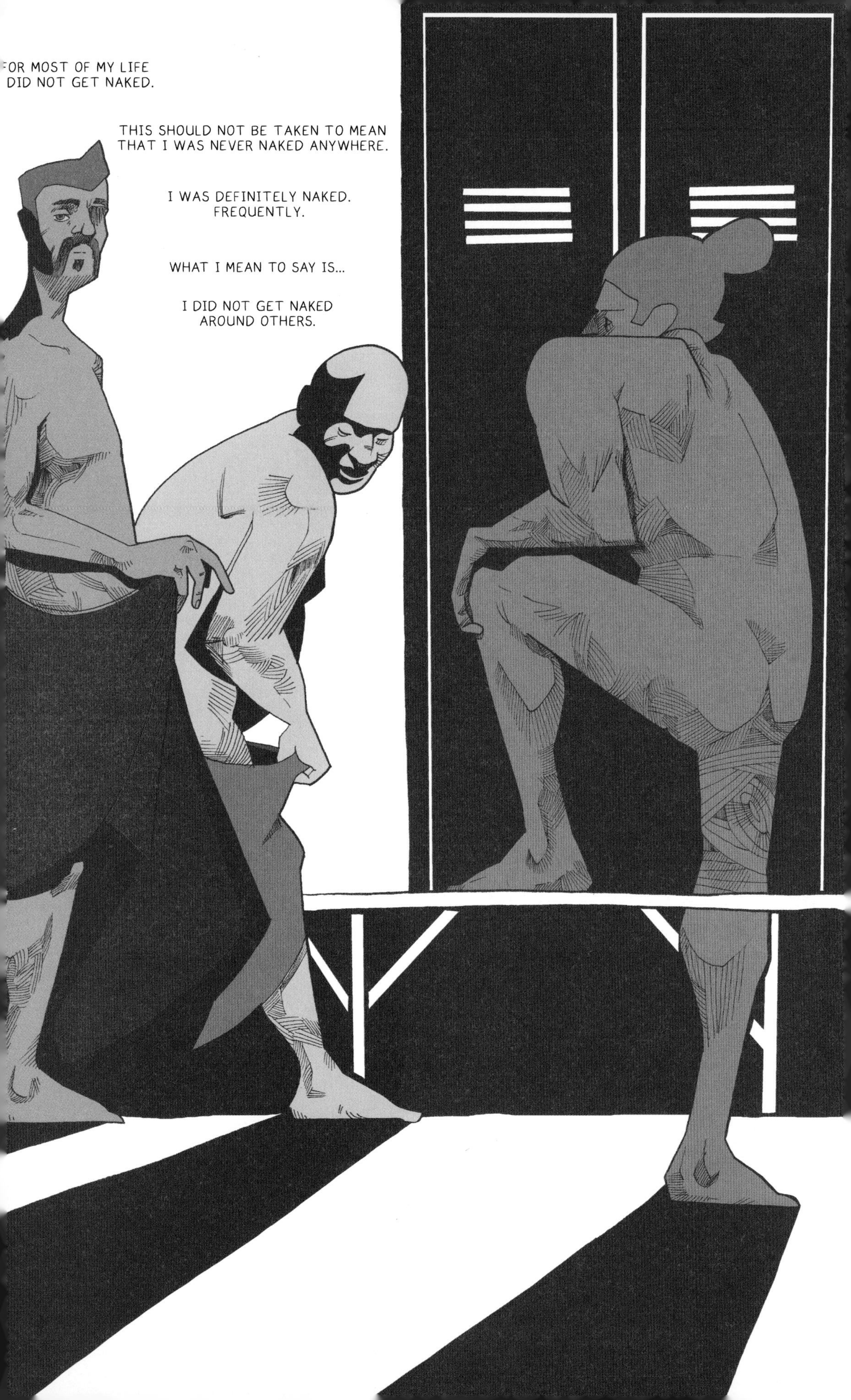
FOR MOST OF MY LIFE
I DID NOT GET NAKED.
THIS SHOULD NOT BE TAKEN TO MEAN THAT I WAS NEVER NAKED ANYWHERE.
I WAS DEFINITELY NAKED. FREQUENTLY.
WHAT I MEAN TO SAY IS...
I DID NOT GET NAKED AROUND OTHERS.

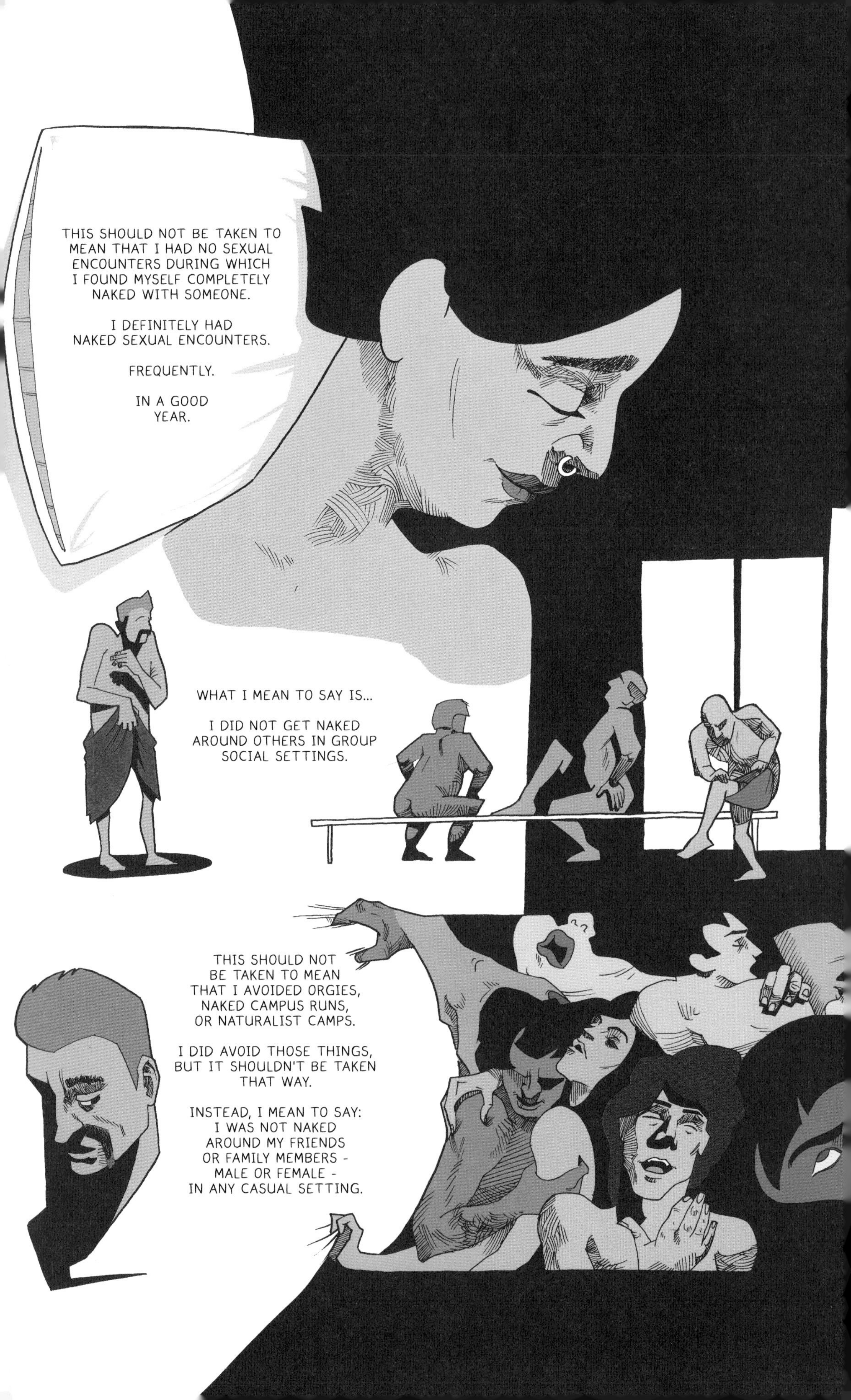
THIS SHOULD NOT BE TAKEN TO MEAN THAT I HAD NO SEXUAL ENCOUNTERS DURING WHICH I FOUND MYSELF COMPLETELY NAKED WITH SOMEONE.
I DEFINITELY HAD NAKED SEXUAL ENCOUNTERS.
FREQUENTLY.
IN A GOOD YEAR.
WHAT I MEAN TO SAY IS...
I DID NOT GET NAKED AROUND OTHERS IN GROUP SOCIAL SETTINGS.
THIS SHOULD NOT BE TAKEN TO MEAN THAT I AVOIDED ORGIES, NAKED CAMPUS RUNS, OR NATURALIST CAMPS.
I DID AVOID THOSE THINGS, BUT IT SHOULDN'T BE TAKEN THAT WAY.
INSTEAD, I MEAN TO SAY: I WAS NOT NAKED AROUND MY FRIENDS OR FAMILY MEMBERS - MALE OR FEMALE - IN ANY CASUAL SETTING.

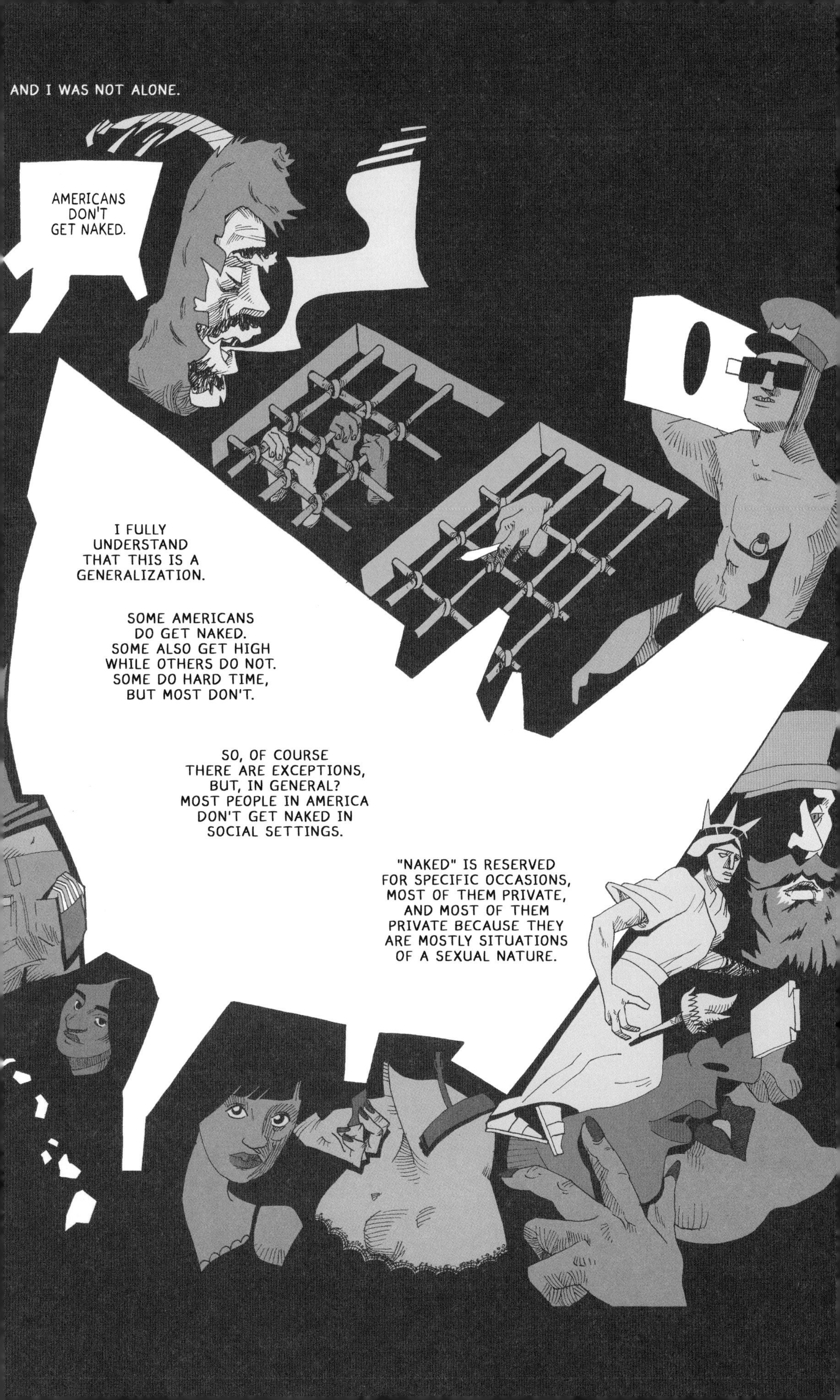
AND I WAS NOT ALONE.
AMERICANS DON'T GET NAKED.
I FULLY UNDERSTAND THAT THIS IS A GENERALIZATION.
SOME AMERICANS DO GET NAKED. SOME ALSO GET HIGH WHILE OTHERS DO NOT. SOME DO HARD TIME, BUT MOST DON'T.
SO, OF COURSE THERE ARE EXCEPTIONS, BUT, IN GENERAL? MOST PEOPLE IN AMERICA DON'T GET NAKED IN SOCIAL SETTINGS.
"NAKED" IS RESERVED FOR SPECIFIC OCCASIONS, MOST OF THEM PRIVATE, AND MOST OF THEM PRIVATE BECAUSE THEY ARE MOSTLY SITUATIONS OF A SEXUAL NATURE.

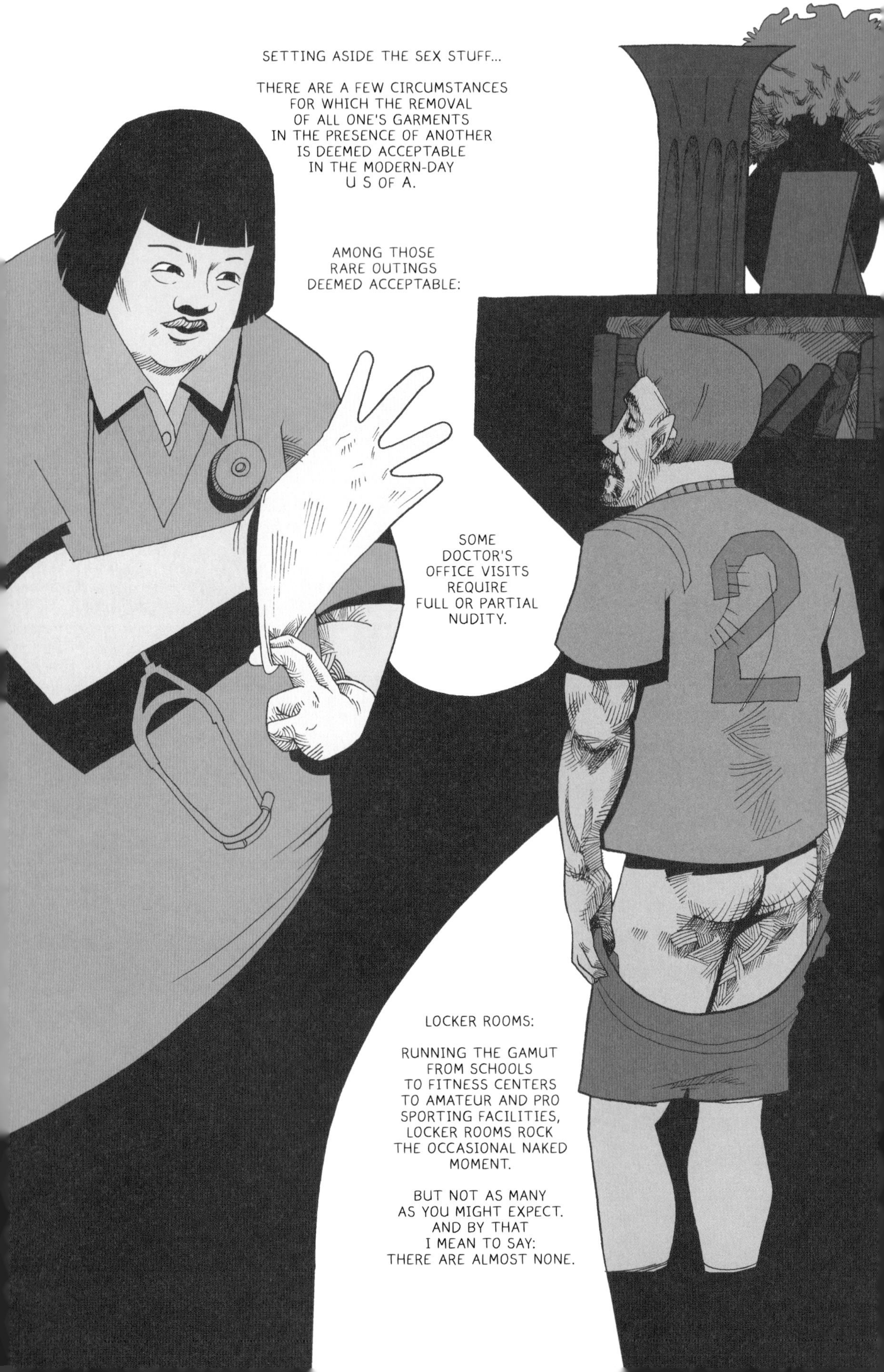
SETTING ASIDE THE SEX STUFF...
THERE ARE A FEW CIRCUMSTANCES FOR WHICH THE REMOVAL OF ALL ONE'S GARMENTS IN THE PRESENCE OF ANOTHER IS DEEMED ACCEPTABLE IN THE MODERN-DAY U S OF A.
AMONG THOSE RARE OUTINGS DEEMED ACCEPTABLE:
SOME DOCTOR'S OFFICE VISITS REQUIRE FULL OR PARTIAL NUDITY.
2
LOCKER ROOMS:
RUNNING THE GAMUT FROM SCHOOLS TO FITNESS CENTERS TO AMATEUR AND PRO SPORTING FACILITIES, LOCKER ROOMS ROCK THE OCCASIONAL NAKED MOMENT.
BUT NOT AS MANY AS YOU MIGHT EXPECT. AND BY THAT I MEAN TO SAY: THERE ARE ALMOST NONE.

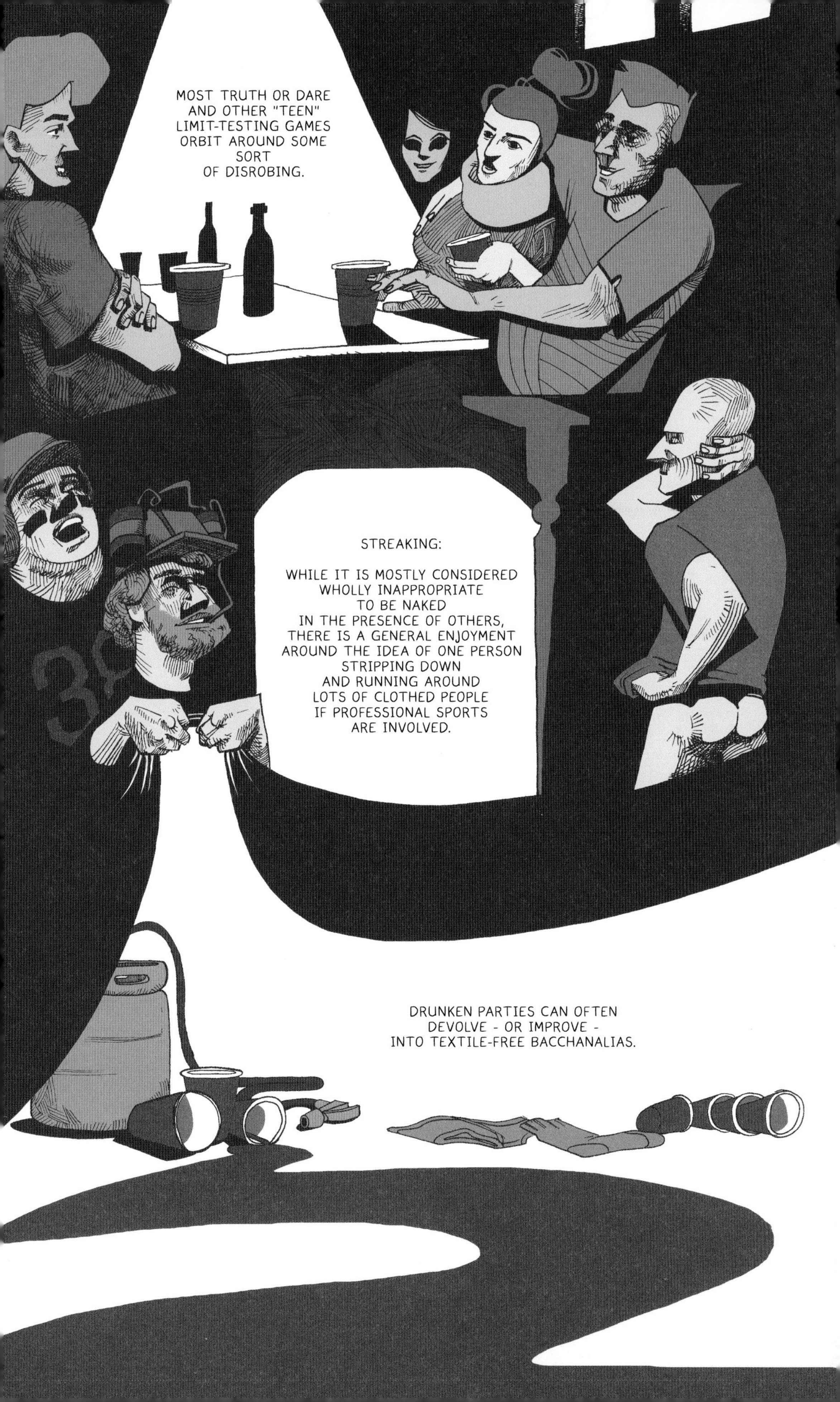
MOST TRUTH OR DARE AND OTHER "TEEN" LIMIT-TESTING GAMES ORBIT AROUND SOME SORT OF DISROBING.
STREAKING:
WHILE IT IS MOSTLY CONSIDERED WHOLLY INAPPROPRIATE TO BE NAKED IN THE PRESENCE OF OTHERS, THERE IS A GENERAL ENJOYMENT AROUND THE IDEA OF ONE PERSON STRIPPING DOWN AND RUNNING AROUND LOTS OF CLOTHED PEOPLE IF PROFESSIONAL SPORTS ARE INVOLVED.
DRUNKEN PARTIES CAN OFTEN DEVOLVE - OR IMPROVE - INTO TEXTILE-FREE BACCHANALIAS.

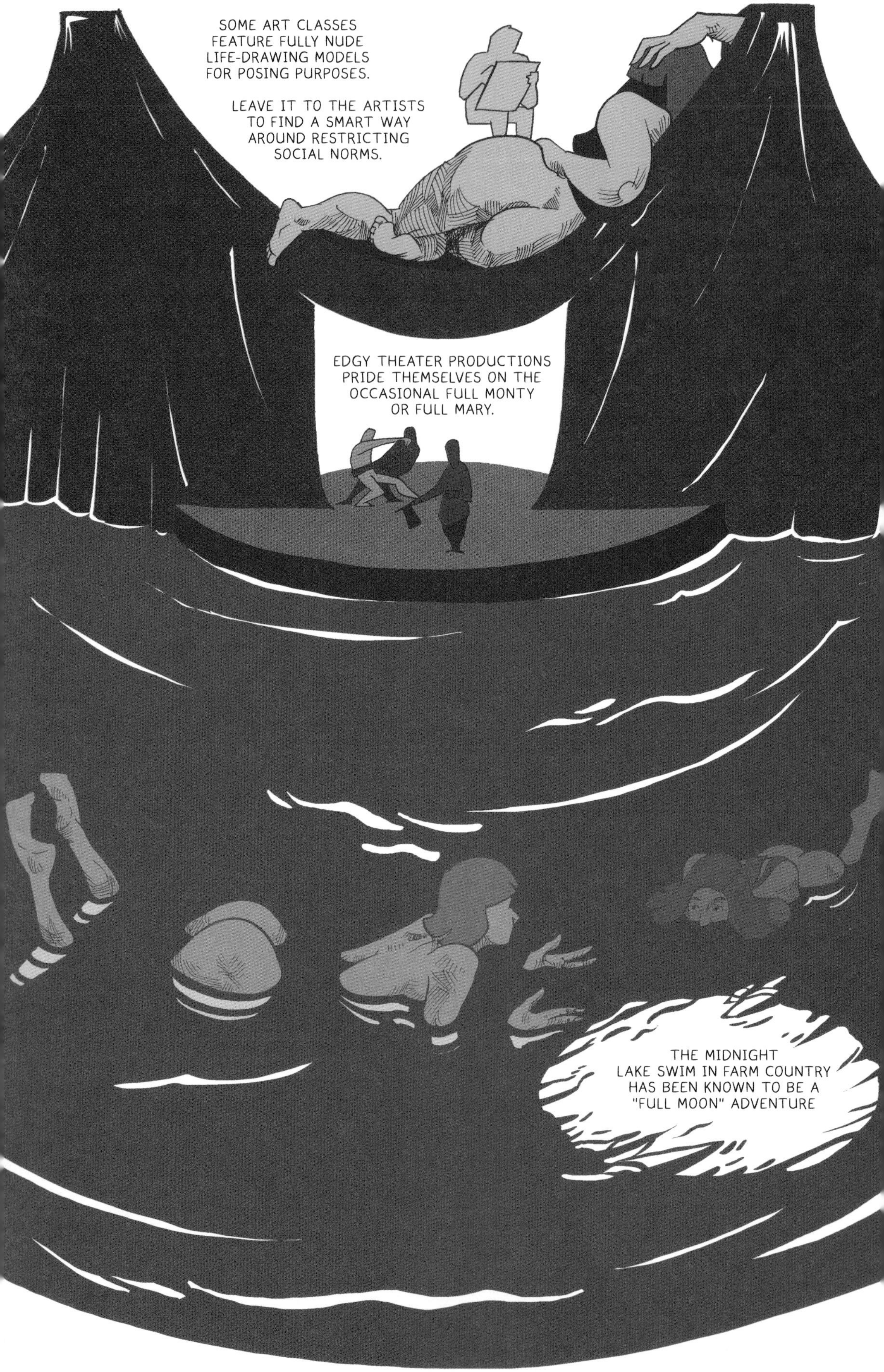
SOME ART CLASSES FEATURE FULLY NUDE LIFE-DRAWING MODELS FOR POSING PURPOSES.
LEAVE IT TO THE ARTISTS TO FIND A SMART WAY AROUND RESTRICTING SOCIAL NORMS.
EDGY THEATER PRODUCTIONS PRIDE THEMSELVES ON THE OCCASIONAL FULL MONTY OR FULL MARY.
THE MIDNIGHT LAKE SWIM IN FARM COUNTRY HAS BEEN KNOWN TO BE A "FULL MOON" ADVENTURE

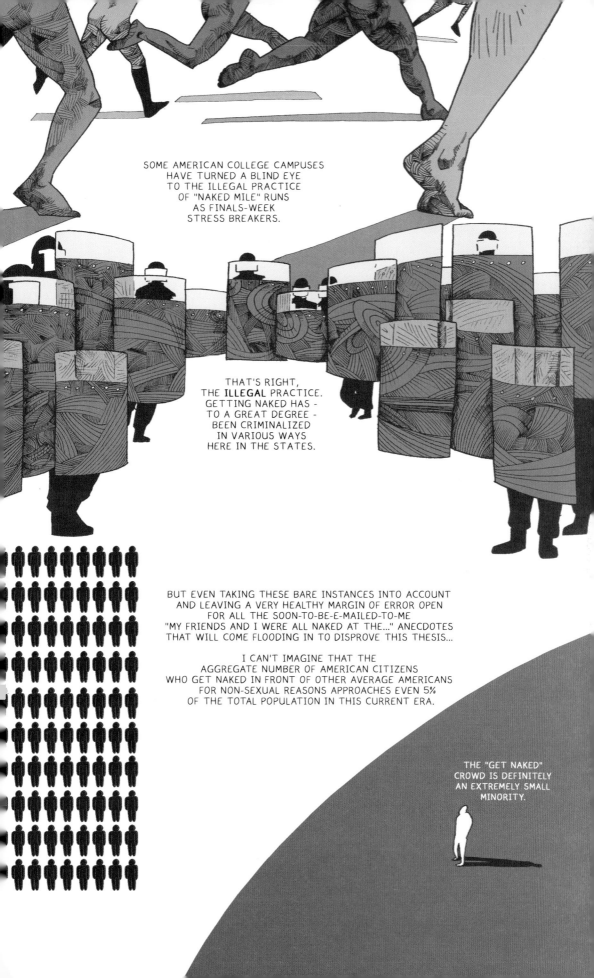

SOME AMERICAN COLLEGE CAMPUSES
HAVE TURNED A BLIND EYE
TO THE ILLEGAL PRACTICE
OF "NAKED MILE" RUNS
AS FINALS-WEEK
STRESS BREAKERS.

THAT'S RIGHT,
THE **ILLEGAL** PRACTICE.
GETTING NAKED HAS -
TO A GREAT DEGREE -
BEEN CRIMINALIZED
IN VARIOUS WAYS
HERE IN THE STATES.

BUT EVEN TAKING THESE BARE INSTANCES INTO ACCOUNT
AND LEAVING A VERY HEALTHY MARGIN OF ERROR OPEN
FOR ALL THE SOON-TO-BE-E-MAILED-TO-ME
"MY FRIENDS AND I WERE ALL NAKED AT THE..." ANECDOTES
THAT WILL COME FLOODING IN TO DISPROVE THIS THESIS...

I CAN'T IMAGINE THAT THE
AGGREGATE NUMBER OF AMERICAN CITIZENS
WHO GET NAKED IN FRONT OF OTHER AVERAGE AMERICANS
FOR NON-SEXUAL REASONS APPROACHES EVEN 5%
OF THE TOTAL POPULATION IN THIS CURRENT ERA.

THE "GET NAKED"
CROWD IS DEFINITELY
AN EXTREMELY SMALL
MINORITY.

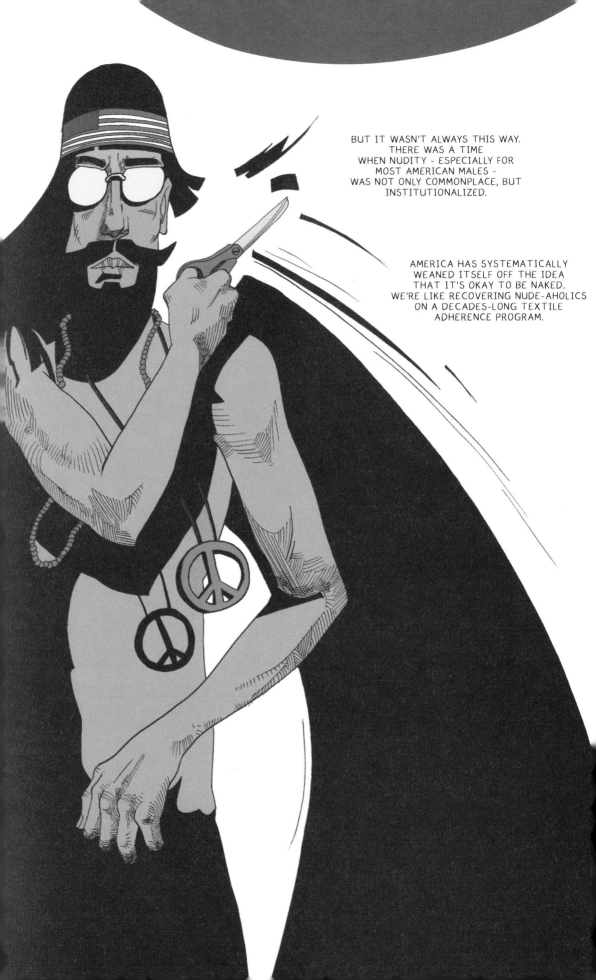

BUT IT WASN'T ALWAYS THIS WAY. THERE WAS A TIME WHEN NUDITY - ESPECIALLY FOR MOST AMERICAN MALES - WAS NOT ONLY COMMONPLACE, BUT INSTITUTIONALIZED.

AMERICA HAS SYSTEMATICALLY WEANED ITSELF OFF THE IDEA THAT IT'S OKAY TO BE NAKED. WE'RE LIKE RECOVERING NUDE-AHOLICS ON A DECADES-LONG TEXTILE ADHERENCE PROGRAM.

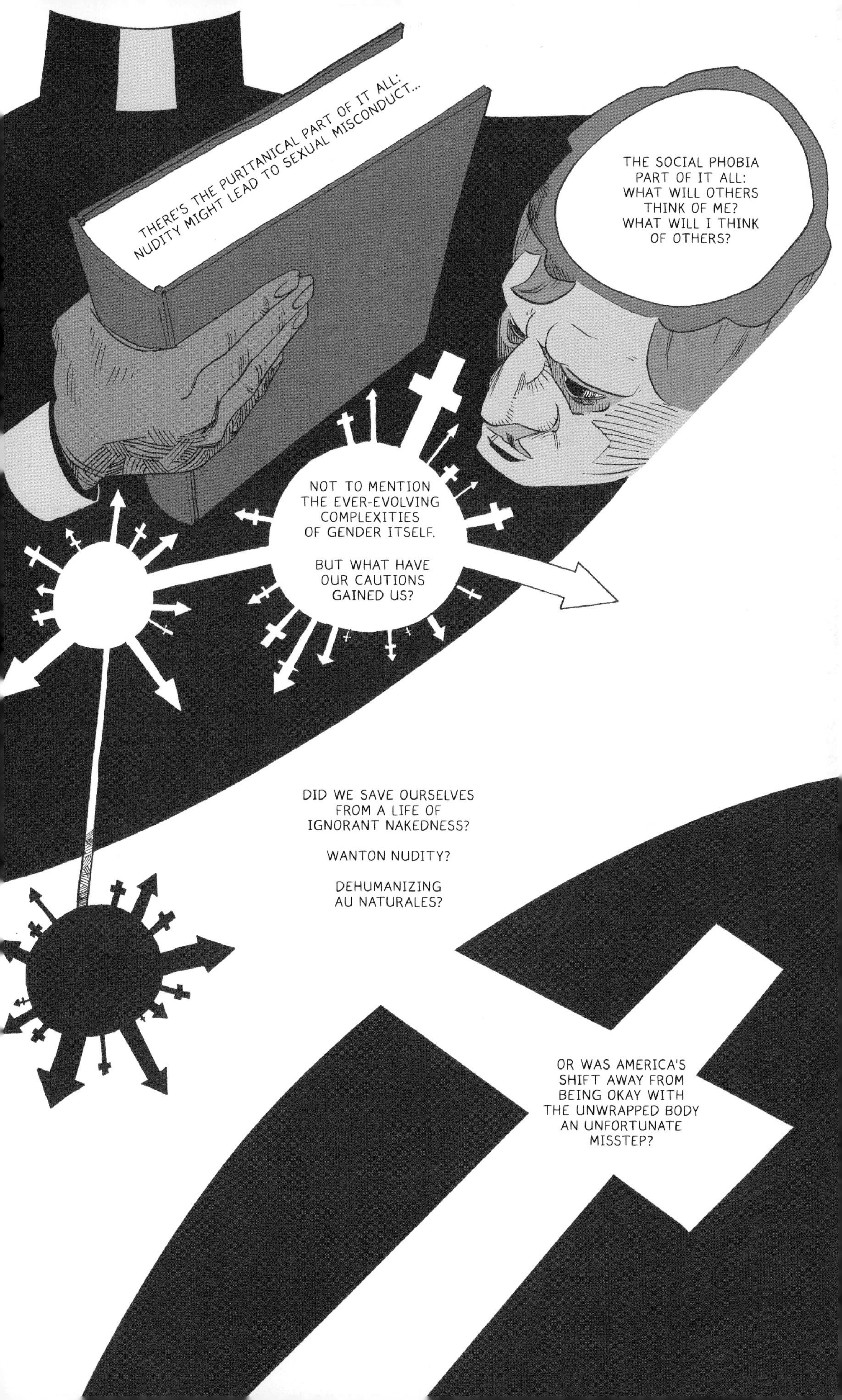

THERE'S THE PURITANICAL PART OF IT ALL: NUDITY MIGHT LEAD TO SEXUAL MISCONDUCT...
THE SOCIAL PHOBIA PART OF IT ALL: WHAT WILL OTHERS THINK OF ME? WHAT WILL I THINK OF OTHERS?
NOT TO MENTION THE EVER-EVOLVING COMPLEXITIES OF GENDER ITSELF.
BUT WHAT HAVE OUR CAUTIONS GAINED US?
DID WE SAVE OURSELVES FROM A LIFE OF IGNORANT NAKEDNESS?
WANTON NUDITY?
DEHUMANIZING AU NATURALES?
OR WAS AMERICA'S SHIFT AWAY FROM BEING OKAY WITH THE UNWRAPPED BODY AN UNFORTUNATE MISSTEP?

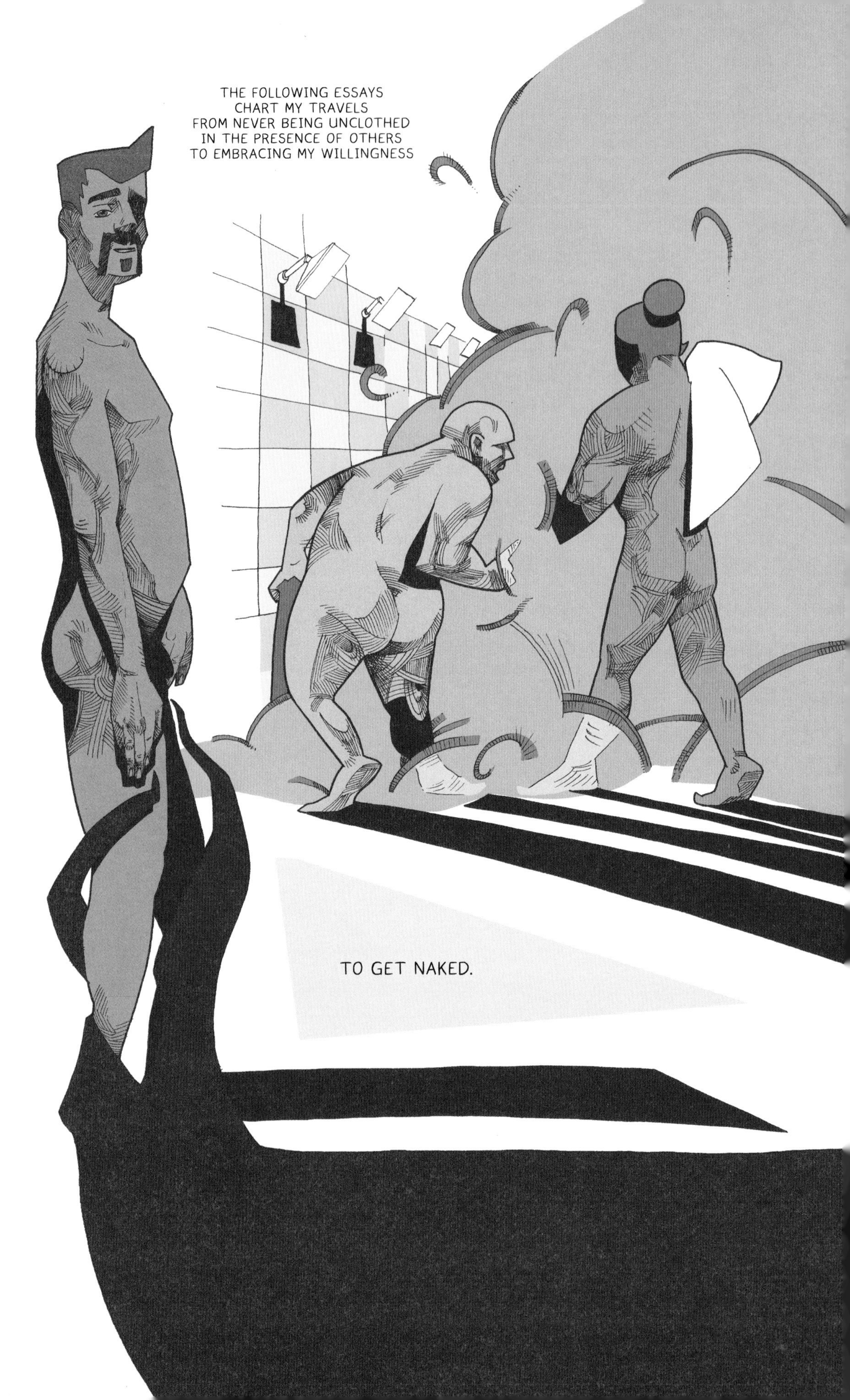
THE FOLLOWING ESSAYS CHART MY TRAVELS FROM NEVER BEING UNCLOTHED IN THE PRESENCE OF OTHERS TO EMBRACING MY WILLINGNESS
TO GET NAKED.

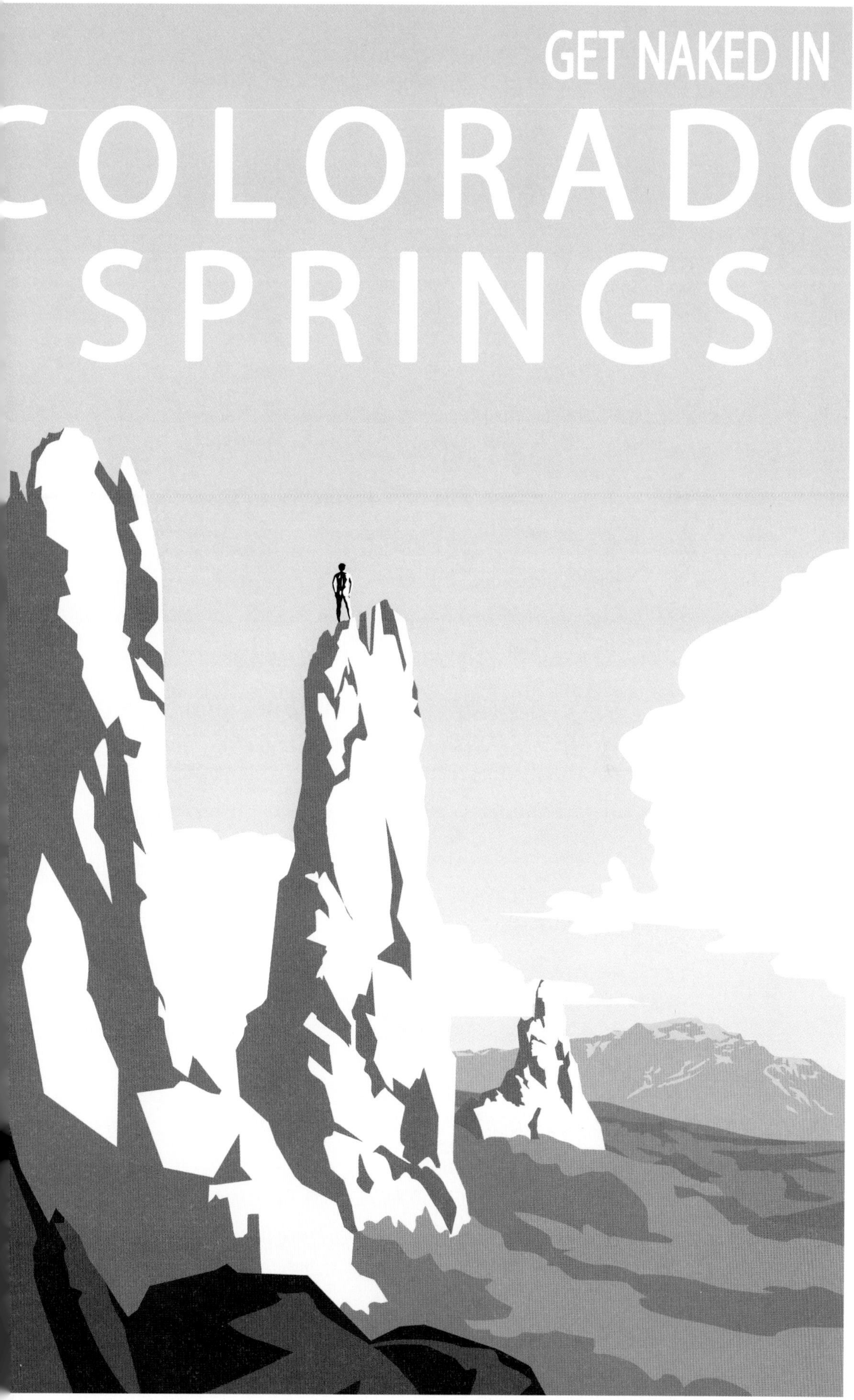
GET NAKED IN
COLORADO
SPRINGS

GUYS USED TO SWIM NAKED IN AMERICAN HIGH SCHOOLS.

BUTT NAKED.

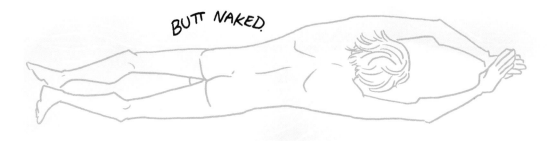

NOT AS SOME ACT OF REBELLION, NOT BECAUSE OF THE FREE LOVE MOVEMENT OF THE 60s, BUT AS DISTRICT-MANDATED POLICY IN MANY CITIES AROUND AMERICA.

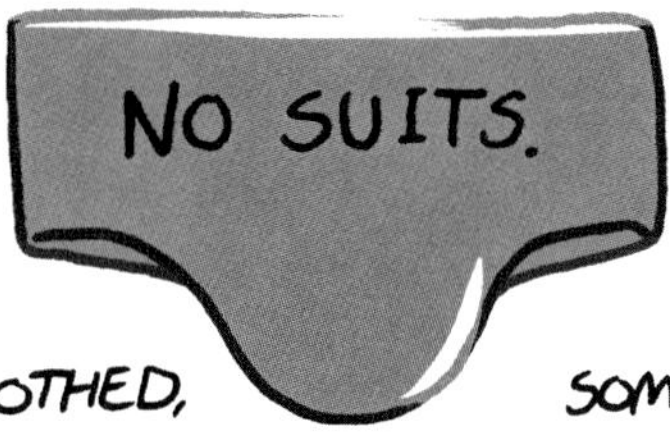

NO SUITS.

THEIR TEACHERS WERE SOMETIMES CLOTHED, SOMETIMES NOT.

THE CLASSES WERE GENDER SEGREGATED AND WOMEN EITHER DID NOT HAVE SWIM CLASS, OR, IF THEY DID, WORE SWIMSUITS.

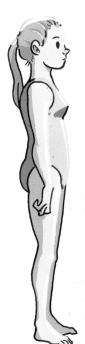

BUT NOT THE GUYS.

IT'S AN ODD PIECE OF AMERICAN HISTORY THAT HAS BEEN EDITED OUT OF THE CULTURAL NARRATIVE AS WE MOVED TO A CULTURE OF BODYSHAME, STRANGER DANGER, AND EVER MORE REPRESSED SEXUALITY.

BUT IT'S TRUE.

GUYS SWAM NAKED IN PUBLIC SCHOOLS.

THERE'S A FAMOUS PICTURE DOCUMENTING THIS FACT IN AN OLD LIFE MAGAZINE.

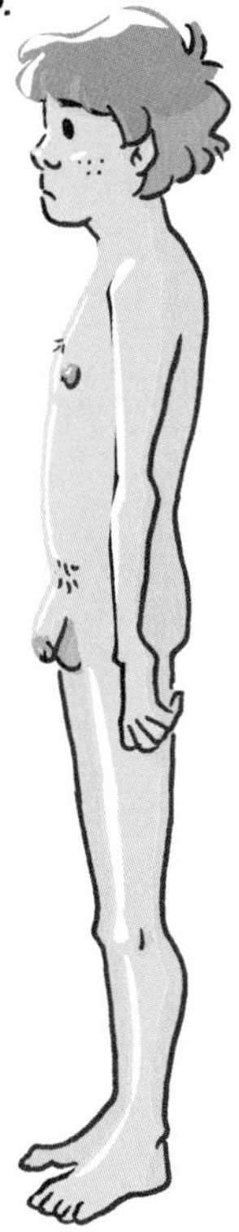

THIS CLAIM IS USUALLY MET WITH DENIAL BY PEOPLE WHO GRADUATED FROM HIGH SCHOOL AFTER 1990...

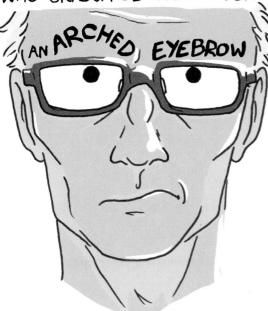

AN ARCHED EYEBROW

FROM PEOPLE WHO GRADUATED IN THE 80s AND 90s...

BUT A KNOWING NOD FOR MANY MEN WHO GRADUATED BEFORE 1979.

I REMEMBER HEARING SOMETIME AROUND 6TH OR 7TH GRADE THAT IN HIGH SCHOOL WE HAD TO TAKE SWIMMING CLASS AND FOR SWIMMING CLASS WE HAD TO GET

NAKED.

I ASSUMED THAT THIS WAS IN REFERENCE TO CHANGING FROM STREET CLOTHES TO SWIMSUITS AND - FOR MY EXPERIENCE AT LEAST - THIS PROVED TO BE TRUE.

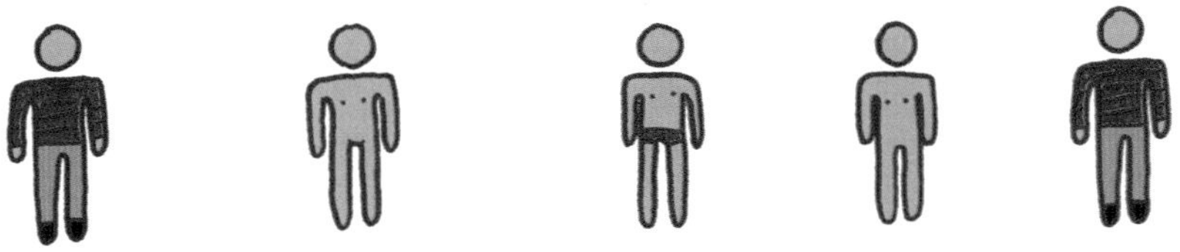

CHANGING LEFT YOU EXPOSED. SHOWERING EVEN MORE SO IF YOU TOOK ONE.

BUT THE NUDITY CLAIM - IF IT WAS EVER TRUE - WAS OVERSTATED FOR

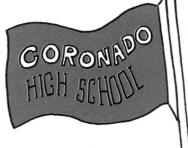

CORONADO HIGH SCHOOL

BY 1982 WHEN I GOT THERE.

NONETHELESS, SWIM CLASS EACH YEAR WAS STILL A VARIATION ON A FAMILIAR, HUMILIATING THEME FOR ME.

I WOULD APPROACH OUR HYPER-MASCULINE GYM TEACHER AND DECLARE A SIMPLE FACT:

I DON'T FLOAT.

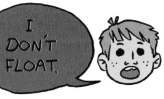

THE HYPER MASCULINE GYM TEACHER - OFTEN A WOMAN - WOULD "SCOFF" AT THIS DECLARATION.

THERE WOULD BE SOME KIND OF TEST ARRANGED - SORT OF A

SALEM

SINK THE WITCH!
EPISODE
UM...

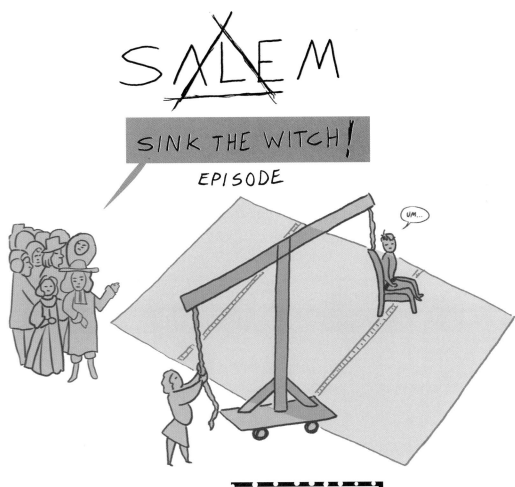

WITH ME IN THE TITLE ROLE.

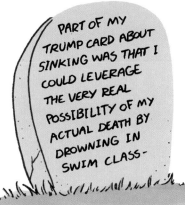

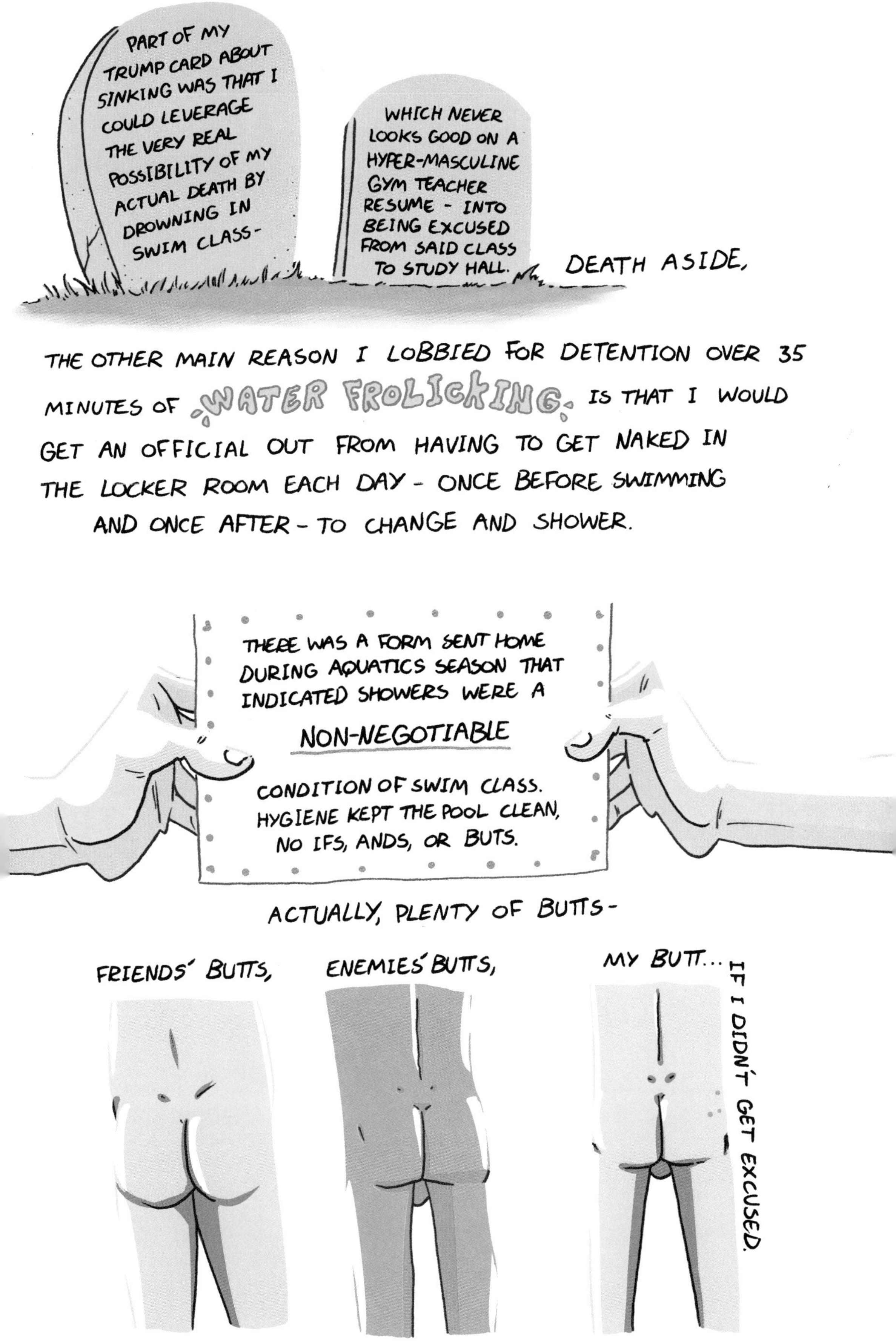

PART OF MY TRUMP CARD ABOUT SINKING WAS THAT I COULD LEVERAGE THE VERY REAL POSSIBILITY OF MY ACTUAL DEATH BY DROWNING IN SWIM CLASS —

WHICH NEVER LOOKS GOOD ON A HYPER-MASCULINE GYM TEACHER RESUME — INTO BEING EXCUSED FROM SAID CLASS TO STUDY HALL.

DEATH ASIDE,

THE OTHER MAIN REASON I LOBBIED FOR DETENTION OVER 35 MINUTES OF *WATER FROLICKING* IS THAT I WOULD GET AN OFFICIAL OUT FROM HAVING TO GET NAKED IN THE LOCKER ROOM EACH DAY — ONCE BEFORE SWIMMING AND ONCE AFTER — TO CHANGE AND SHOWER.

THERE WAS A FORM SENT HOME DURING AQUATICS SEASON THAT INDICATED SHOWERS WERE A

NON-NEGOTIABLE

CONDITION OF SWIM CLASS. HYGIENE KEPT THE POOL CLEAN, NO IFS, ANDS, OR BUTS.

ACTUALLY, PLENTY OF BUTTS —

FRIENDS' BUTTS,   ENEMIES' BUTTS,

MY BUTT...

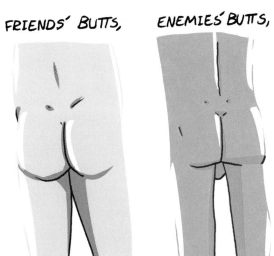

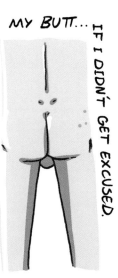

IF I DIDN'T GET EXCUSED.

AFTER TWO SEMESTERS OF NEAR

HYDRO-ASPHYXIATION,

I WAS SURPRISINGLY ADEPT AT THE PROCESS OF PROVING MY LACK OF *BUOYANCY* BY SENIOR YEAR. I WAS DIRECTED TO JUMP INTO THE DEEP END, RETRIEVE A  FROM THE BOTTOM OF THE POOL, AND RETURN TO THE SURFACE WITH SAID BRICK.

I ASKED THE HYPER-MASCULINE GYM TEACHER TO HAVE SOMEONE STAND BY TO JUMP IN AND RESCUE ME WHEN I DIDN'T COME BACK UP.

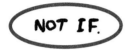 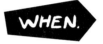

WITHOUT HESITATION, I HELD MY BREATH, JUMPED IN AND MADE MY WAY TO THE BOTTOM. I GRABBED THE TWENTY-POUND BRICK - MORE THAN ONE - SIXTH OF MY TOTAL BODY WEIGHT AT THE TIME - AND PUSHED OFF FROM THE SHARP-EDGED TILES BELOW. I WENT TOWARD THE LIGHT TEN FEET ABOVE - ROSE ABOUT THREE AND A HALF OF THOSE FEET -

THEN SANK STRAIGHT BACK DOWN TO THE BOTTOM. I DROPPED THE BRICK - PUSHED OFF - MADE IT ABOUT SIX OF THE TEN FEET UP FROM THE FORCE OF MY KICK - THEN - AGAIN - SANK BACK DOWN.

I LOOKED UP AND WAVED FOR RESCUE.

RESCUE WAS DISPATCHED.

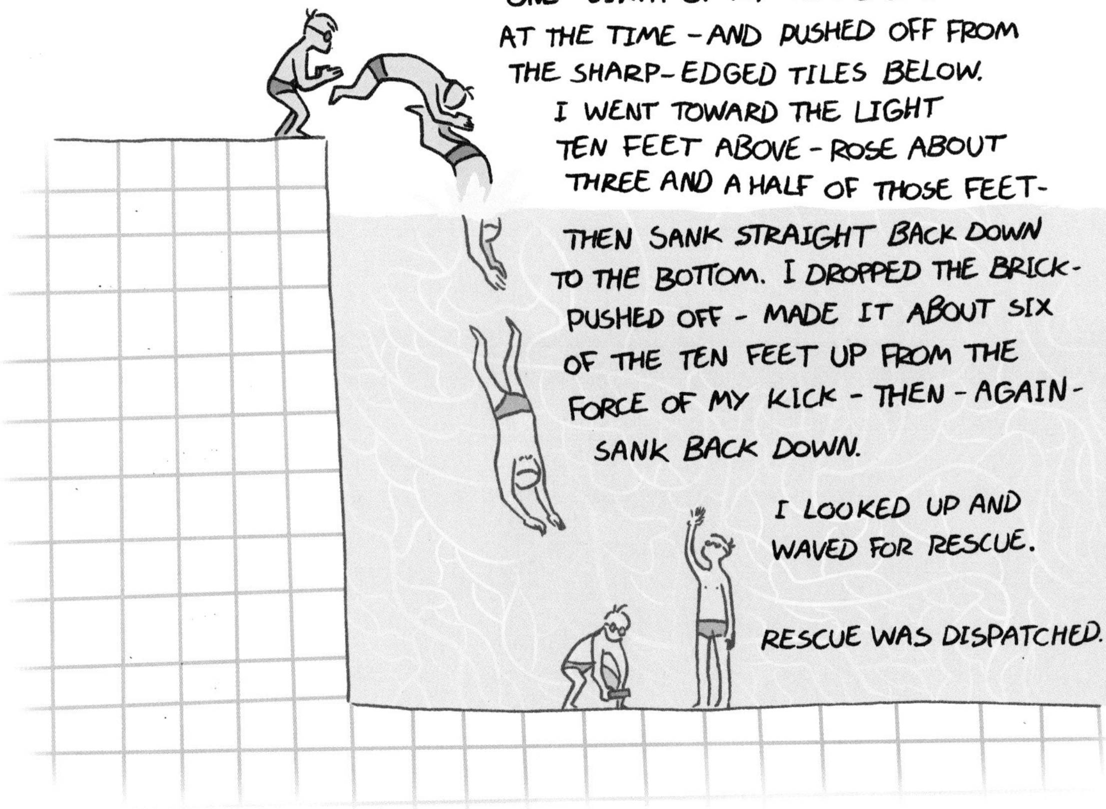

I SAT GASPING AND DRIPPING ON THE POOL'S EDGE, WAITING TO BE AWARDED MY TRIUMPHANT DISMISSAL TO STUDY HALL FOR THE REST OF THE QUARTER.

UNFORTUNATELY,

THE HYPER-MASCULINE TEACHER HAD, AFTER 25 YEARS IN THE PROFESSION,

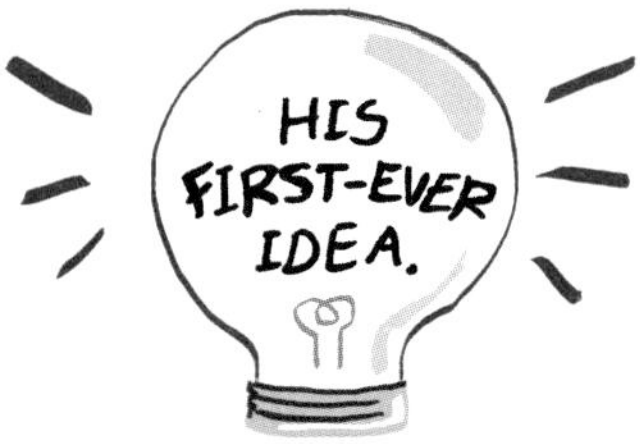

HIS FIRST-EVER IDEA.

HE SUSSED OUT THAT MY FRIEND AND BAND-MATE KARI, A TRAINED LIFEGUARD AT THE LOCAL PRIVATE CLUB POOL BY MY HOUSE, DIDN'T NEED THIS SWIM CLASS ALMOST AS MUCH AS I DID.

HE ASSIGNED HER TO TEACH ME THE BASICS IN THE SHALLOW END EACH DAY WHILE THE NORMAL FLOATING HUMANS DID THE STANDARD DRILLS IN THE DEEP END.

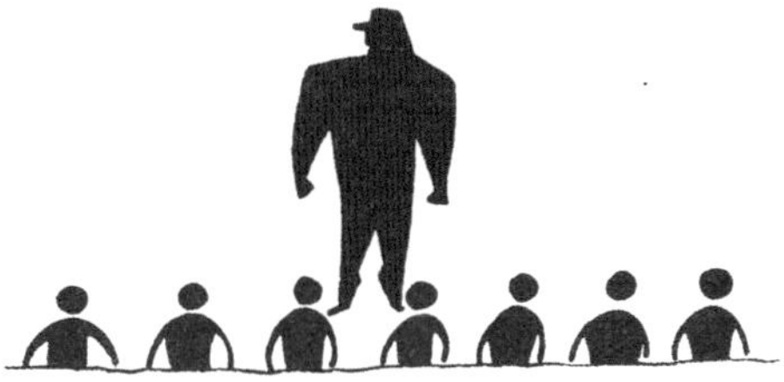

I HAD GOTTEN OUT OF SWIMMING BUT I HADN'T GOTTEN OUT OF GETTING OUT OF MY CLOTHES TWICE A DAY.

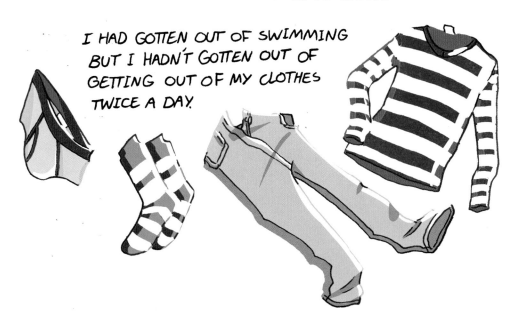

MY RELUCTANCE TO GET NAKED IN SCHOOL DIDN'T START AT THE FULL MONTY LEVEL. IT WELLED UP AND INCLUDED EVERY PART OF ME EXCEPT MY 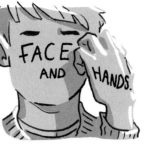 FACE AND HANDS.

I NEVER WORE SHORTS.

I WAS NEVER A "SKIN" FOR A GYM CLASS BASKETBALL GAME.

I NEVER EVEN WORE SANDAL STYLE SHOES.

I COVERED AS MUCH OF ME AS WAS POSSIBLE IN THE EARLY 80s AND IF I'D KNOWN ABOUT BEE KEEPER OUTFITS BACK THEN, I WOULD HAVE BEEN AN ADOPTER.

THIS WAS ALL BECAUSE A COUPLE OF YEARS PRIOR,

I'D BEEN CALLED CUTE.

THE CALLEE WAS

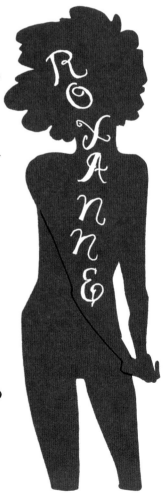

ROXANNE

GENERALLY REGARDED AS THE MOST ATTRACTIVE GIRL IN THE EIGHTH GRADE.

AND AS A 7TH GRADER

I RELISHED IN THIS MILFY KIND OF ATTENTION.

THERE WERE OLDER JOCKS SHE WOULDN'T GIVE THE TIME OF DAY TO, BUT SHE REGULARLY TALKED TO ME AND CALLED ME CUTE.

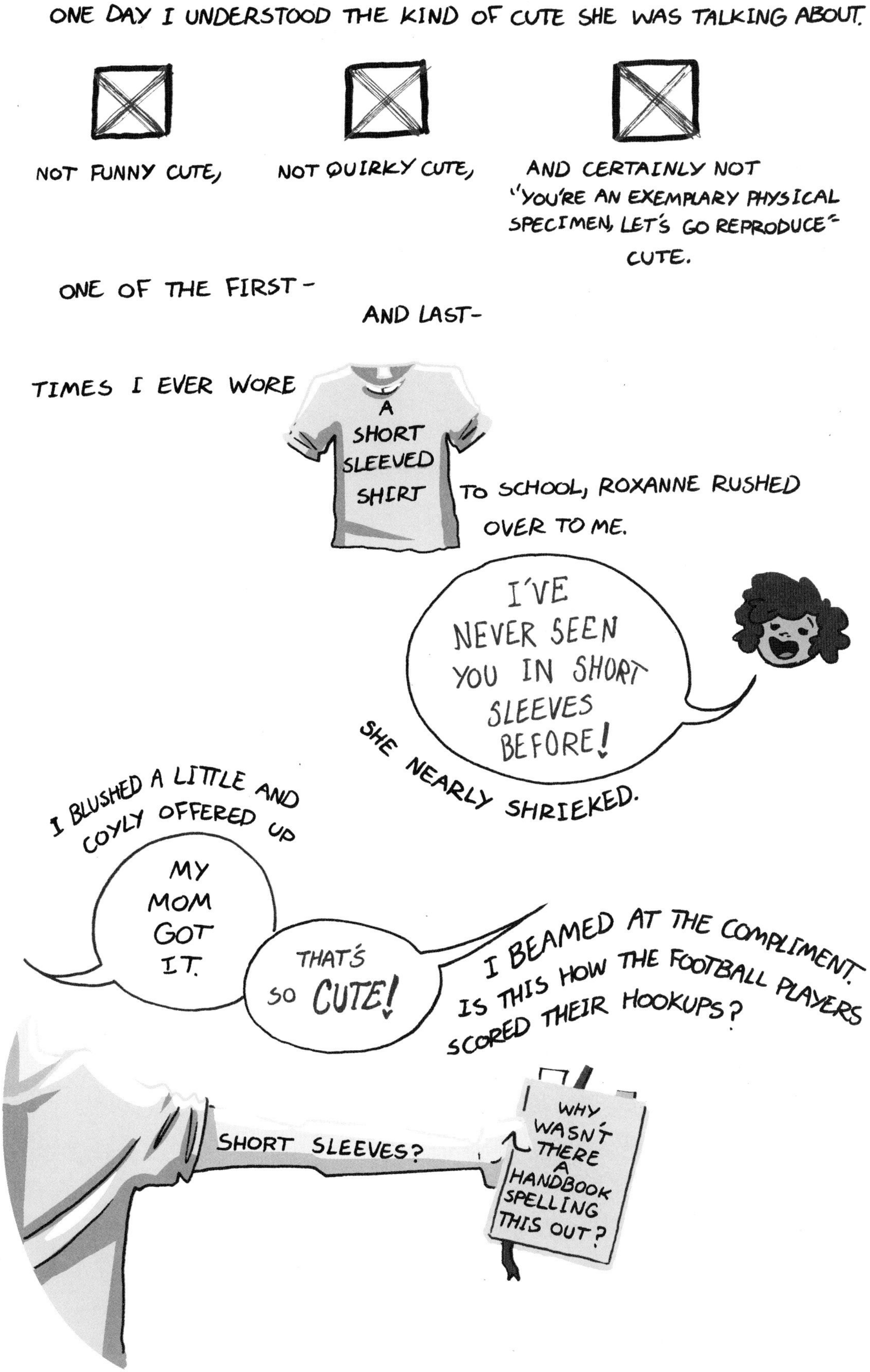
ONE DAY I UNDERSTOOD THE KIND OF CUTE SHE WAS TALKING ABOUT.
NOT FUNNY CUTE,
NOT QUIRKY CUTE,
AND CERTAINLY NOT "YOU'RE AN EXEMPLARY PHYSICAL SPECIMEN, LET'S GO REPRODUCE" CUTE.
ONE OF THE FIRST -
AND LAST -
TIMES I EVER WORE
A SHORT SLEEVED SHIRT
TO SCHOOL, ROXANNE RUSHED OVER TO ME.
I'VE NEVER SEEN YOU IN SHORT SLEEVES BEFORE!
SHE NEARLY SHRIEKED.
I BLUSHED A LITTLE AND COYLY OFFERED UP
MY MOM GOT IT.
THAT'S SO CUTE!
I BEAMED AT THE COMPLIMENT. IS THIS HOW THE FOOTBALL PLAYERS SCORED THEIR HOOKUPS?
SHORT SLEEVES?
WHY WASN'T THERE A HANDBOOK SPELLING THIS OUT?

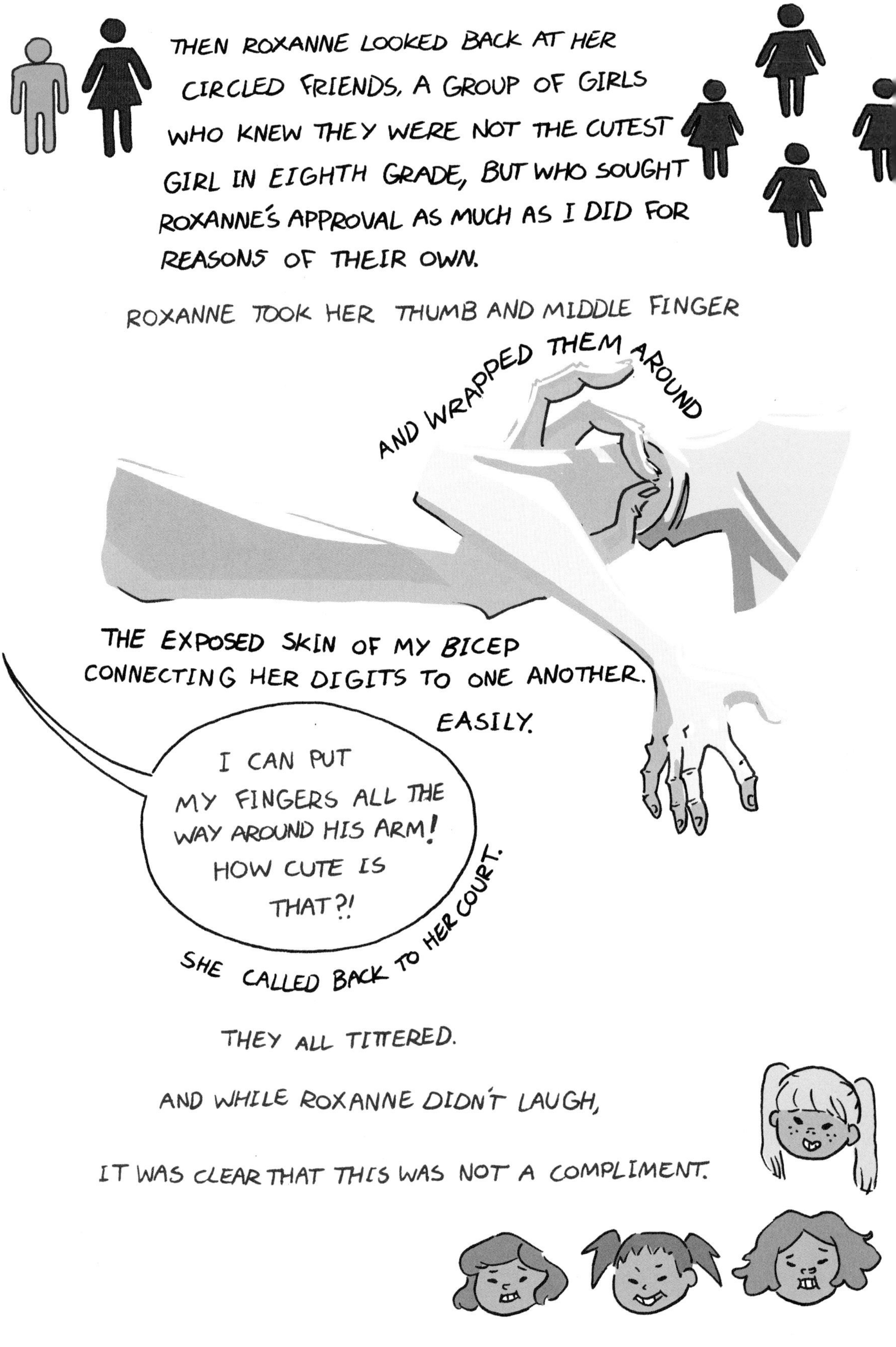
THEN ROXANNE LOOKED BACK AT HER CIRCLED FRIENDS, A GROUP OF GIRLS WHO KNEW THEY WERE NOT THE CUTEST GIRL IN EIGHTH GRADE, BUT WHO SOUGHT ROXANNE'S APPROVAL AS MUCH AS I DID FOR REASONS OF THEIR OWN.
ROXANNE TOOK HER THUMB AND MIDDLE FINGER
AND WRAPPED THEM AROUND
THE EXPOSED SKIN OF MY BICEP CONNECTING HER DIGITS TO ONE ANOTHER.
EASILY.
I CAN PUT MY FINGERS ALL THE WAY AROUND HIS ARM! HOW CUTE IS THAT?!
SHE CALLED BACK TO HER COURT.
THEY ALL TITTERED.
AND WHILE ROXANNE DIDN'T LAUGH,
IT WAS CLEAR THAT THIS WAS NOT A COMPLIMENT.

THAT MOMENT MORE THAN ANY OTHER SENT ME INTO A BURQA-ESQUE PERIOD.

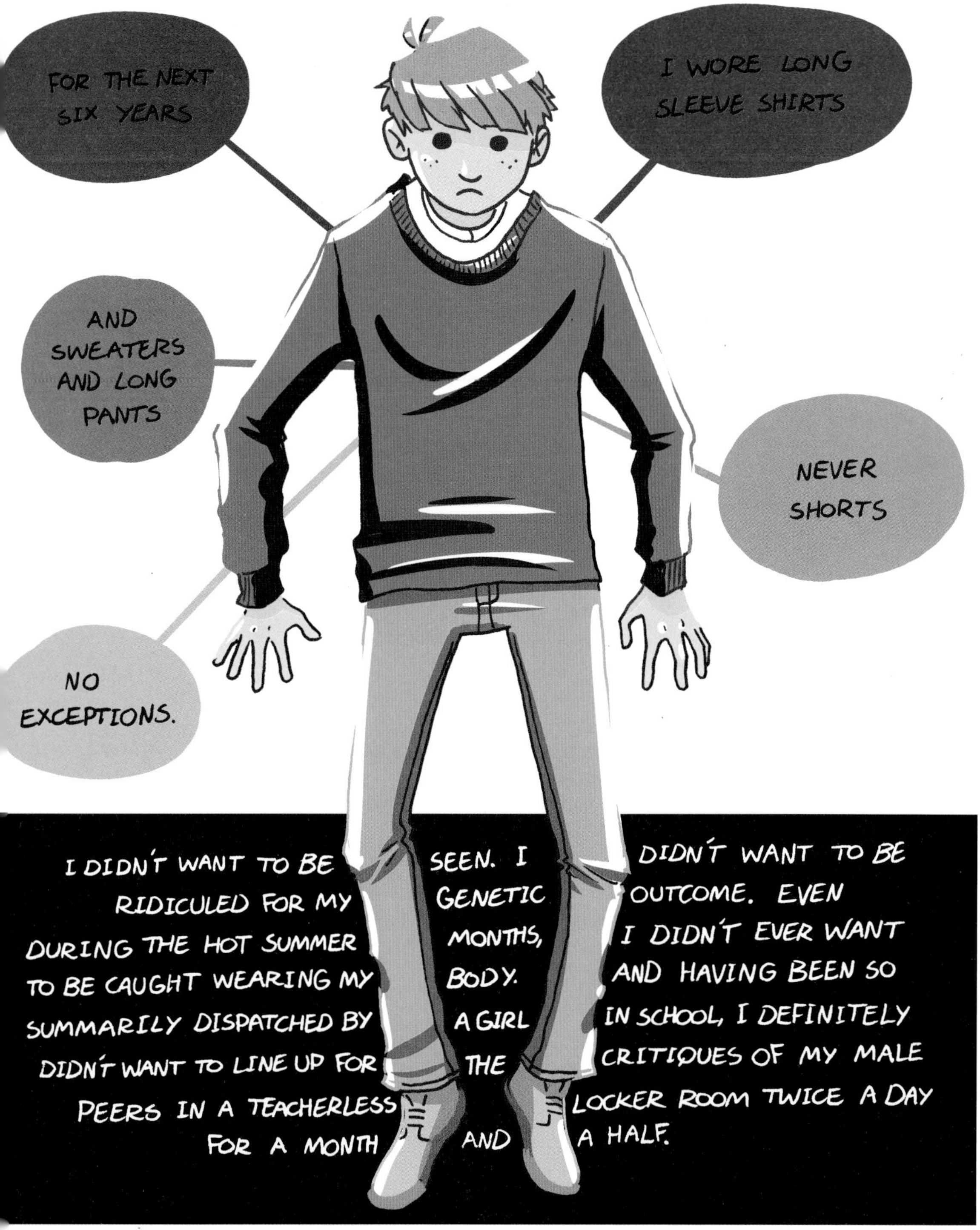
FOR THE NEXT SIX YEARS
I WORE LONG SLEEVE SHIRTS
AND SWEATERS AND LONG PANTS
NEVER SHORTS
NO EXCEPTIONS.
I DIDN'T WANT TO BE SEEN. I DIDN'T WANT TO BE RIDICULED FOR MY GENETIC OUTCOME. EVEN DURING THE HOT SUMMER MONTHS, I DIDN'T EVER WANT TO BE CAUGHT WEARING MY BODY. AND HAVING BEEN SO SUMMARILY DISPATCHED BY A GIRL IN SCHOOL, I DEFINITELY DIDN'T WANT TO LINE UP FOR THE CRITIQUES OF MY MALE PEERS IN A TEACHERLESS LOCKER ROOM TWICE A DAY FOR A MONTH AND A HALF.

BUT WITHOUT MY SWIM CLASS EXCUSED...

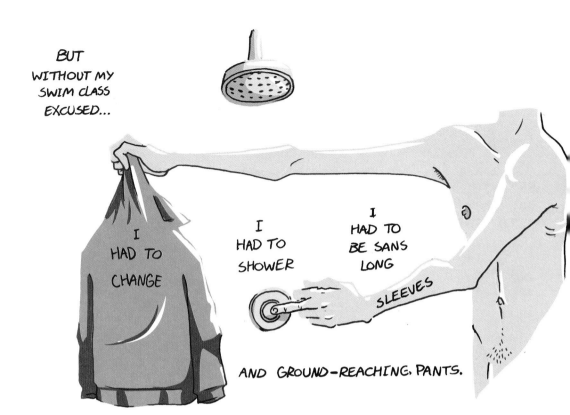

I HAD TO CHANGE

I HAD TO SHOWER

I HAD TO BE SANS LONG SLEEVES

AND GROUND-REACHING PANTS.

IT WAS MY WORST NIGHTMARE REALIZED.

AND WHILE I THINK BACK ON IT AS THE WORST SINGLE SEMESTER OF MY HIGH SCHOOL LIFE, IN RETROSPECT THERE WAS A TRUTH TO IT THAT I ONLY MUCH LATER PROCESSED.

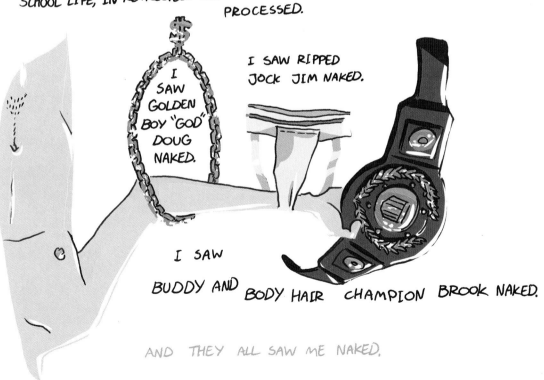

I SAW GOLDEN BOY "GOD" DOUG NAKED.

I SAW RIPPED JOCK JIM NAKED.

I SAW BUDDY AND BODY HAIR CHAMPION BROOK NAKED.

AND THEY ALL SAW ME NAKED.

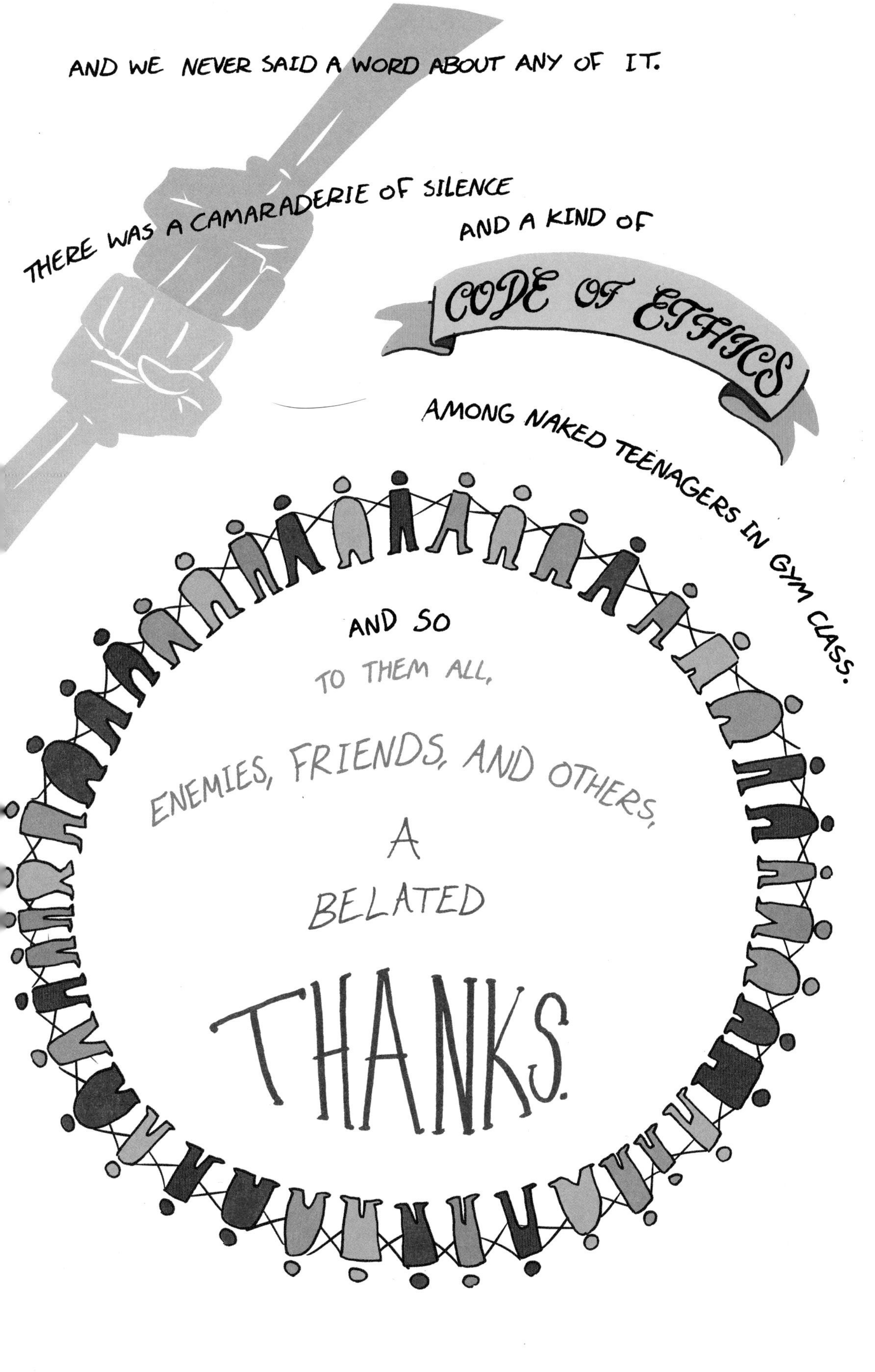
AND WE NEVER SAID A WORD ABOUT ANY OF IT.
THERE WAS A CAMARADERIE OF SILENCE
AND A KIND OF
CODE OF ETHICS
AMONG NAKED TEENAGERS IN GYM CLASS.
AND SO
TO THEM ALL,
ENEMIES, FRIENDS, AND OTHERS,
A
BELATED
THANKS.

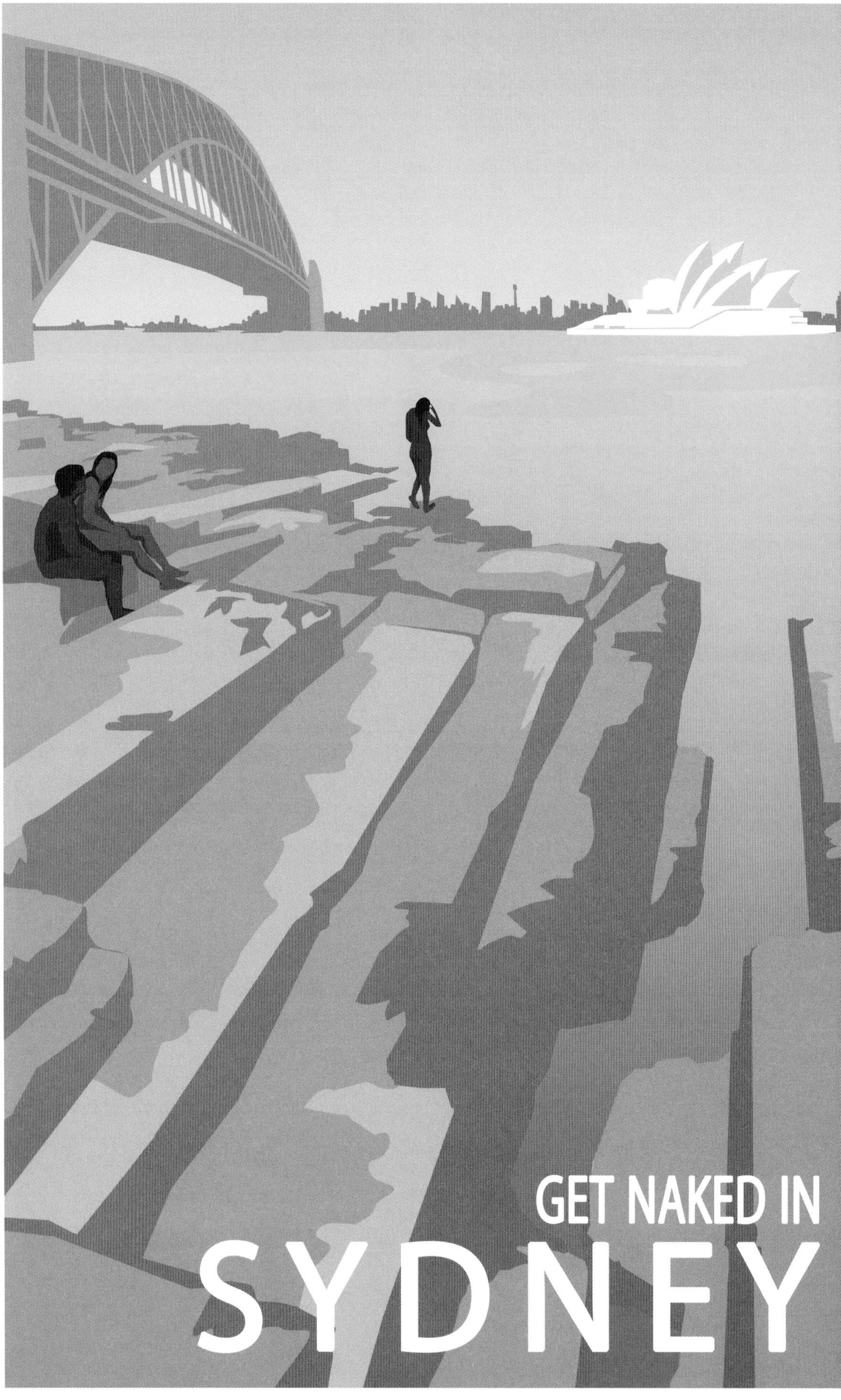
GET NAKED IN
SYDNEY

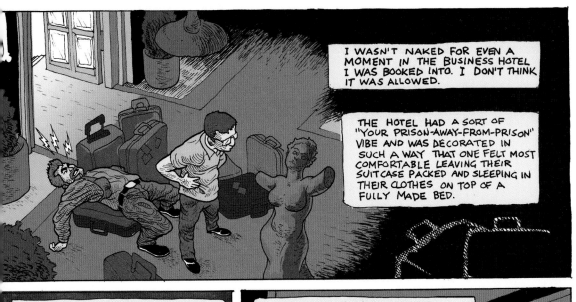

I WASN'T NAKED FOR EVEN A MOMENT IN THE BUSINESS HOTEL I WAS BOOKED INTO. I DON'T THINK IT WAS ALLOWED.

THE HOTEL HAD A SORT OF "YOUR PRISON-AWAY-FROM-PRISON" VIBE AND WAS DECORATED IN SUCH A WAY THAT ONE FELT MOST COMFORTABLE LEAVING THEIR SUITCASE PACKED AND SLEEPING IN THEIR CLOTHES ON TOP OF A FULLY MADE BED.

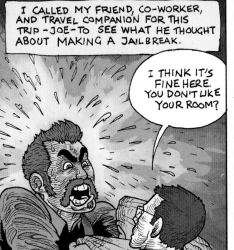

I CALLED MY FRIEND, CO-WORKER, AND TRAVEL COMPANION FOR THIS TRIP -JOE- TO SEE WHAT HE THOUGHT ABOUT MAKING A JAILBREAK.

I THINK IT'S FINE HERE. YOU DON'T LIKE YOUR ROOM?

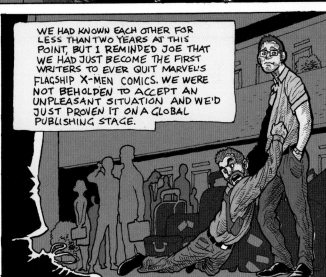

WE HAD KNOWN EACH OTHER FOR LESS THAN TWO YEARS AT THIS POINT, BUT I REMINDED JOE THAT WE HAD JUST BECOME THE FIRST WRITERS TO EVER QUIT MARVEL'S FLAGSHIP X-MEN COMICS. WE WERE NOT BEHOLDEN TO ACCEPT AN UNPLEASANT SITUATION AND WE'D JUST PROVEN IT ON A GLOBAL PUBLISHING STAGE.

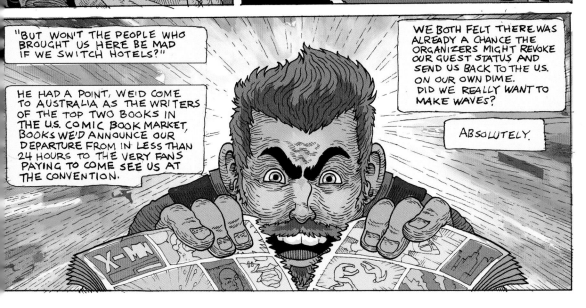

"BUT WON'T THE PEOPLE WHO BROUGHT US HERE BE MAD IF WE SWITCH HOTELS?"

HE HAD A POINT. WE'D COME TO AUSTRALIA AS THE WRITERS OF THE TOP TWO BOOKS IN THE U.S. COMIC BOOK MARKET, BOOKS WE'D ANNOUNCE OUR DEPARTURE FROM IN LESS THAN 24 HOURS TO THE VERY FANS PAYING TO COME SEE US AT THE CONVENTION.

WE BOTH FELT THERE WAS ALREADY A CHANCE THE ORGANIZERS MIGHT REVOKE OUR GUEST STATUS AND SEND US BACK TO THE U.S. ON OUR OWN DIME. DID WE REALLY WANT TO MAKE WAVES?

ABSOLUTELY.

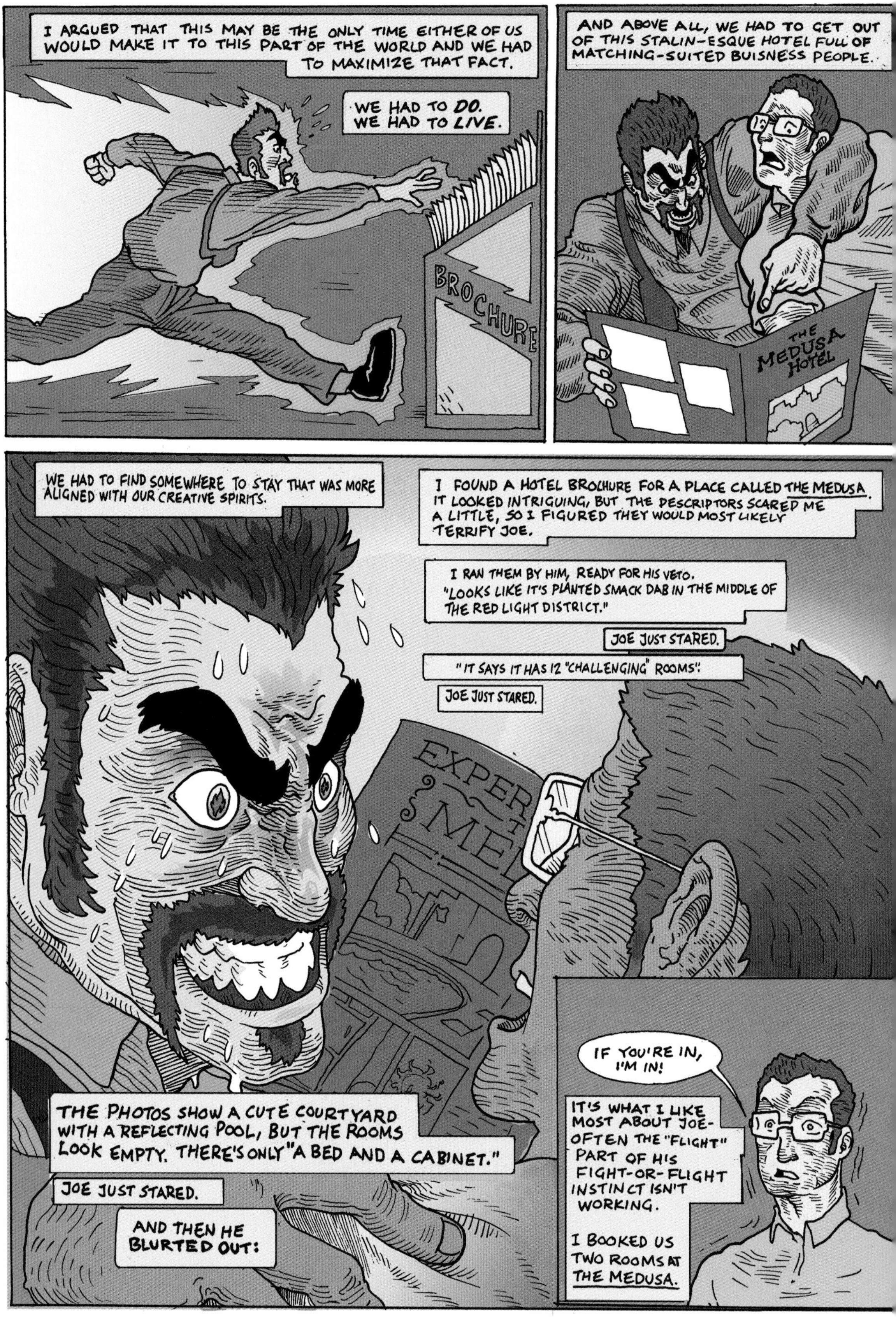
I ARGUED THAT THIS MAY BE THE ONLY TIME EITHER OF US WOULD MAKE IT TO THIS PART OF THE WORLD AND WE HAD TO MAXIMIZE THAT FACT.
WE HAD TO DO. WE HAD TO LIVE.
BROCHURE
AND ABOVE ALL, WE HAD TO GET OUT OF THIS STALIN-ESQUE HOTEL FULL OF MATCHING-SUITED BUISNESS PEOPLE.
THE MEDUSA HOTEL
WE HAD TO FIND SOMEWHERE TO STAY THAT WAS MORE ALIGNED WITH OUR CREATIVE SPIRITS.
I FOUND A HOTEL BROCHURE FOR A PLACE CALLED THE MEDUSA. IT LOOKED INTRIGUING, BUT THE DESCRIPTORS SCARED ME A LITTLE, SO I FIGURED THEY WOULD MOST LIKELY TERRIFY JOE.
I RAN THEM BY HIM, READY FOR HIS VETO. "LOOKS LIKE IT'S PLANTED SMACK DAB IN THE MIDDLE OF THE RED LIGHT DISTRICT."
JOE JUST STARED.
"IT SAYS IT HAS 12 "CHALLENGING" ROOMS".
JOE JUST STARED.
THE PHOTOS SHOW A CUTE COURTYARD WITH A REFLECTING POOL, BUT THE ROOMS LOOK EMPTY. THERE'S ONLY "A BED AND A CABINET."
JOE JUST STARED.
AND THEN HE BLURTED OUT:
IF YOU'RE IN, I'M IN!
IT'S WHAT I LIKE MOST ABOUT JOE- OFTEN THE "FLIGHT" PART OF HIS FIGHT-OR-FLIGHT INSTINCT ISN'T WORKING.
I BOOKED US TWO ROOMS AT THE MEDUSA.

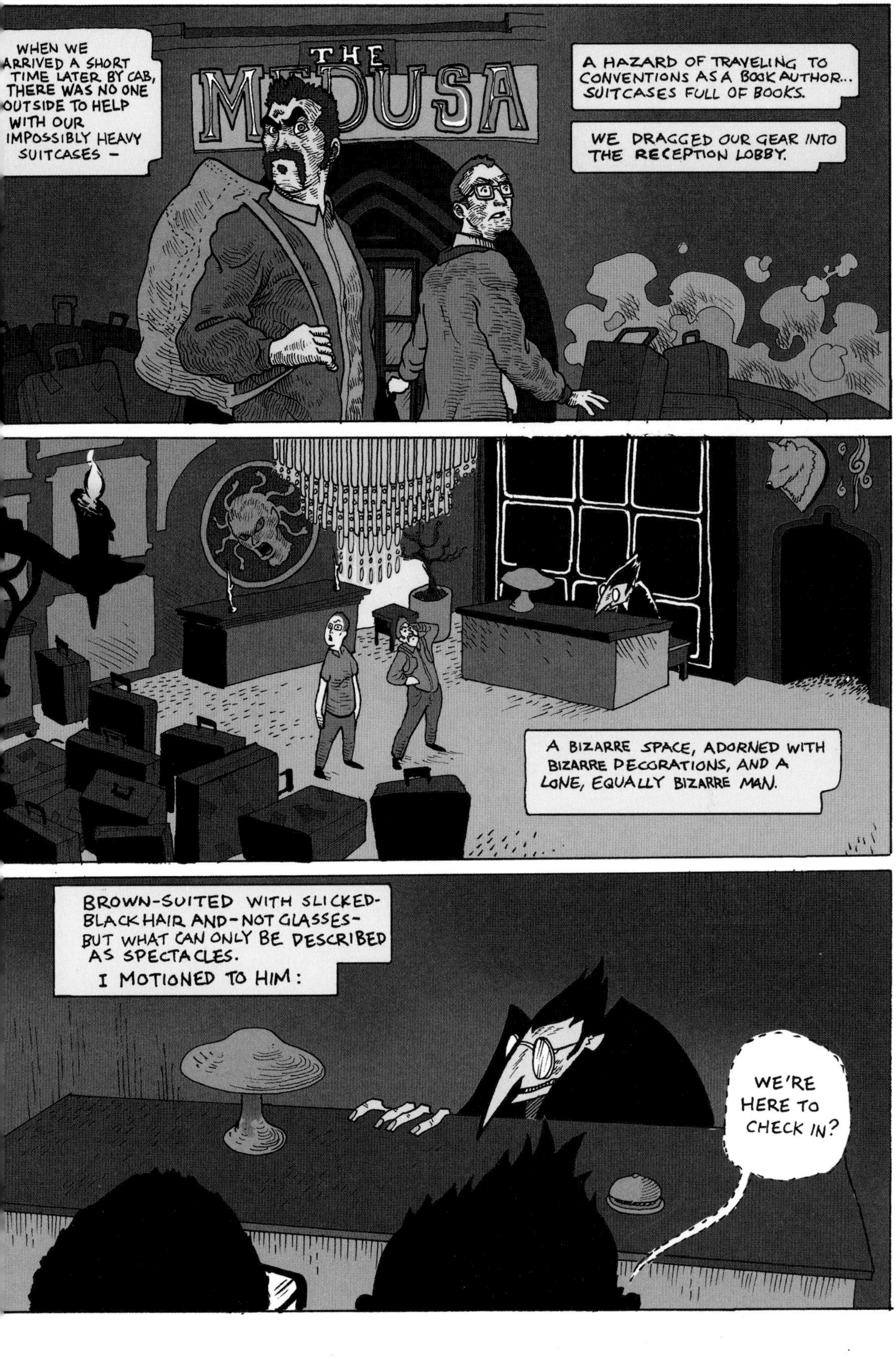
THE MEDUSA
WHEN WE ARRIVED A SHORT TIME LATER BY CAB, THERE WAS NO ONE OUTSIDE TO HELP WITH OUR IMPOSSIBLY HEAVY SUITCASES –
A HAZARD OF TRAVELING TO CONVENTIONS AS A BOOK AUTHOR... SUITCASES FULL OF BOOKS.
WE DRAGGED OUR GEAR INTO THE RECEPTION LOBBY.
A BIZARRE SPACE, ADORNED WITH BIZARRE DECORATIONS, AND A LONE, EQUALLY BIZARRE MAN.
BROWN-SUITED WITH SLICKED-BLACK HAIR AND – NOT GLASSES – BUT WHAT CAN ONLY BE DESCRIBED AS SPECTACLES.
I MOTIONED TO HIM:
WE'RE HERE TO CHECK IN?

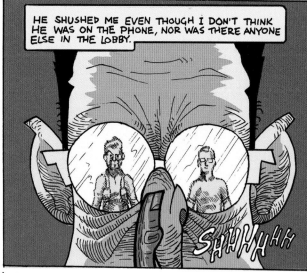

HE SHUSHED ME EVEN THOUGH I DON'T THINK HE WAS ON THE PHONE, NOR WAS THERE ANYONE ELSE IN THE LOBBY.

SHHHHHH

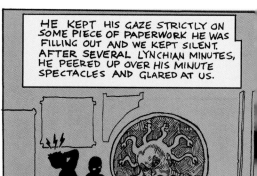

HE KEPT HIS GAZE STRICTLY ON SOME PIECE OF PAPERWORK HE WAS FILLING OUT AND WE KEPT SILENT. AFTER SEVERAL LYNCHIAN MINUTES, HE PEERED UP OVER HIS MINUTE SPECTACLES AND GLARED AT US.

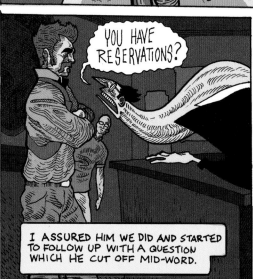

YOU HAVE RESERVATIONS?

I ASSURED HIM WE DID AND STARTED TO FOLLOW UP WITH A QUESTION WHICH HE CUT OFF MID-WORD.

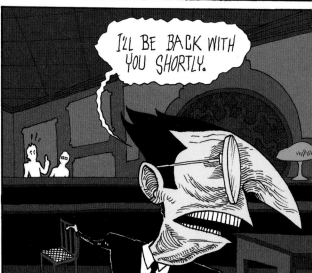

I'LL BE BACK WITH YOU SHORTLY.

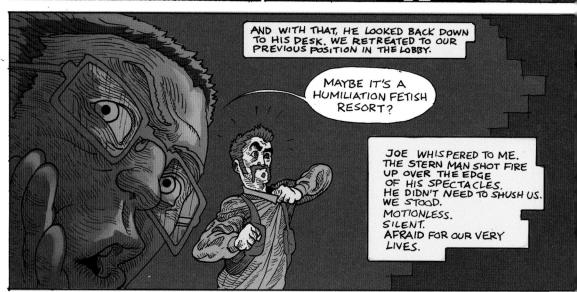

AND WITH THAT, HE LOOKED BACK DOWN TO HIS DESK. WE RETREATED TO OUR PREVIOUS POSITION IN THE LOBBY.

MAYBE IT'S A HUMILIATION FETISH RESORT?

JOE WHISPERED TO ME. THE STERN MAN SHOT FIRE UP OVER THE EDGE OF HIS SPECTACLES. HE DIDN'T NEED TO SHUSH US. WE STOOD.
MOTIONLESS.
SILENT.
AFRAID FOR OUR VERY LIVES.

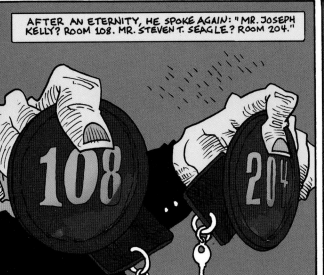

AFTER AN ETERNITY, HE SPOKE AGAIN: "MR. JOSEPH KELLY? ROOM 108. MR. STEVEN T. SEAGLE? ROOM 204."

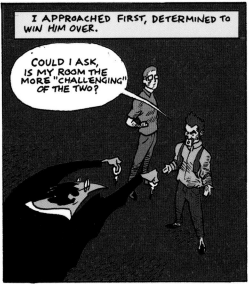

I APPROACHED FIRST, DETERMINED TO WIN HIM OVER.

COULD I ASK, IS MY ROOM THE MORE "CHALLENGING" OF THE TWO?

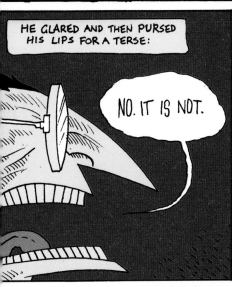

HE GLARED AND THEN PURSED HIS LIPS FOR A TERSE:

NO. IT IS NOT.

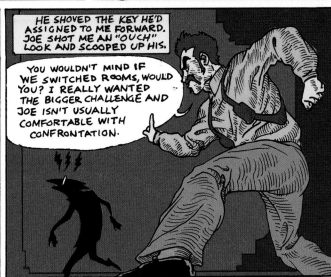

HE SHOVED THE KEY HE'D ASSIGNED TO ME FORWARD. JOE SHOT ME AN "OUCH" LOOK AND SCOOPED UP HIS.

YOU WOULDN'T MIND IF WE SWITCHED ROOMS, WOULD YOU? I REALLY WANTED THE BIGGER CHALLENGE AND JOE ISN'T USUALLY COMFORTABLE WITH CONFRONTATION.

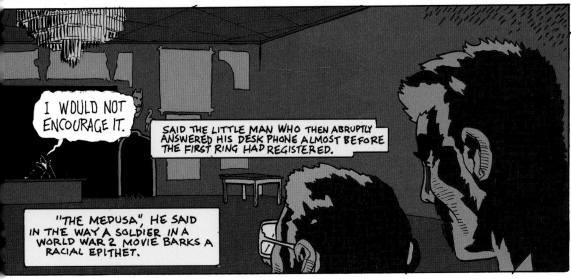

I WOULD NOT ENCOURAGE IT.

SAID THE LITTLE MAN WHO THEN ABRUPTLY ANSWERED HIS DESK PHONE ALMOST BEFORE THE FIRST RING HAD REGISTERED.

"THE MEDUSA", HE SAID IN THE WAY A SOLDIER IN A WORLD WAR 2 MOVIE BARKS A RACIAL EPITHET.

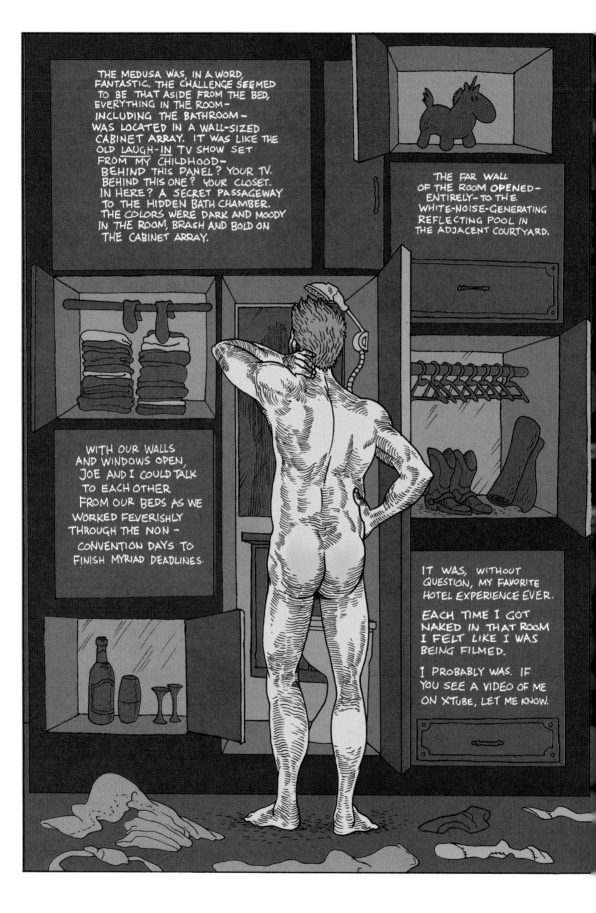

THE MEDUSA WAS, IN A WORD, FANTASTIC. THE CHALLENGE SEEMED TO BE THAT ASIDE FROM THE BED, EVERYTHING IN THE ROOM— INCLUDING THE BATHROOM— WAS LOCATED IN A WALL-SIZED CABINET ARRAY. IT WAS LIKE THE OLD LAUGH-IN TV SHOW SET FROM MY CHILDHOOD— BEHIND THIS PANEL? YOUR TV. BEHIND THIS ONE? YOUR CLOSET. IN HERE? A SECRET PASSAGEWAY TO THE HIDDEN BATH CHAMBER. THE COLORS WERE DARK AND MOODY IN THE ROOM, BRASH AND BOLD ON THE CABINET ARRAY.

THE FAR WALL OF THE ROOM OPENED— ENTIRELY—TO THE WHITE-NOISE-GENERATING REFLECTING POOL IN THE ADJACENT COURTYARD.

WITH OUR WALLS AND WINDOWS OPEN, JOE AND I COULD TALK TO EACH OTHER FROM OUR BEDS AS WE WORKED FEVERISHLY THROUGH THE NON- CONVENTION DAYS TO FINISH MYRIAD DEADLINES.

IT WAS, WITHOUT QUESTION, MY FAVORITE HOTEL EXPERIENCE EVER.

EACH TIME I GOT NAKED IN THAT ROOM I FELT LIKE I WAS BEING FILMED.

I PROBABLY WAS. IF YOU SEE A VIDEO OF ME ON XTUBE, LET ME KNOW.

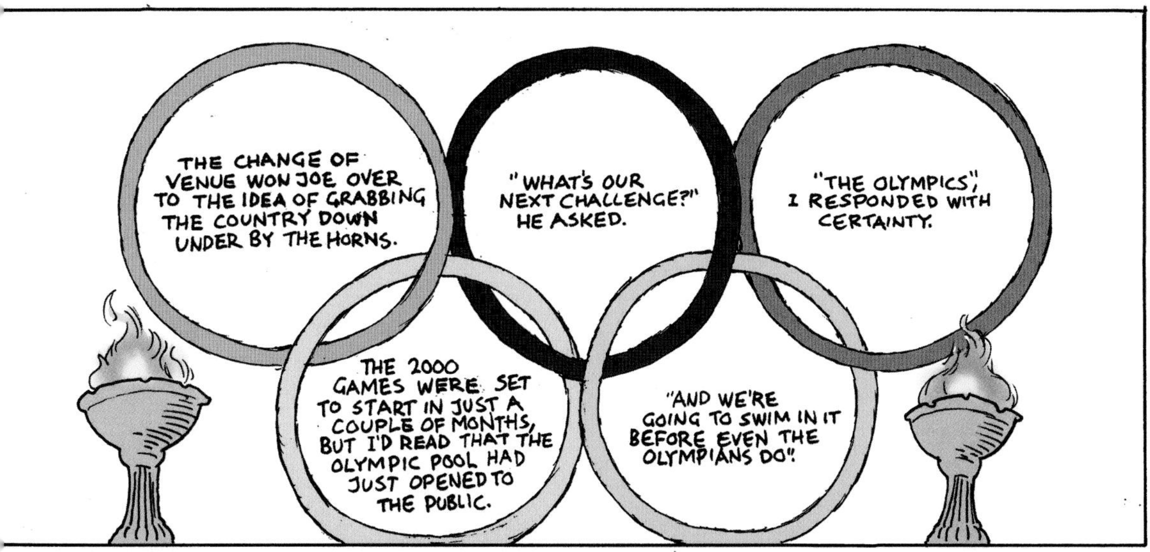
THE CHANGE OF VENUE WON JOE OVER TO THE IDEA OF GRABBING THE COUNTRY DOWN UNDER BY THE HORNS.
THE 2000 GAMES WERE SET TO START IN JUST A COUPLE OF MONTHS, BUT I'D READ THAT THE OLYMPIC POOL HAD JUST OPENED TO THE PUBLIC.
"WHAT'S OUR NEXT CHALLENGE?" HE ASKED.
"AND WE'RE GOING TO SWIM IN IT BEFORE EVEN THE OLYMPIANS DO".
"THE OLYMPICS", I RESPONDED WITH CERTAINTY.

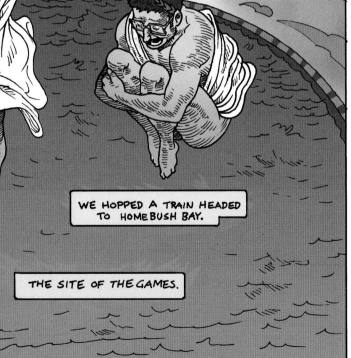

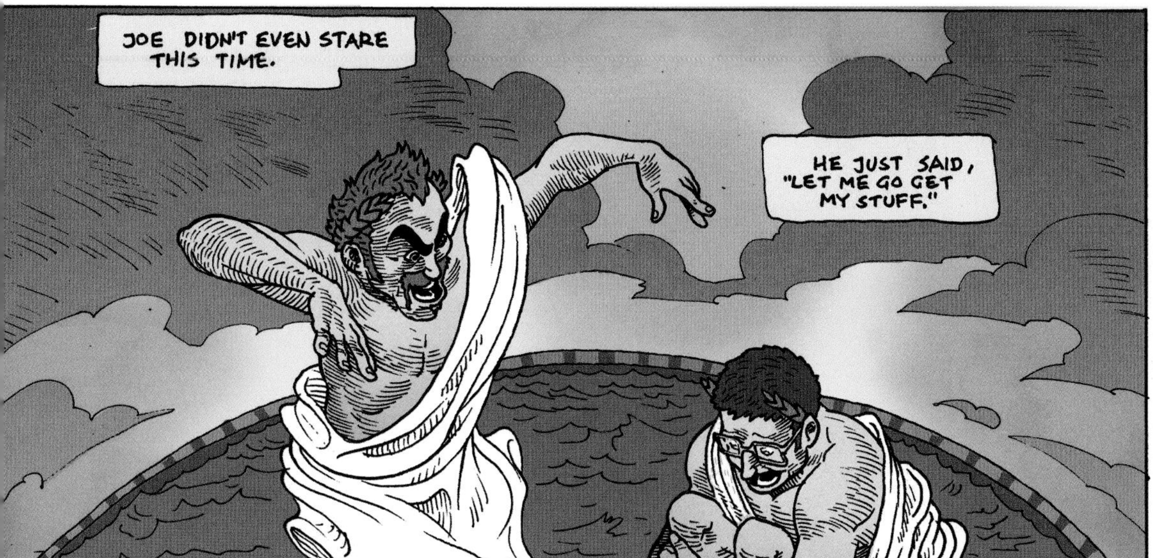
JOE DIDN'T EVEN STARE THIS TIME.
HE JUST SAID, "LET ME GO GET MY STUFF."
WE HOPPED A TRAIN HEADED TO HOMEBUSH BAY.
THE SITE OF THE GAMES.

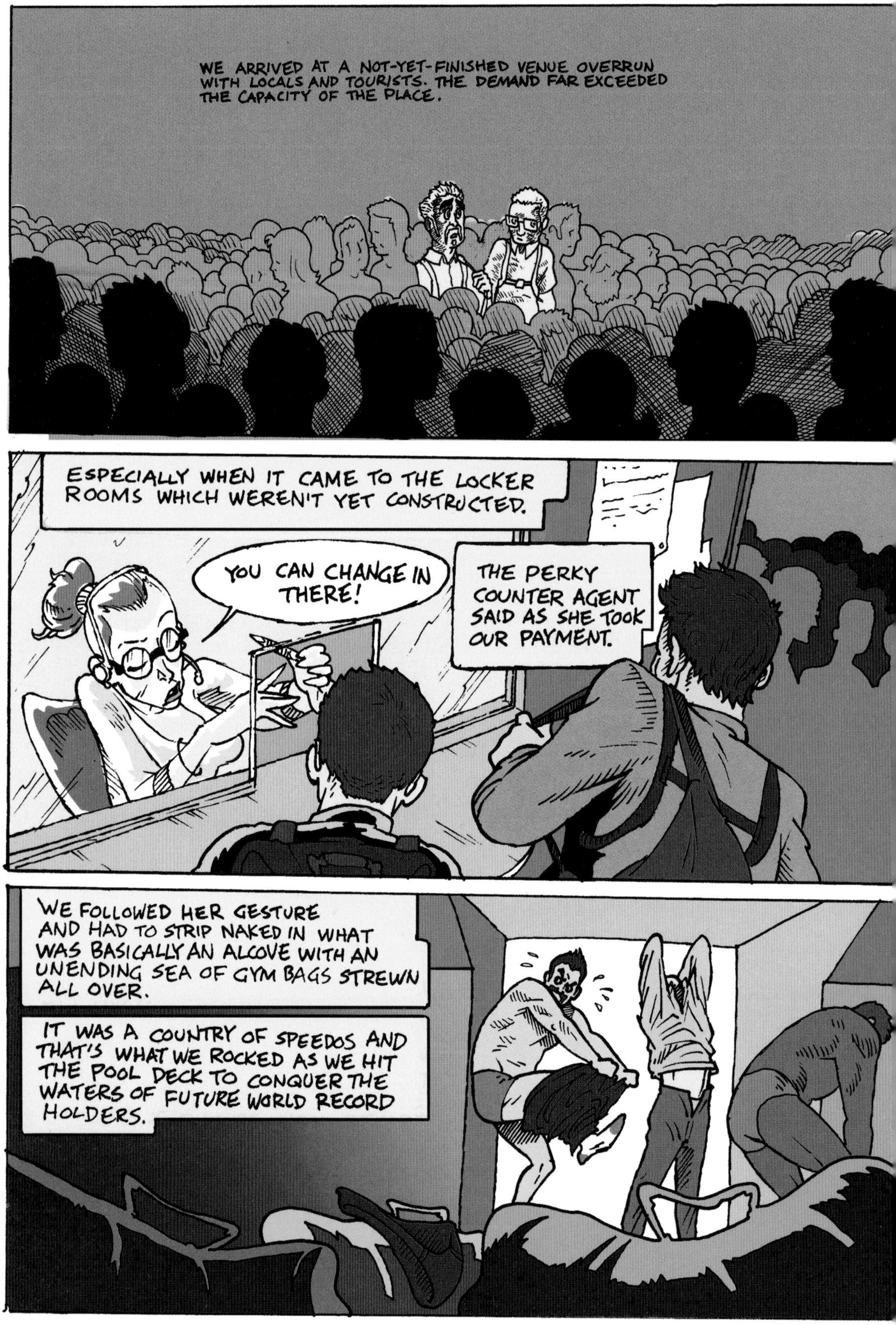
WE ARRIVED AT A NOT-YET-FINISHED VENUE OVERRUN WITH LOCALS AND TOURISTS. THE DEMAND FAR EXCEEDED THE CAPACITY OF THE PLACE.
ESPECIALLY WHEN IT CAME TO THE LOCKER ROOMS WHICH WEREN'T YET CONSTRUCTED.
YOU CAN CHANGE IN THERE!
THE PERKY COUNTER AGENT SAID AS SHE TOOK OUR PAYMENT.
WE FOLLOWED HER GESTURE AND HAD TO STRIP NAKED IN WHAT WAS BASICALLY AN ALCOVE WITH AN UNENDING SEA OF GYM BAGS STREWN ALL OVER.
IT WAS A COUNTRY OF SPEEDOS AND THAT'S WHAT WE ROCKED AS WE HIT THE POOL DECK TO CONQUER THE WATERS OF FUTURE WORLD RECORD HOLDERS.

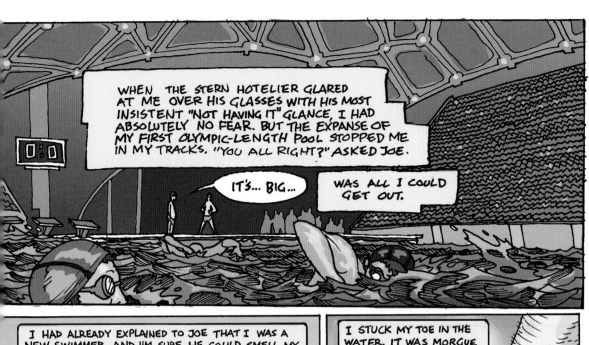

WHEN THE STERN HOTELIER GLARED AT ME OVER HIS GLASSES WITH HIS MOST INSISTENT "NOT HAVING IT" GLANCE, I HAD ABSOLUTELY NO FEAR. BUT THE EXPANSE OF MY FIRST OLYMPIC-LENGTH POOL STOPPED ME IN MY TRACKS. "YOU ALL RIGHT?" ASKED JOE.

IT'S... BIG...

WAS ALL I COULD GET OUT.

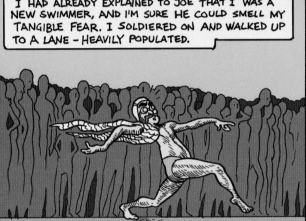

I HAD ALREADY EXPLAINED TO JOE THAT I WAS A NEW SWIMMER, AND I'M SURE HE COULD SMELL MY TANGIBLE FEAR. I SOLDIERED ON AND WALKED UP TO A LANE - HEAVILY POPULATED.

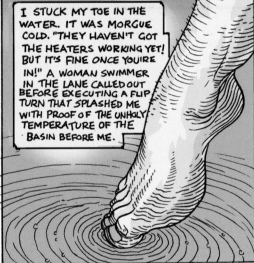

I STUCK MY TOE IN THE WATER. IT WAS MORGUE COLD. "THEY HAVEN'T GOT THE HEATERS WORKING YET! BUT IT'S FINE ONCE YOU'RE IN!" A WOMAN SWIMMER IN THE LANE CALLED OUT BEFORE EXECUTING A FLIP TURN THAT SPLASHED ME WITH PROOF OF THE UNHOLY TEMPERATURE OF THE BASIN BEFORE ME.

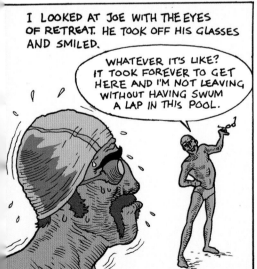

I LOOKED AT JOE WITH THE EYES OF RETREAT. HE TOOK OFF HIS GLASSES AND SMILED.

WHATEVER IT'S LIKE? IT TOOK FOREVER TO GET HERE AND I'M NOT LEAVING WITHOUT HAVING SWUM A LAP IN THIS POOL.

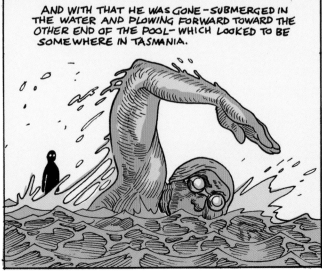

AND WITH THAT HE WAS GONE - SUBMERGED IN THE WATER AND PLOWING FORWARD TOWARD THE OTHER END OF THE POOL - WHICH LOOKED TO BE SOMEWHERE IN TASMANIA.

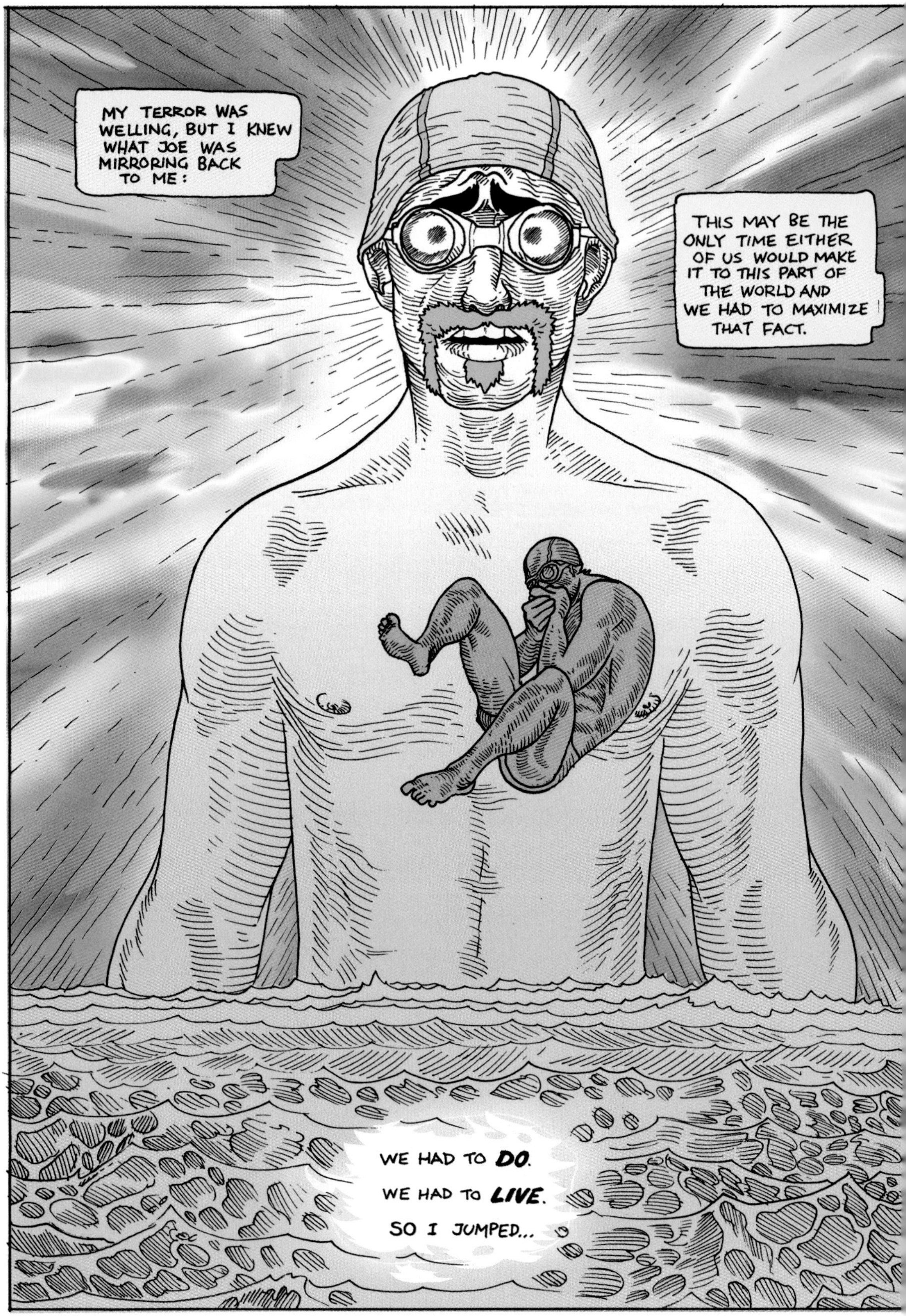
MY TERROR WAS WELLING, BUT I KNEW WHAT JOE WAS MIRRORING BACK TO ME:
THIS MAY BE THE ONLY TIME EITHER OF US WOULD MAKE IT TO THIS PART OF THE WORLD AND WE HAD TO MAXIMIZE THAT FACT.
WE HAD TO DO.
WE HAD TO LIVE.
SO I JUMPED...

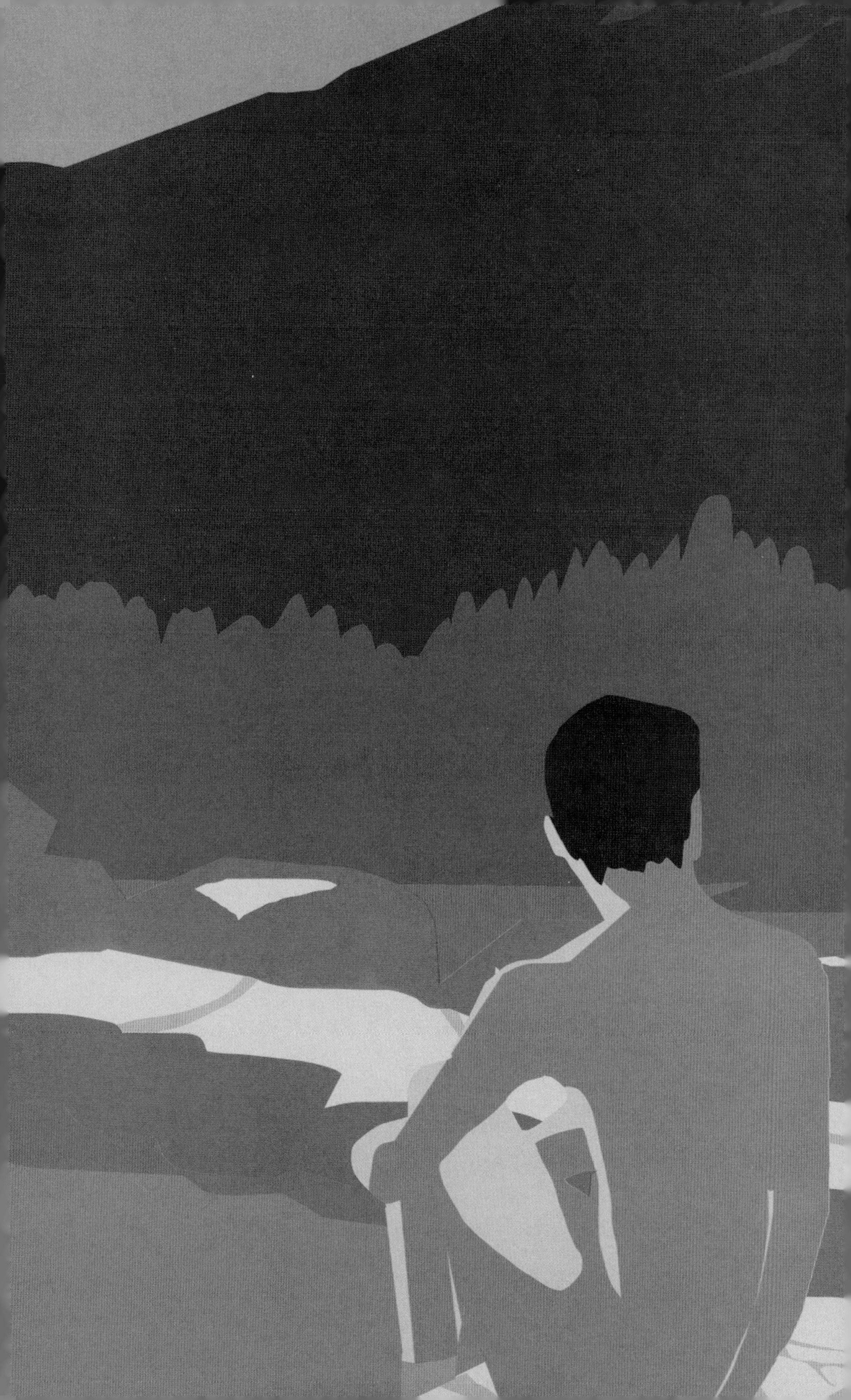

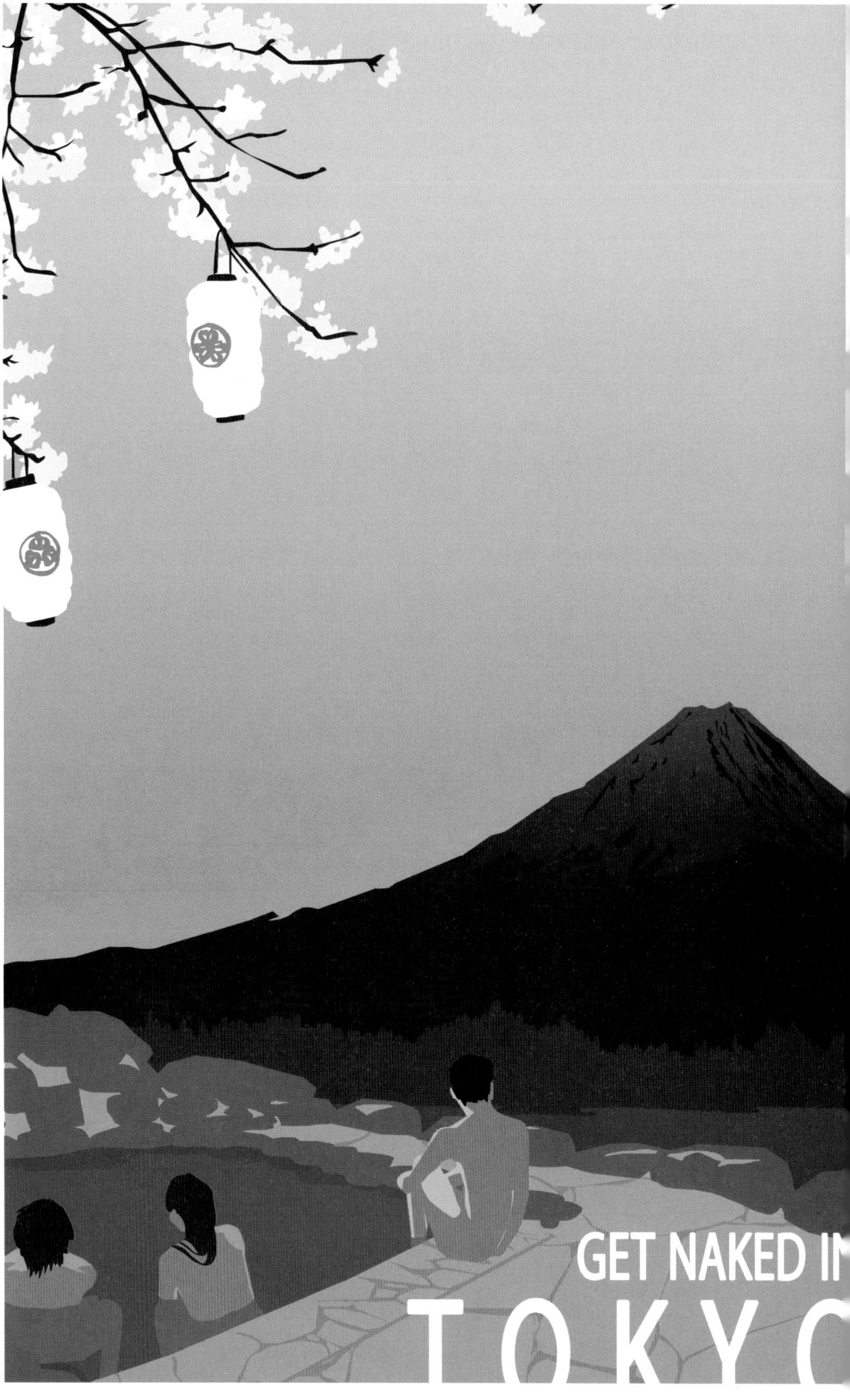
GET NAKED IN
TOKYO

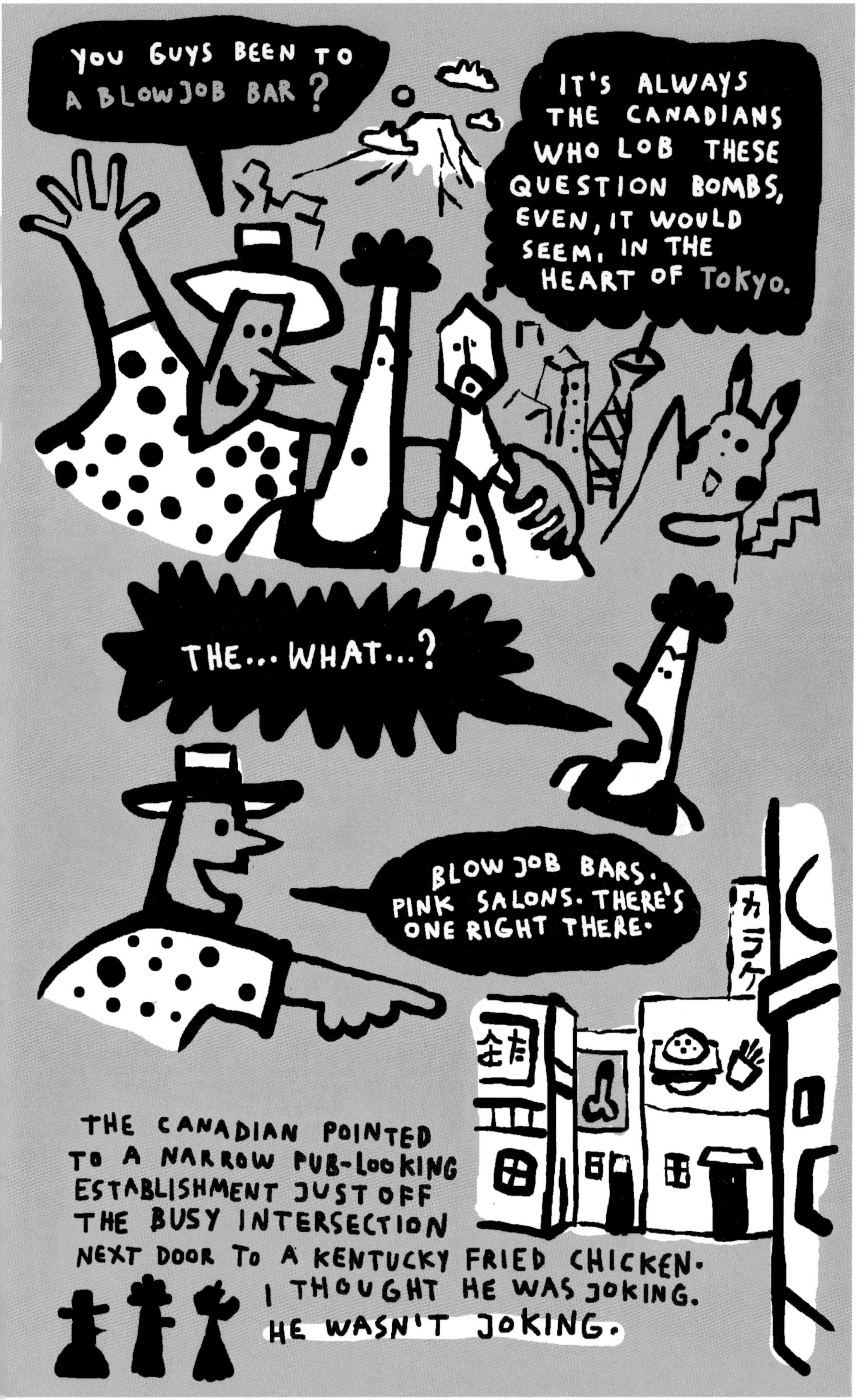

YOU GUYS BEEN TO A BLOWJOB BAR?
IT'S ALWAYS THE CANADIANS WHO LOB THESE QUESTION BOMBS, EVEN, IT WOULD SEEM, IN THE HEART OF TOKYO.
THE... WHAT...?
BLOW JOB BARS. PINK SALONS. THERE'S ONE RIGHT THERE.
カラケ
THE CANADIAN POINTED TO A NARROW PUB-LOOKING ESTABLISHMENT JUST OFF THE BUSY INTERSECTION NEXT DOOR TO A KENTUCKY FRIED CHICKEN.
I THOUGHT HE WAS JOKING.
HE WASN'T JOKING.

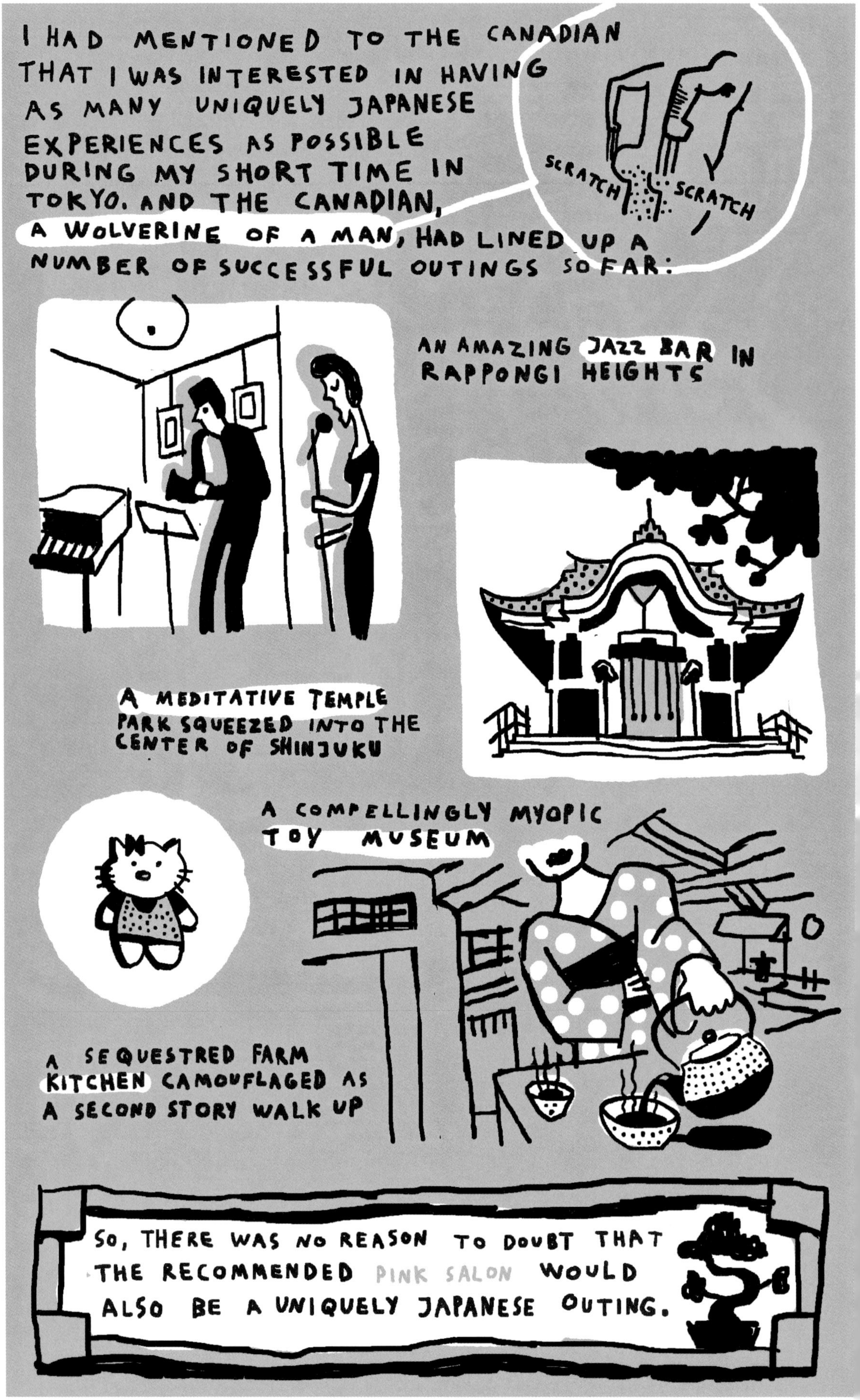
I HAD MENTIONED TO THE CANADIAN THAT I WAS INTERESTED IN HAVING AS MANY UNIQUELY JAPANESE EXPERIENCES AS POSSIBLE DURING MY SHORT TIME IN TOKYO. AND THE CANADIAN, A WOLVERINE OF A MAN, HAD LINED UP A NUMBER OF SUCCESSFUL OUTINGS SO FAR:
SCRATCH
SCRATCH
AN AMAZING JAZZ BAR IN RAPPONGI HEIGHTS
A MEDITATIVE TEMPLE PARK SQUEEZED INTO THE CENTER OF SHINJUKU
A COMPELLINGLY MYOPIC TOY MUSEUM
A SEQUESTRED FARM KITCHEN CAMOUFLAGED AS A SECOND STORY WALK UP
SO, THERE WAS NO REASON TO DOUBT THAT THE RECOMMENDED PINK SALON WOULD ALSO BE A UNIQUELY JAPANESE OUTING.

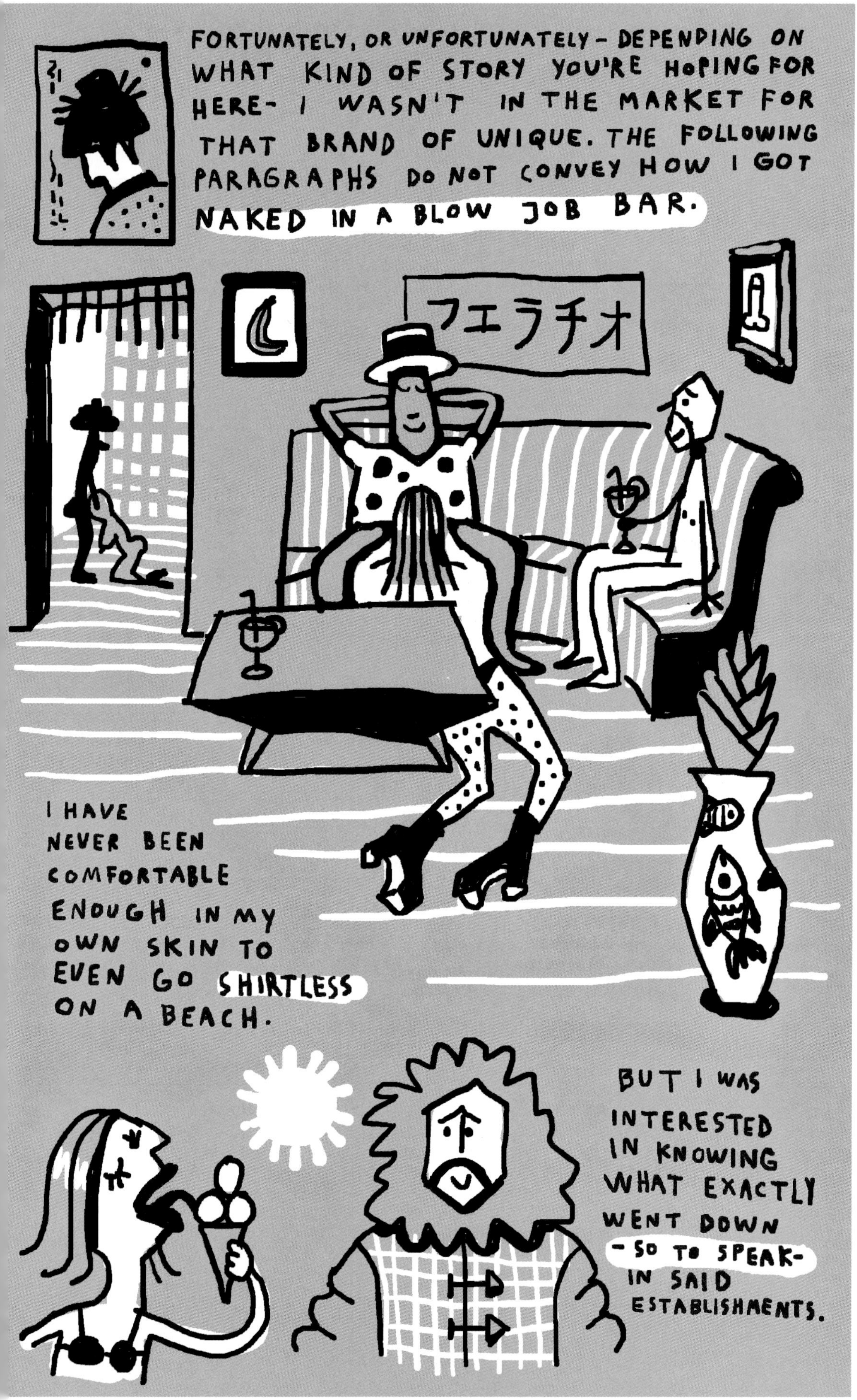
FORTUNATELY, OR UNFORTUNATELY - DEPENDING ON WHAT KIND OF STORY YOU'RE HOPING FOR HERE - I WASN'T IN THE MARKET FOR THAT BRAND OF UNIQUE. THE FOLLOWING PARAGRAPHS DO NOT CONVEY HOW I GOT NAKED IN A BLOW JOB BAR.
フェラチオ
I HAVE NEVER BEEN COMFORTABLE ENOUGH IN MY OWN SKIN TO EVEN GO SHIRTLESS ON A BEACH.
BUT I WAS INTERESTED IN KNOWING WHAT EXACTLY WENT DOWN - SO TO SPEAK - IN SAID ESTABLISHMENTS.

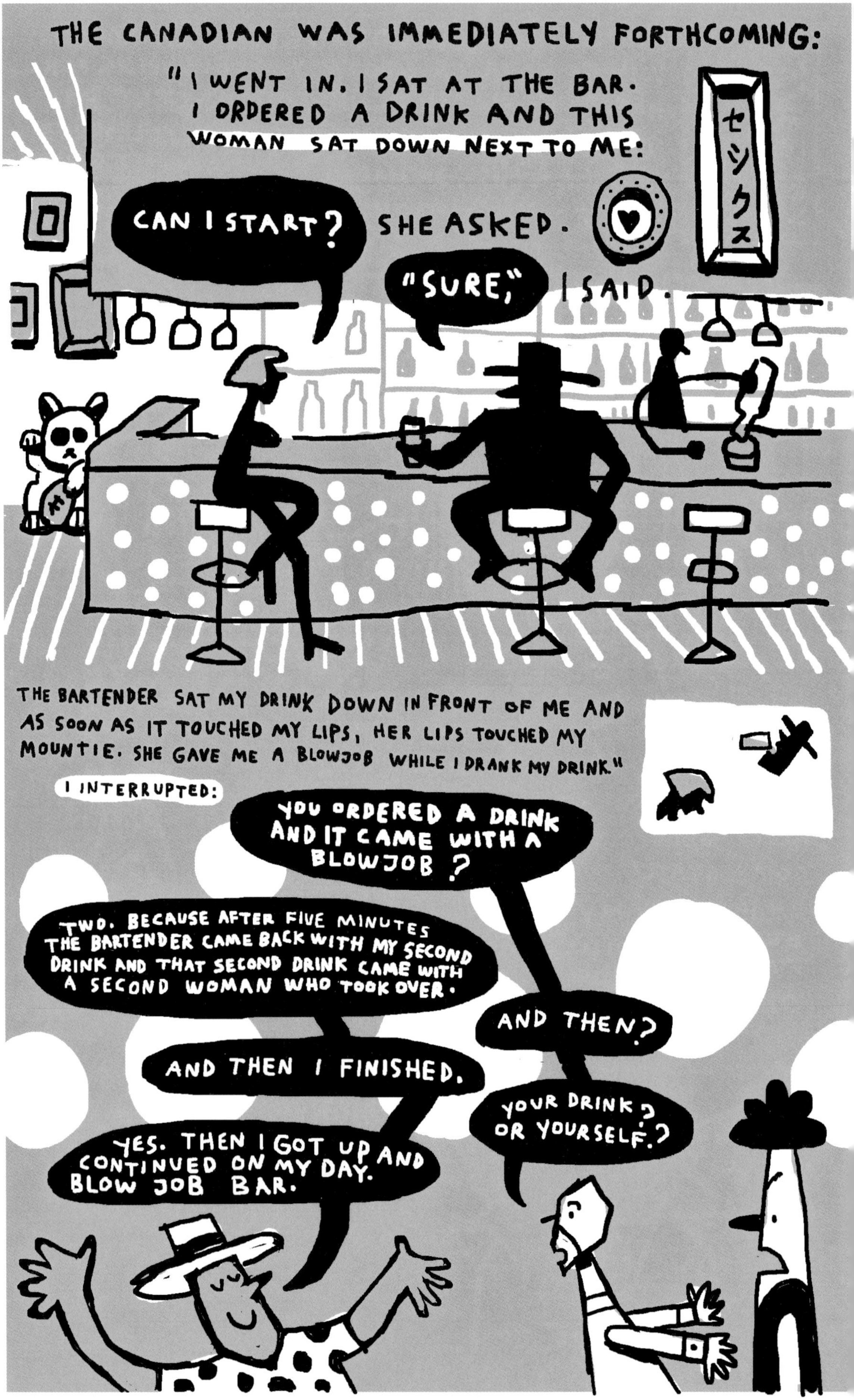

THE CANADIAN WAS IMMEDIATELY FORTHCOMING:
"I WENT IN. I SAT AT THE BAR. I ORDERED A DRINK AND THIS WOMAN SAT DOWN NEXT TO ME:
CAN I START?
SHE ASKED.
セシクス
"SURE,"
I SAID.
THE BARTENDER SAT MY DRINK DOWN IN FRONT OF ME AND AS SOON AS IT TOUCHED MY LIPS, HER LIPS TOUCHED MY MOUNTIE. SHE GAVE ME A BLOWJOB WHILE I DRANK MY DRINK."
I INTERRUPTED:
YOU ORDERED A DRINK AND IT CAME WITH A BLOWJOB?
TWO. BECAUSE AFTER FIVE MINUTES THE BARTENDER CAME BACK WITH MY SECOND DRINK AND THAT SECOND DRINK CAME WITH A SECOND WOMAN WHO TOOK OVER.
AND THEN?
AND THEN I FINISHED.
YOUR DRINK? OR YOURSELF?
YES. THEN I GOT UP AND CONTINUED ON MY DAY. BLOW JOB BAR.

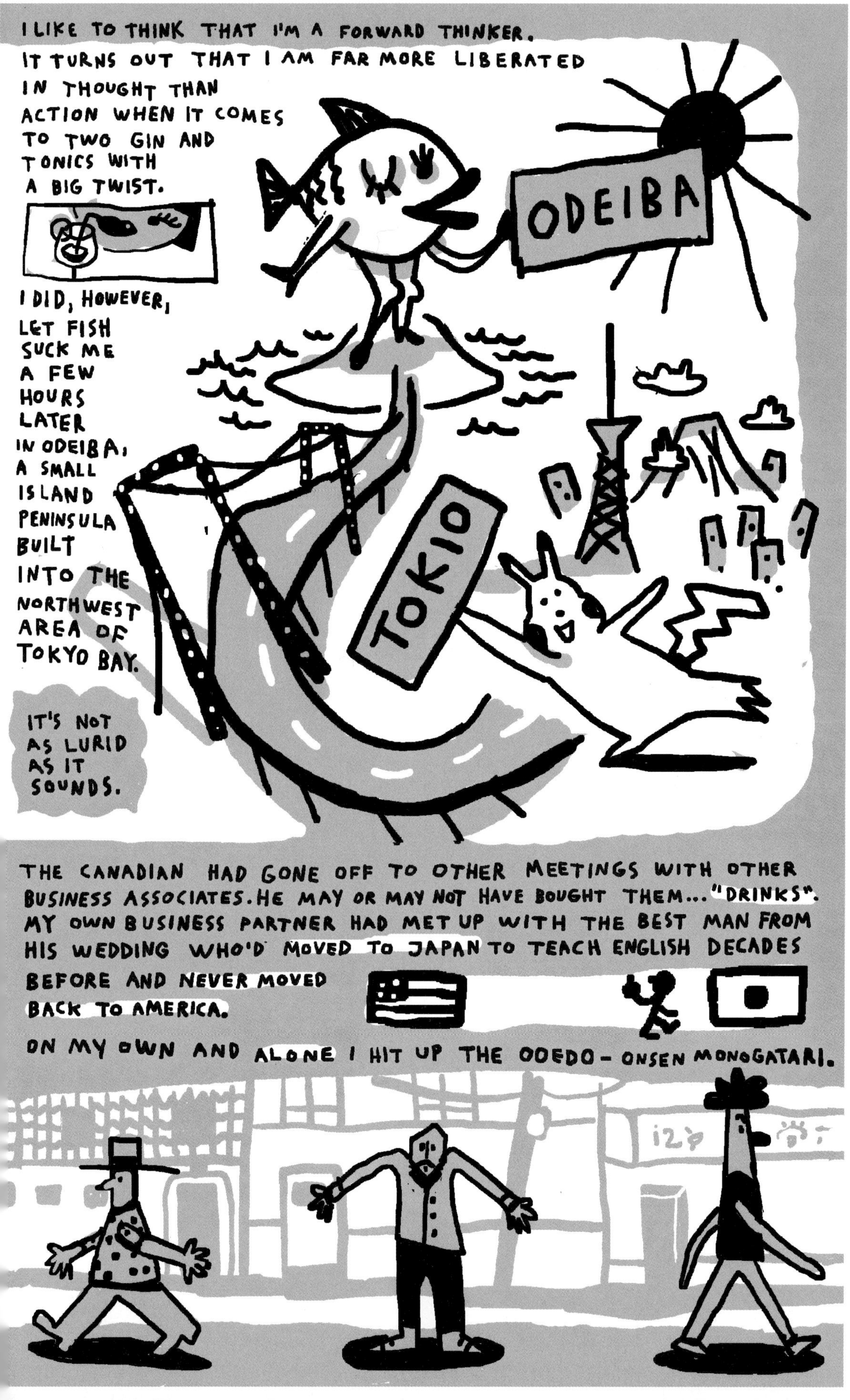
I LIKE TO THINK THAT I'M A FORWARD THINKER. IT TURNS OUT THAT I AM FAR MORE LIBERATED IN THOUGHT THAN ACTION WHEN IT COMES TO TWO GIN AND TONICS WITH A BIG TWIST.
ODEIBA
I DID, HOWEVER, LET FISH SUCK ME A FEW HOURS LATER IN ODEIBA, A SMALL ISLAND PENINSULA BUILT INTO THE NORTHWEST AREA OF TOKYO BAY.
TOKIO
IT'S NOT AS LURID AS IT SOUNDS.
THE CANADIAN HAD GONE OFF TO OTHER MEETINGS WITH OTHER BUSINESS ASSOCIATES. HE MAY OR MAY NOT HAVE BOUGHT THEM... "DRINKS". MY OWN BUSINESS PARTNER HAD MET UP WITH THE BEST MAN FROM HIS WEDDING WHO'D MOVED TO JAPAN TO TEACH ENGLISH DECADES BEFORE AND NEVER MOVED BACK TO AMERICA.
ON MY OWN AND ALONE I HIT UP THE ODEDO-ONSEN MONOGATARI.

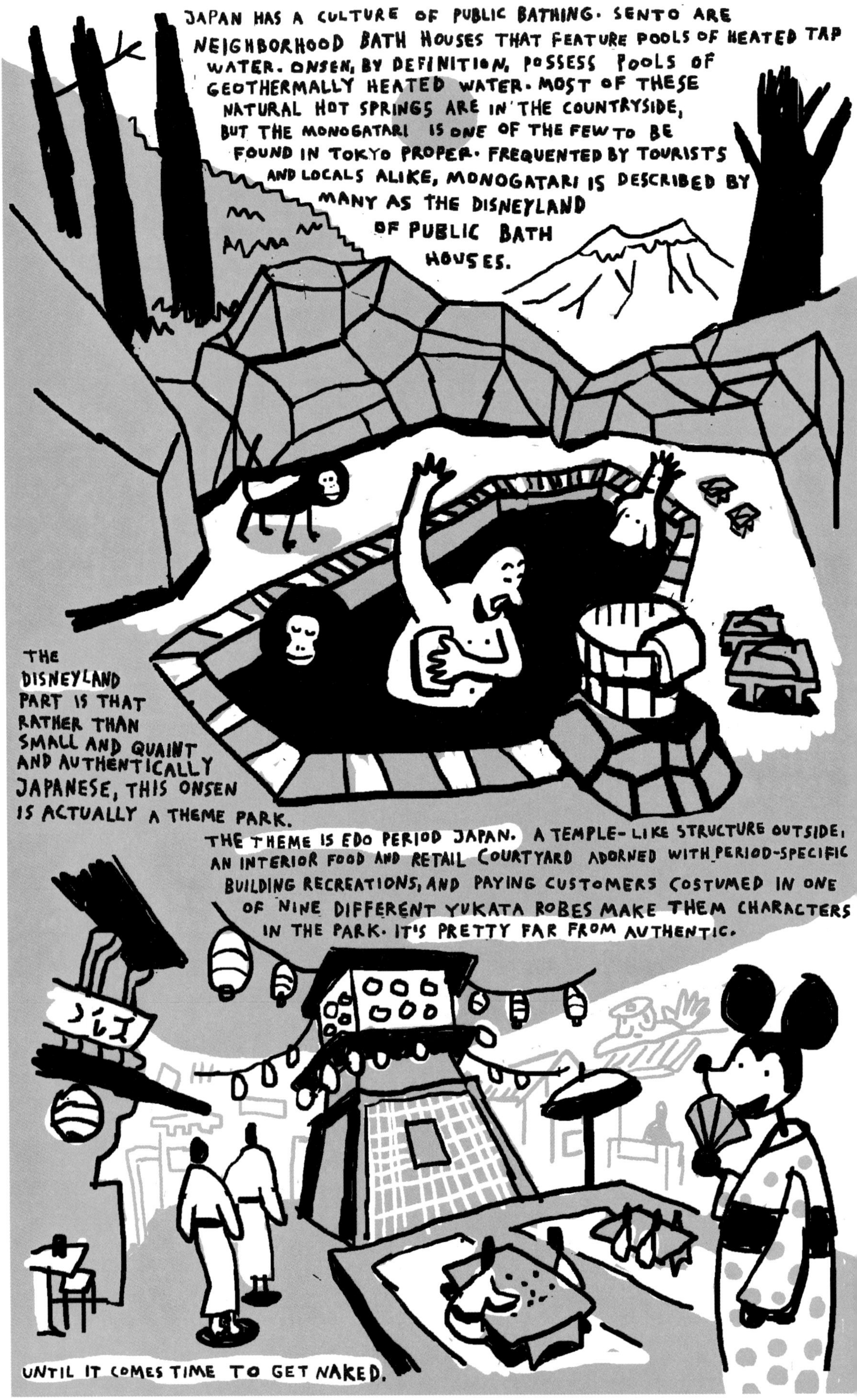
JAPAN HAS A CULTURE OF PUBLIC BATHING. SENTO ARE NEIGHBORHOOD BATH HOUSES THAT FEATURE POOLS OF HEATED TAP WATER. ONSEN, BY DEFINITION, POSSESS POOLS OF GEOTHERMALLY HEATED WATER. MOST OF THESE NATURAL HOT SPRINGS ARE IN THE COUNTRYSIDE, BUT THE MONOGATARI IS ONE OF THE FEW TO BE FOUND IN TOKYO PROPER. FREQUENTED BY TOURISTS AND LOCALS ALIKE, MONOGATARI IS DESCRIBED BY MANY AS THE DISNEYLAND OF PUBLIC BATH HOUSES.
THE DISNEYLAND PART IS THAT RATHER THAN SMALL AND QUAINT AND AUTHENTICALLY JAPANESE, THIS ONSEN IS ACTUALLY A THEME PARK.
THE THEME IS EDO PERIOD JAPAN. A TEMPLE-LIKE STRUCTURE OUTSIDE, AN INTERIOR FOOD AND RETAIL COURTYARD ADORNED WITH PERIOD-SPECIFIC BUILDING RECREATIONS, AND PAYING CUSTOMERS COSTUMED IN ONE OF NINE DIFFERENT YUKATA ROBES MAKE THEM CHARACTERS IN THE PARK. IT'S PRETTY FAR FROM AUTHENTIC.
UNTIL IT COMES TIME TO GET NAKED.

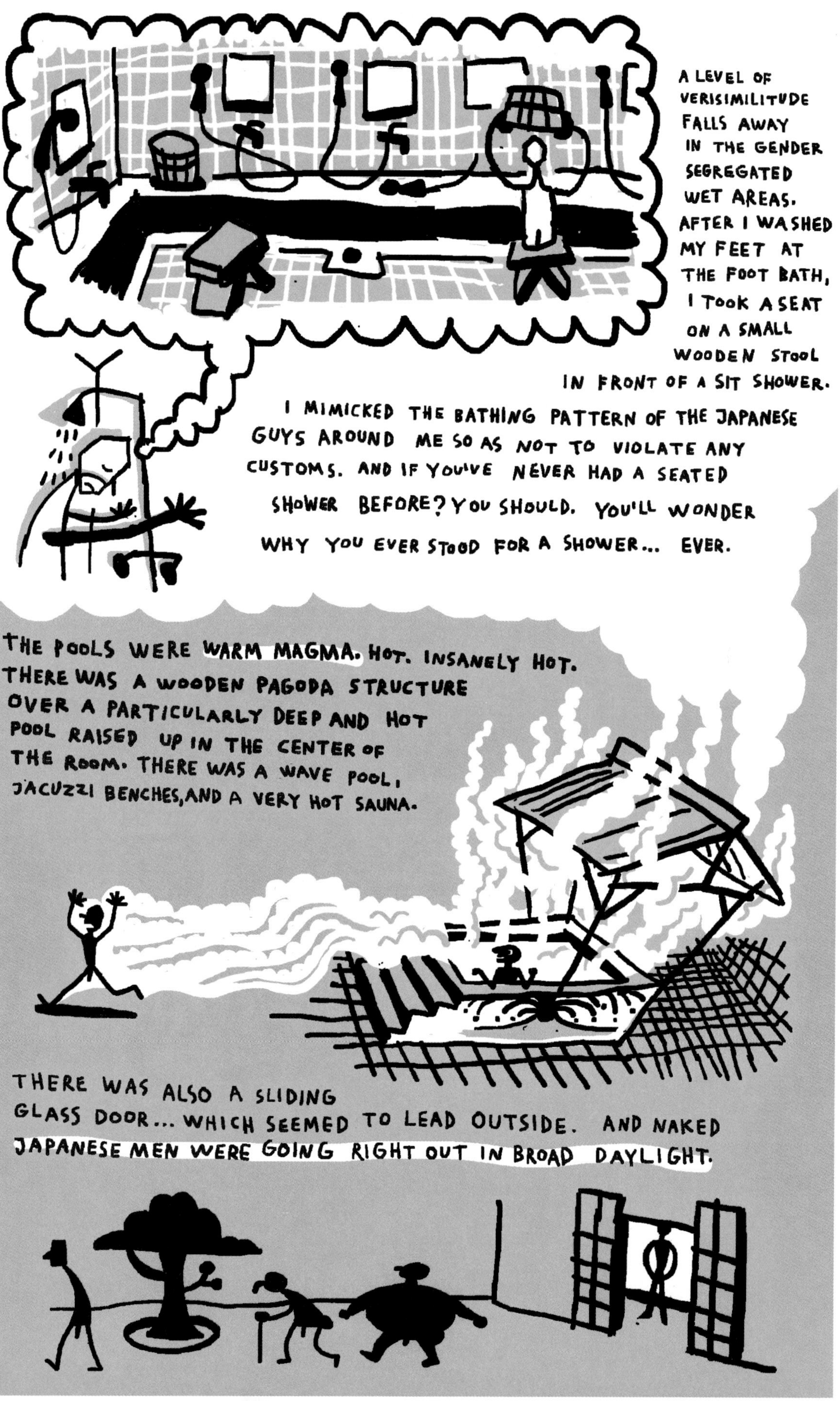
A LEVEL OF VERISIMILITUDE FALLS AWAY IN THE GENDER SEGREGATED WET AREAS. AFTER I WASHED MY FEET AT THE FOOT BATH, I TOOK A SEAT ON A SMALL WOODEN STOOL IN FRONT OF A SIT SHOWER.
I MIMICKED THE BATHING PATTERN OF THE JAPANESE GUYS AROUND ME SO AS NOT TO VIOLATE ANY CUSTOMS. AND IF YOU'VE NEVER HAD A SEATED SHOWER BEFORE? YOU SHOULD. YOU'LL WONDER WHY YOU EVER STOOD FOR A SHOWER... EVER.
THE POOLS WERE WARM MAGMA. HOT. INSANELY HOT. THERE WAS A WOODEN PAGODA STRUCTURE OVER A PARTICULARLY DEEP AND HOT POOL RAISED UP IN THE CENTER OF THE ROOM. THERE WAS A WAVE POOL, JACUZZI BENCHES, AND A VERY HOT SAUNA.
THERE WAS ALSO A SLIDING GLASS DOOR... WHICH SEEMED TO LEAD OUTSIDE. AND NAKED JAPANESE MEN WERE GOING RIGHT OUT IN BROAD DAYLIGHT.

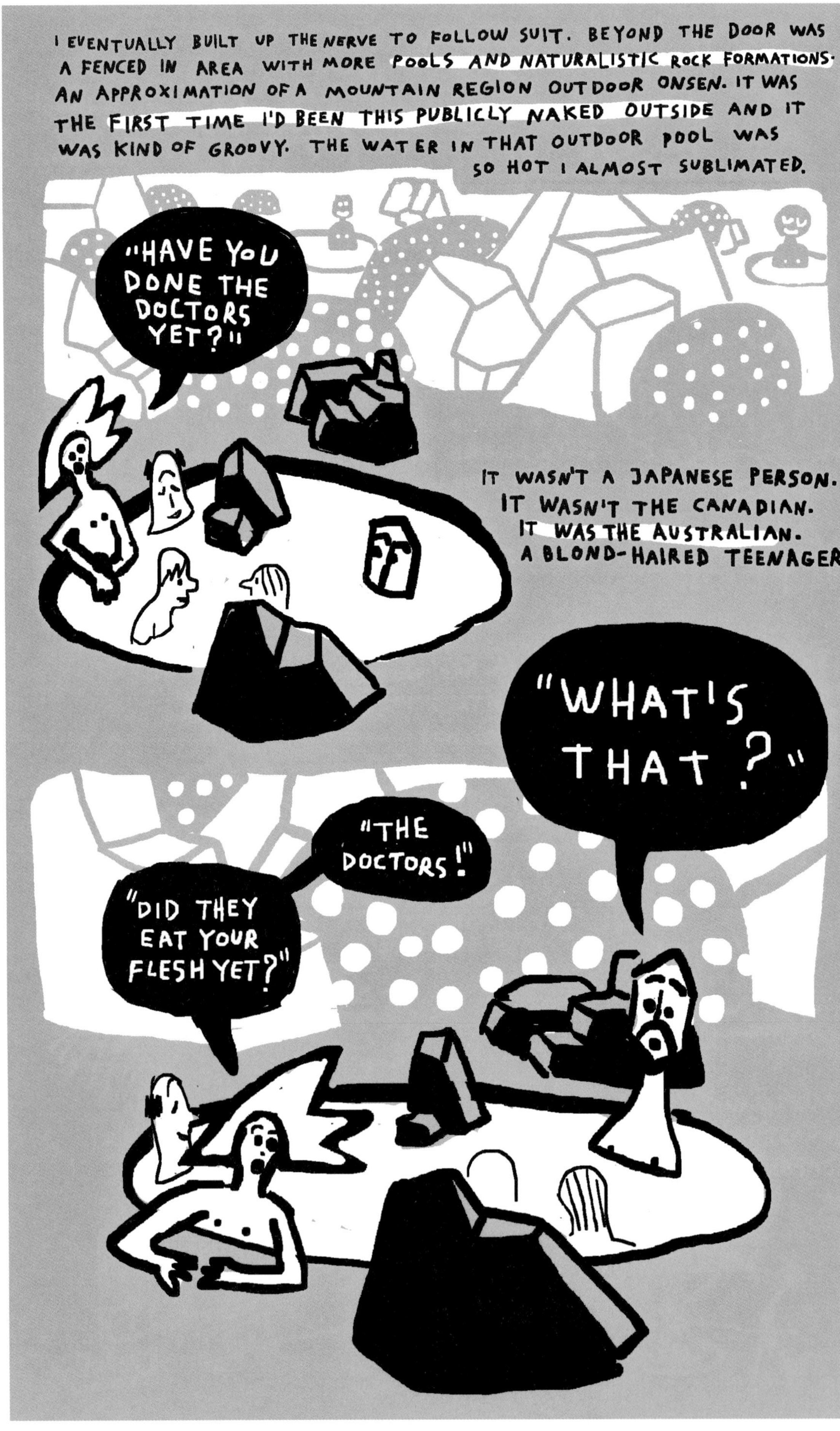
I EVENTUALLY BUILT UP THE NERVE TO FOLLOW SUIT. BEYOND THE DOOR WAS A FENCED IN AREA WITH MORE POOLS AND NATURALISTIC ROCK FORMATIONS. AN APPROXIMATION OF A MOUNTAIN REGION OUTDOOR ONSEN. IT WAS THE FIRST TIME I'D BEEN THIS PUBLICLY NAKED OUTSIDE AND IT WAS KIND OF GROOVY. THE WATER IN THAT OUTDOOR POOL WAS SO HOT I ALMOST SUBLIMATED.
"HAVE YOU DONE THE DOCTORS YET?"
IT WASN'T A JAPANESE PERSON. IT WASN'T THE CANADIAN. IT WAS THE AUSTRALIAN. A BLOND-HAIRED TEENAGER.
"WHAT'S THAT?"
"THE DOCTORS!"
"DID THEY EAT YOUR FLESH YET?"

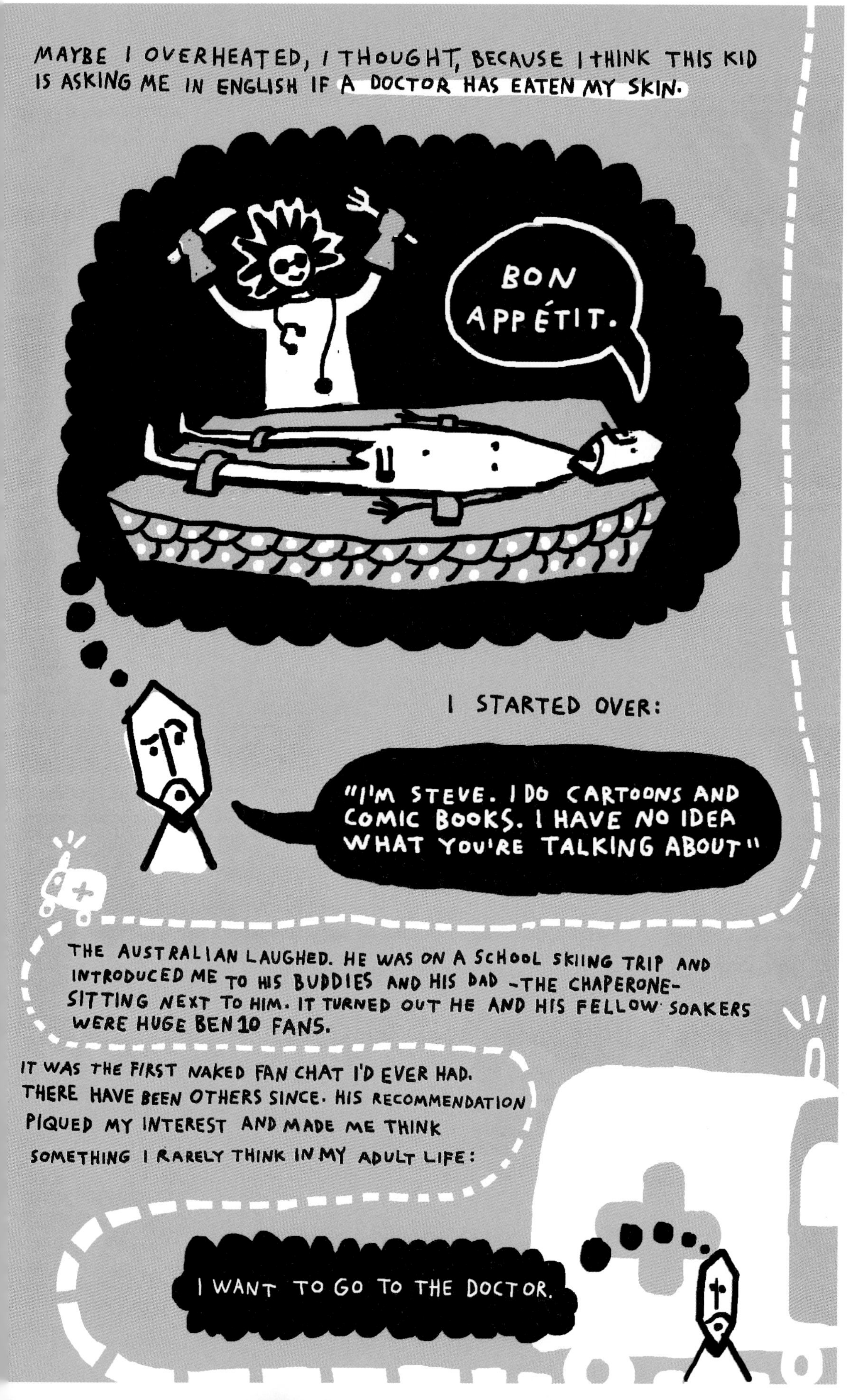
MAYBE I OVERHEATED, I THOUGHT, BECAUSE I THINK THIS KID IS ASKING ME IN ENGLISH IF A DOCTOR HAS EATEN MY SKIN.
BON APPÉTIT.
I STARTED OVER:
"I'M STEVE. I DO CARTOONS AND COMIC BOOKS. I HAVE NO IDEA WHAT YOU'RE TALKING ABOUT"
THE AUSTRALIAN LAUGHED. HE WAS ON A SCHOOL SKIING TRIP AND INTRODUCED ME TO HIS BUDDIES AND HIS DAD -THE CHAPERONE- SITTING NEXT TO HIM. IT TURNED OUT HE AND HIS FELLOW SOAKERS WERE HUGE BEN 10 FANS.
IT WAS THE FIRST NAKED FAN CHAT I'D EVER HAD. THERE HAVE BEEN OTHERS SINCE. HIS RECOMMENDATION PIQUED MY INTEREST AND MADE ME THINK SOMETHING I RARELY THINK IN MY ADULT LIFE:
I WANT TO GO TO THE DOCTOR.

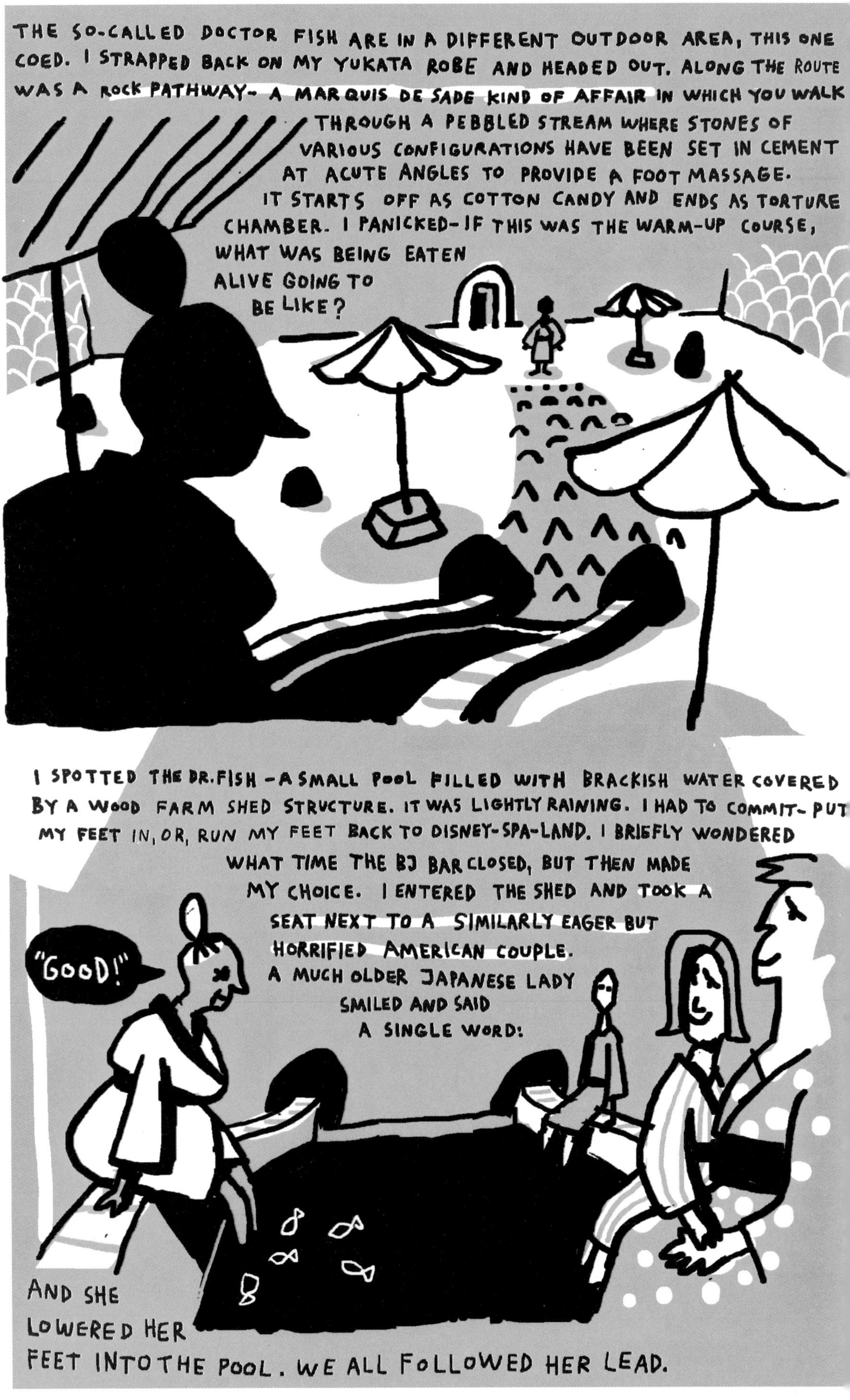
THE SO-CALLED DOCTOR FISH ARE IN A DIFFERENT OUTDOOR AREA, THIS ONE COED. I STRAPPED BACK ON MY YUKATA ROBE AND HEADED OUT. ALONG THE ROUTE WAS A ROCK PATHWAY- A MARQUIS DE SADE KIND OF AFFAIR IN WHICH YOU WALK THROUGH A PEBBLED STREAM WHERE STONES OF VARIOUS CONFIGURATIONS HAVE BEEN SET IN CEMENT AT ACUTE ANGLES TO PROVIDE A FOOT MASSAGE. IT STARTS OFF AS COTTON CANDY AND ENDS AS TORTURE CHAMBER. I PANICKED- IF THIS WAS THE WARM-UP COURSE, WHAT WAS BEING EATEN ALIVE GOING TO BE LIKE?
I SPOTTED THE DR. FISH - A SMALL POOL FILLED WITH BRACKISH WATER COVERED BY A WOOD FARM SHED STRUCTURE. IT WAS LIGHTLY RAINING. I HAD TO COMMIT- PUT MY FEET IN, OR, RUN MY FEET BACK TO DISNEY-SPA-LAND. I BRIEFLY WONDERED WHAT TIME THE BJ BAR CLOSED, BUT THEN MADE MY CHOICE. I ENTERED THE SHED AND TOOK A SEAT NEXT TO A SIMILARLY EAGER BUT HORRIFIED AMERICAN COUPLE. A MUCH OLDER JAPANESE LADY SMILED AND SAID A SINGLE WORD:
"GOOD!"
AND SHE LOWERED HER FEET INTO THE POOL. WE ALL FOLLOWED HER LEAD.

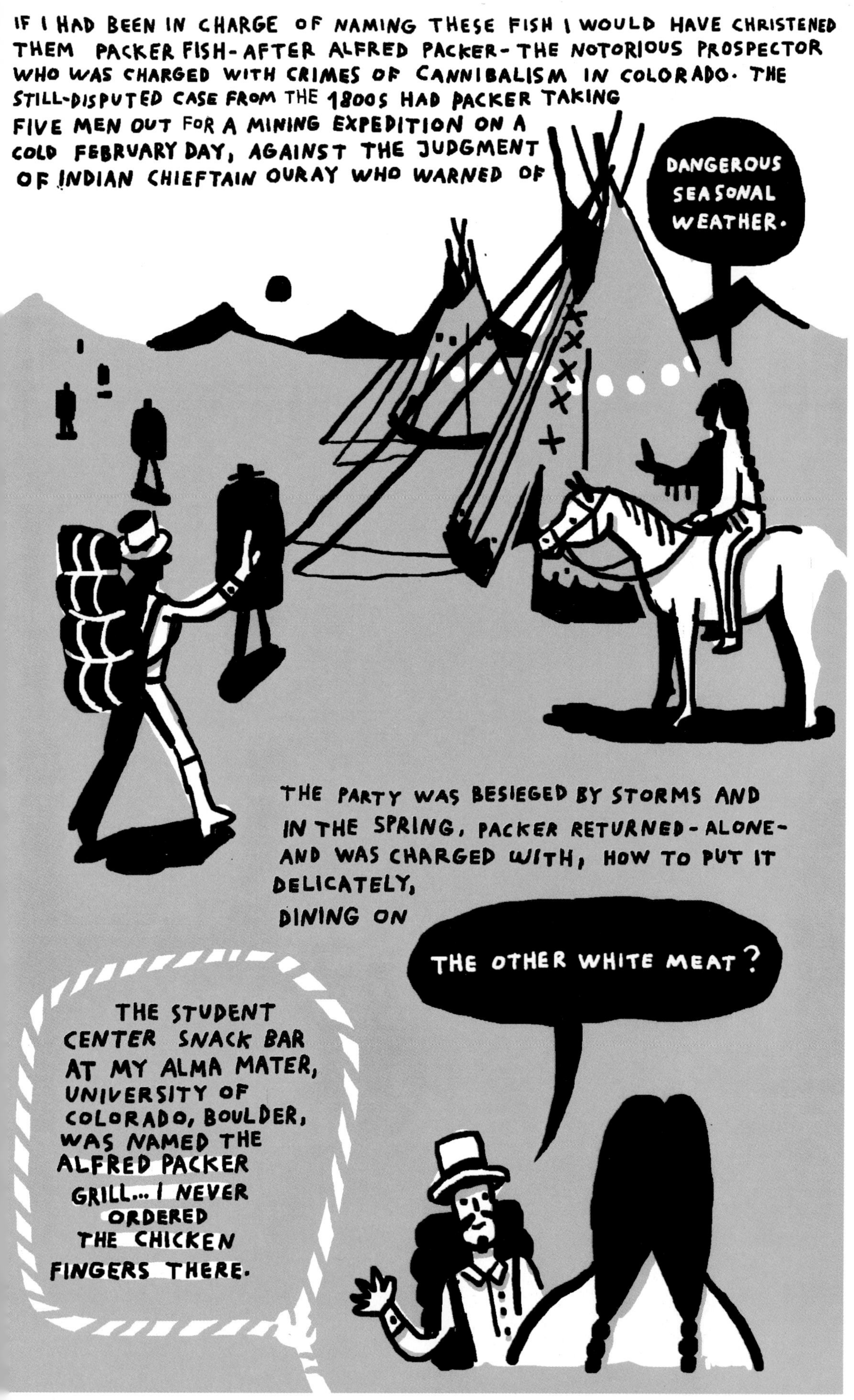
IF I HAD BEEN IN CHARGE OF NAMING THESE FISH I WOULD HAVE CHRISTENED THEM PACKER FISH - AFTER ALFRED PACKER - THE NOTORIOUS PROSPECTOR WHO WAS CHARGED WITH CRIMES OF CANNIBALISM IN COLORADO. THE STILL-DISPUTED CASE FROM THE 1800S HAD PACKER TAKING FIVE MEN OUT FOR A MINING EXPEDITION ON A COLD FEBRUARY DAY, AGAINST THE JUDGMENT OF INDIAN CHIEFTAIN OURAY WHO WARNED OF
DANGEROUS SEASONAL WEATHER.
THE PARTY WAS BESIEGED BY STORMS AND IN THE SPRING, PACKER RETURNED - ALONE - AND WAS CHARGED WITH, HOW TO PUT IT DELICATELY, DINING ON
THE OTHER WHITE MEAT?
THE STUDENT CENTER SNACK BAR AT MY ALMA MATER, UNIVERSITY OF COLORADO, BOULDER, WAS NAMED THE ALFRED PACKER GRILL... I NEVER ORDERED THE CHICKEN FINGERS THERE.

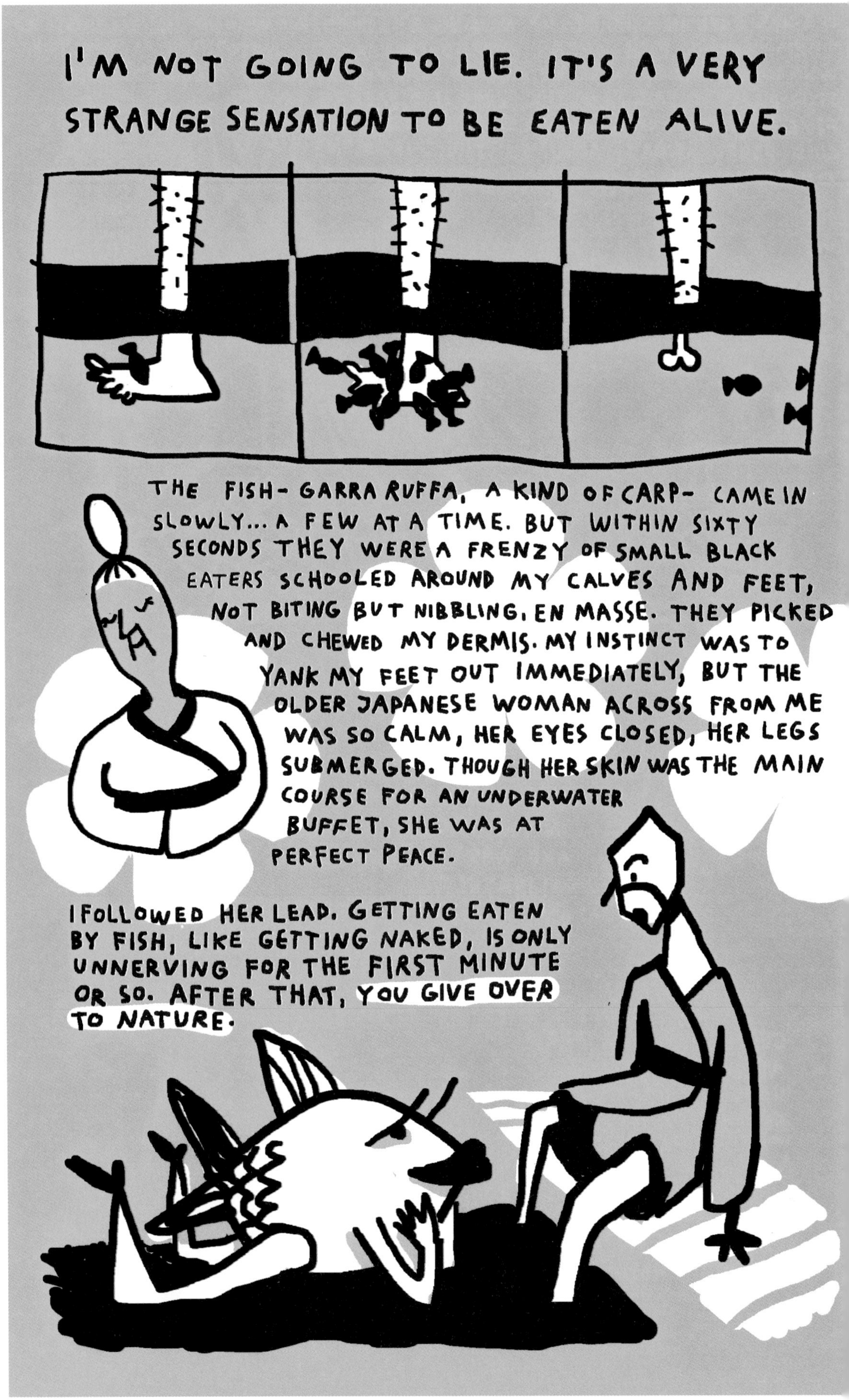
I'M NOT GOING TO LIE. IT'S A VERY STRANGE SENSATION TO BE EATEN ALIVE.
THE FISH- GARRA RUFFA, A KIND OF CARP- CAME IN SLOWLY... A FEW AT A TIME. BUT WITHIN SIXTY SECONDS THEY WERE A FRENZY OF SMALL BLACK EATERS SCHOOLED AROUND MY CALVES AND FEET, NOT BITING BUT NIBBLING, EN MASSE. THEY PICKED AND CHEWED MY DERMIS. MY INSTINCT WAS TO YANK MY FEET OUT IMMEDIATELY, BUT THE OLDER JAPANESE WOMAN ACROSS FROM ME WAS SO CALM, HER EYES CLOSED, HER LEGS SUBMERGED. THOUGH HER SKIN WAS THE MAIN COURSE FOR AN UNDERWATER BUFFET, SHE WAS AT PERFECT PEACE.
I FOLLOWED HER LEAD. GETTING EATEN BY FISH, LIKE GETTING NAKED, IS ONLY UNNERVING FOR THE FIRST MINUTE OR SO. AFTER THAT, YOU GIVE OVER TO NATURE.

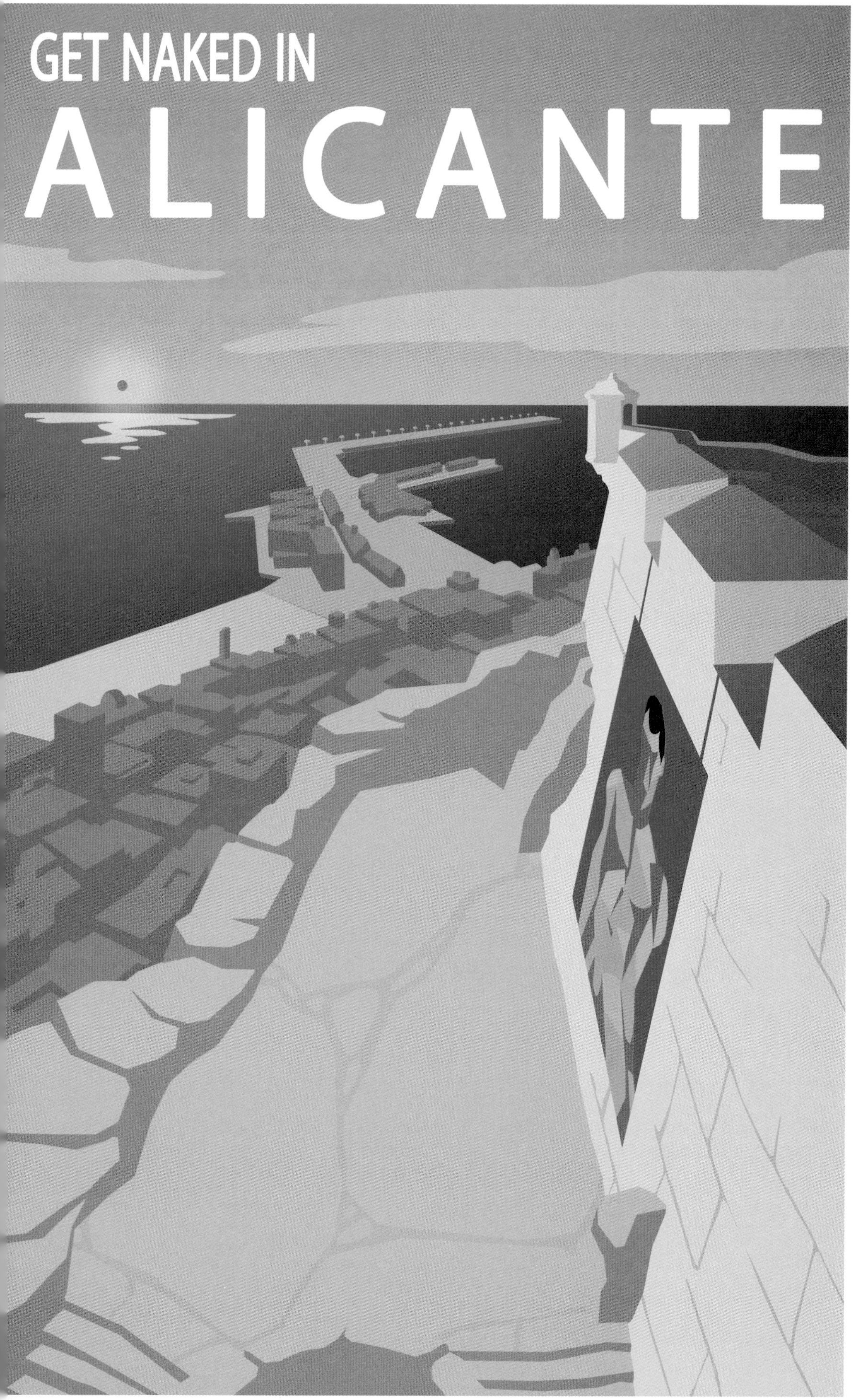
GET NAKED IN
ALICANTE

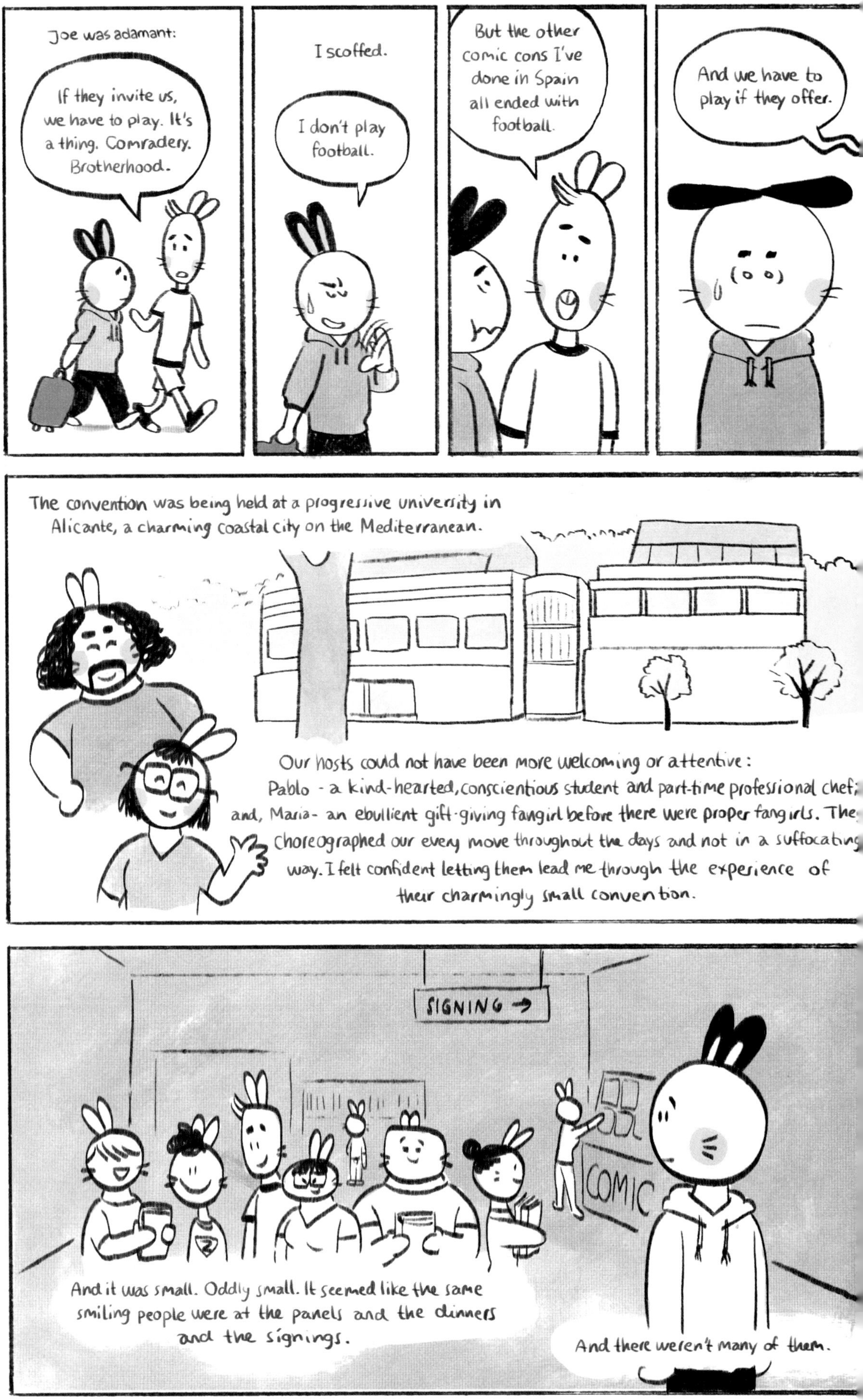
Joe was adamant:
If they invite us, we have to play. It's a thing. Comradery. Brotherhood.
I scoffed.
I don't play football.
But the other comic cons I've done in Spain all ended with football.
And we have to play if they offer.
The convention was being held at a progressive university in Alicante, a charming coastal city on the Mediterranean.
Our hosts could not have been more welcoming or attentive: Pablo - a kind-hearted, conscientious student and part-time professional chef; and, Maria- an ebullient gift-giving fangirl before there were proper fangirls. They choreographed our every move throughout the days and not in a suffocating way. I felt confident letting them lead me through the experience of their charmingly small convention.
SIGNING →
COMIC
And it was small. Oddly small. It seemed like the same smiling people were at the panels and the dinners and the signings.
And there weren't many of them.

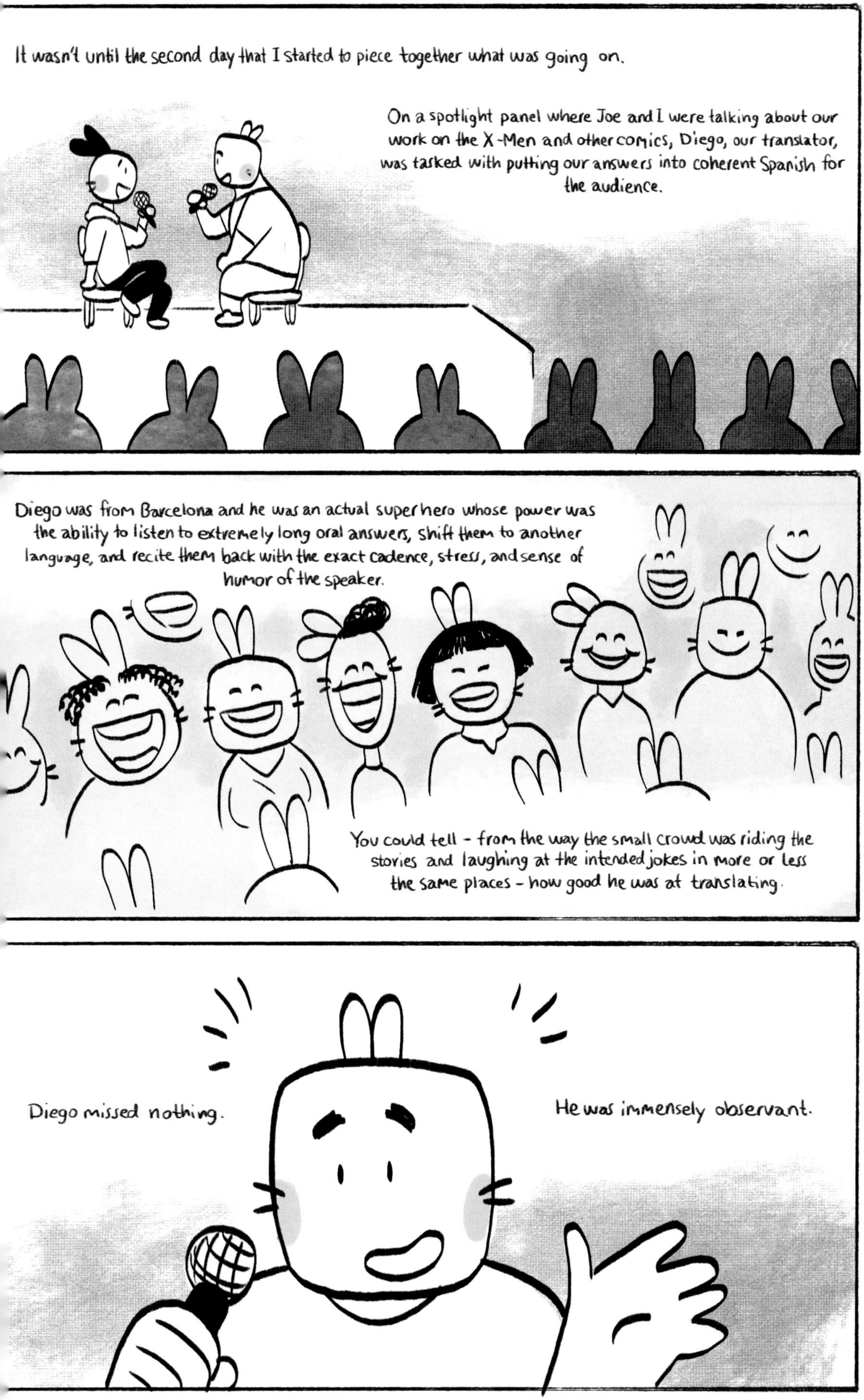
It wasn't until the second day that I started to piece together what was going on.
On a spotlight panel where Joe and I were talking about our work on the X-Men and other comics, Diego, our translator, was tasked with putting our answers into coherent Spanish for the audience.
Diego was from Barcelona and he was an actual superhero whose power was the ability to listen to extremely long oral answers, shift them to another language, and recite them back with the exact cadence, stress, and sense of humor of the speaker.
You could tell - from the way the small crowd was riding the stories and laughing at the intended jokes in more or less the same places - how good he was at translating.
Diego missed nothing.
He was immensely observant.

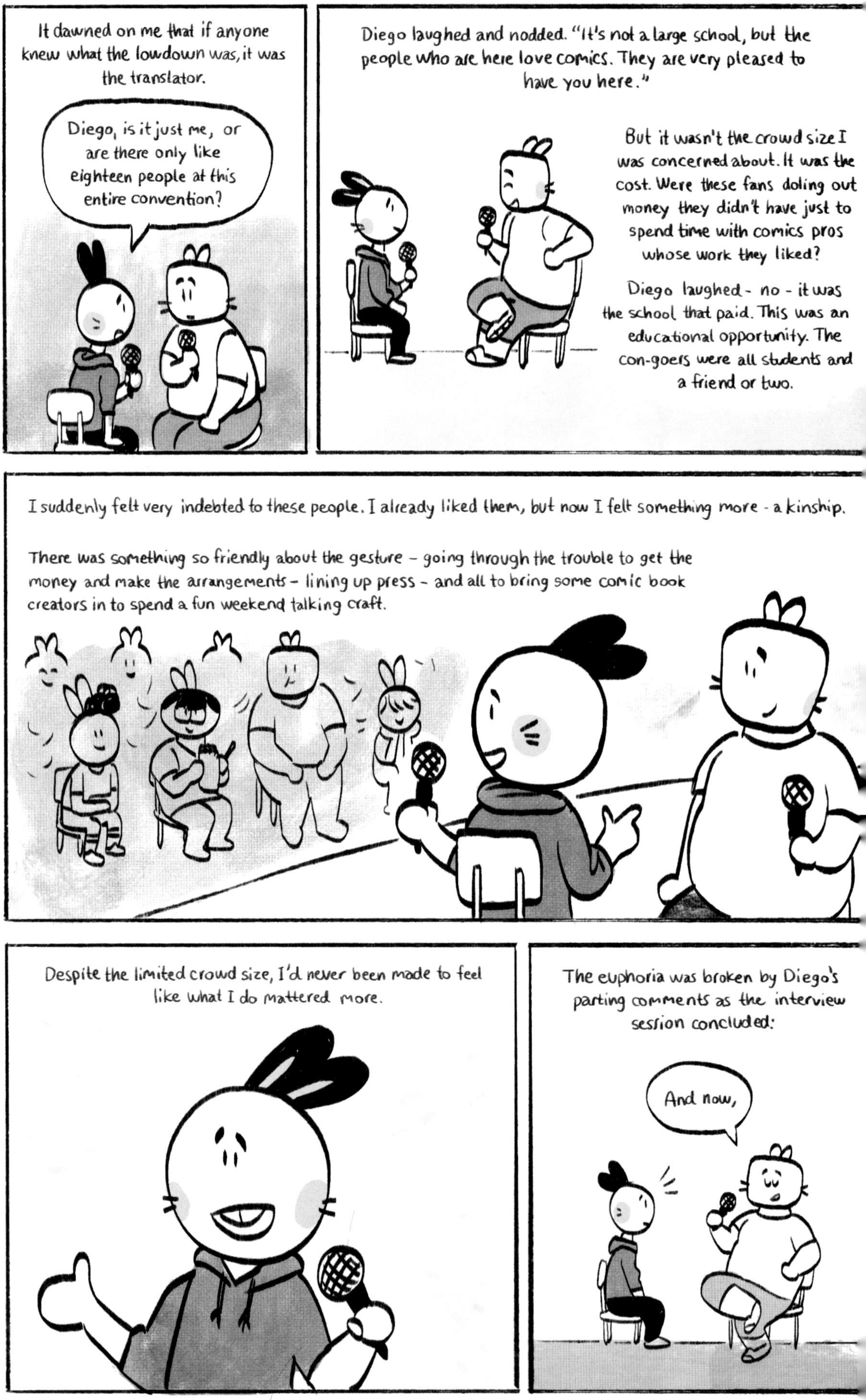

It dawned on me that if anyone knew what the lowdown was, it was the translator.
Diego, is it just me, or are there only like eighteen people at this entire convention?
Diego laughed and nodded. "It's not a large school, but the people who are here love comics. They are very pleased to have you here."
But it wasn't the crowd size I was concerned about. It was the cost. Were these fans doling out money they didn't have just to spend time with comics pros whose work they liked?
Diego laughed - no - it was the school that paid. This was an educational opportunity. The con-goers were all students and a friend or two.
I suddenly felt very indebted to these people. I already liked them, but now I felt something more - a kinship.
There was something so friendly about the gesture - going through the trouble to get the money and make the arrangements - lining up press - and all to bring some comic book creators in to spend a fun weekend talking craft.
Despite the limited crowd size, I'd never been made to feel like what I do mattered more.
The euphoria was broken by Diego's parting comments as the interview session concluded:
And now,

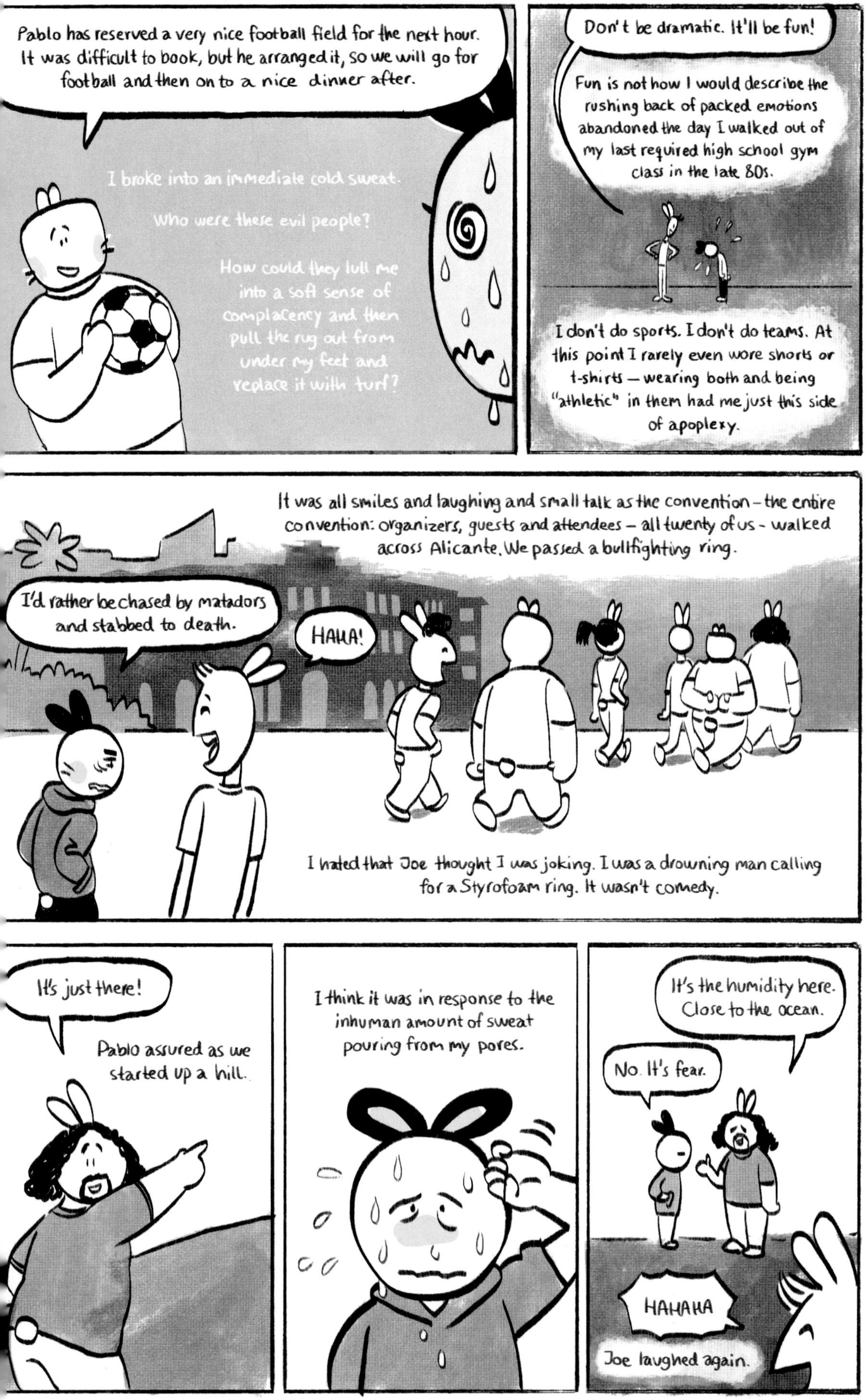

Pablo has reserved a very nice football field for the next hour. It was difficult to book, but he arranged it, so we will go for football and then on to a nice dinner after.
I broke into an immediate cold sweat.
Who were these evil people?
How could they lull me into a soft sense of complacency and then pull the rug out from under my feet and replace it with turf?
Don't be dramatic. It'll be fun!
Fun is not how I would describe the rushing back of packed emotions abandoned the day I walked out of my last required high school gym class in the late 80s.
I don't do sports. I don't do teams. At this point I rarely even wore shorts or t-shirts — wearing both and being "athletic" in them had me just this side of apoplexy.
It was all smiles and laughing and small talk as the convention – the entire convention: organizers, guests and attendees – all twenty of us – walked across Alicante. We passed a bullfighting ring.
I'd rather be chased by matadors and stabbed to death.
HAHA!
I hated that Joe thought I was joking. I was a drowning man calling for a Styrofoam ring. It wasn't comedy.
It's just there!
Pablo assured as we started up a hill.
I think it was in response to the inhuman amount of sweat pouring from my pores.
It's the humidity here. Close to the ocean.
No. It's fear.
HAHAHA
Joe laughed again.

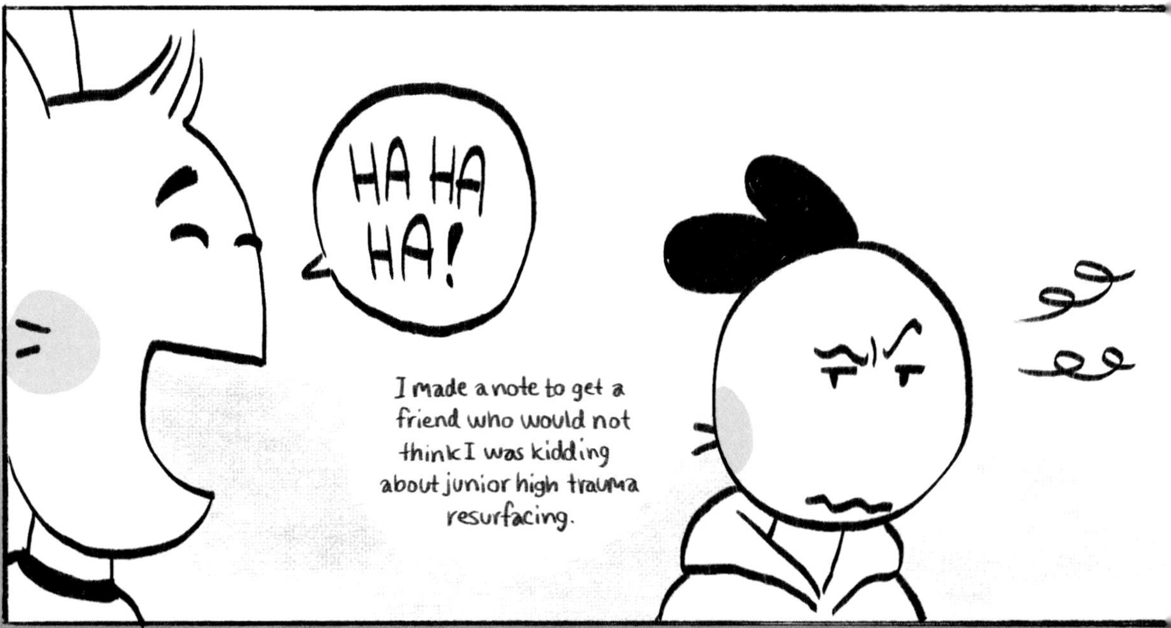
HA HA HA!
I made a note to get a friend who would not think I was kidding about junior high trauma resurfacing.

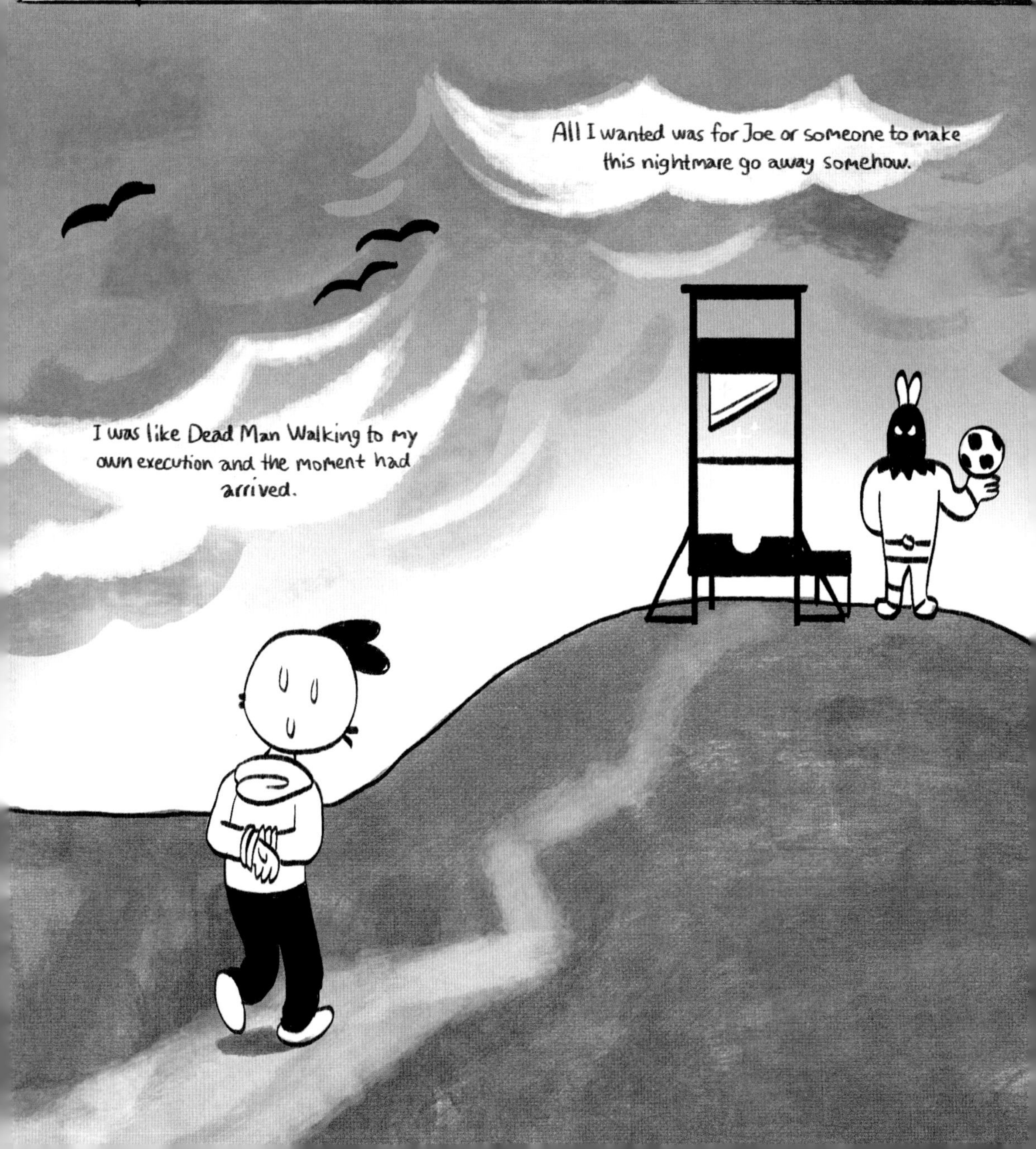
All I wanted was for Joe or someone to make this nightmare go away somehow.
I was like Dead Man Walking to my own execution and the moment had arrived.

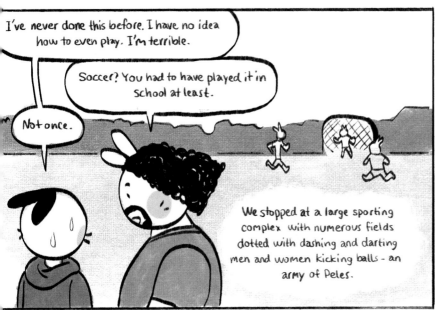

I've never done this before. I have no idea how to even play. I'm terrible.

Soccer? You had to have played it in school at least.

Not once.

We stopped at a large sporting complex with numerous fields dotted with dashing and darting men and women kicking balls - an army of Peles.

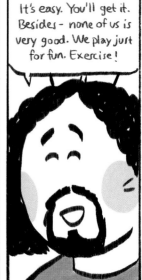

It's easy. You'll get it. Besides - none of us is very good. We play just for fun. Exercise!

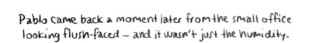

Pablo came back a moment later from the small office looking flush-faced — and it wasn't just the humidity.

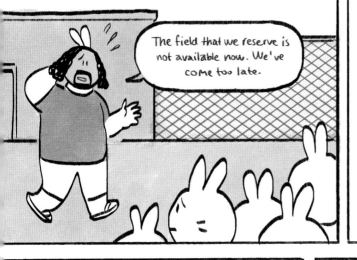

The field that we reserve is not available now. We've come too late.

I might have accidentally smiled before quickly flipping my lips over to form a sad face. I feigned genuine disappointment.

"No football? Well that's not fair!"

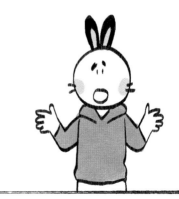

I paused to wonder why I don't use positive imaging more often. The secret to getting what we want is to see it, feel it, believe it, and materialize it into being—

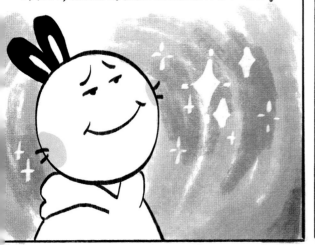

But we got the backup field so it's okay! It's just not the nice grass one.

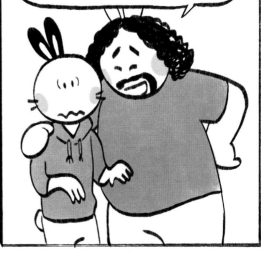

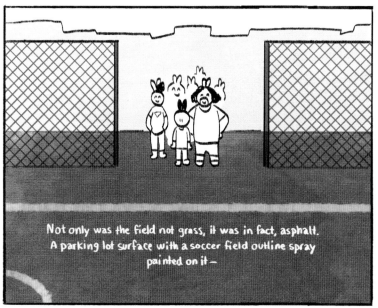

Not only was the field not grass, it was in fact, asphalt. A parking lot surface with a soccer field outline spray painted on it —

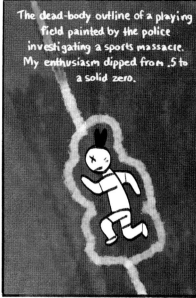

The dead-body outline of a playing field painted by the police investigating a sports massacre. My enthusiasm dipped from .5 to a solid zero.

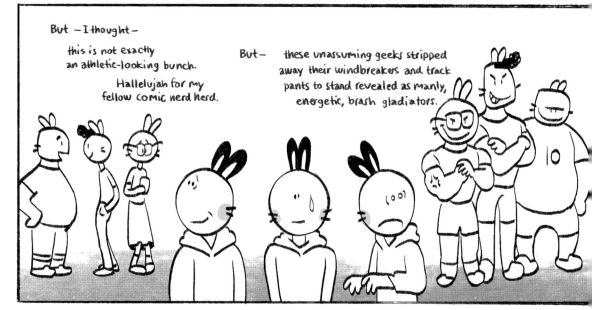

But — I thought —

this is not exactly an athletic-looking bunch.

Hallelujah for my fellow comic nerd herd.

But — these unassuming geeks stripped away their windbreakers and track pants to stand revealed as manly, energetic, brash gladiators.

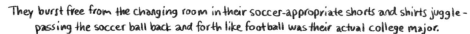

They burst free from the changing room in their soccer-appropriate shorts and shirts juggle-passing the soccer ball back and forth like football was their actual college major.

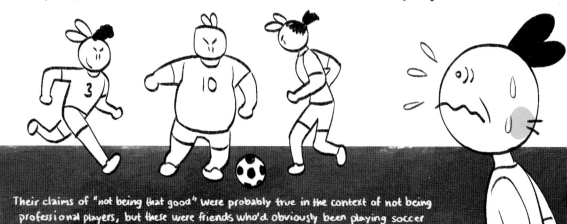

Their claims of "not being that good" were probably true in the context of not being professional players, but these were friends who'd obviously been playing soccer since they were infants.

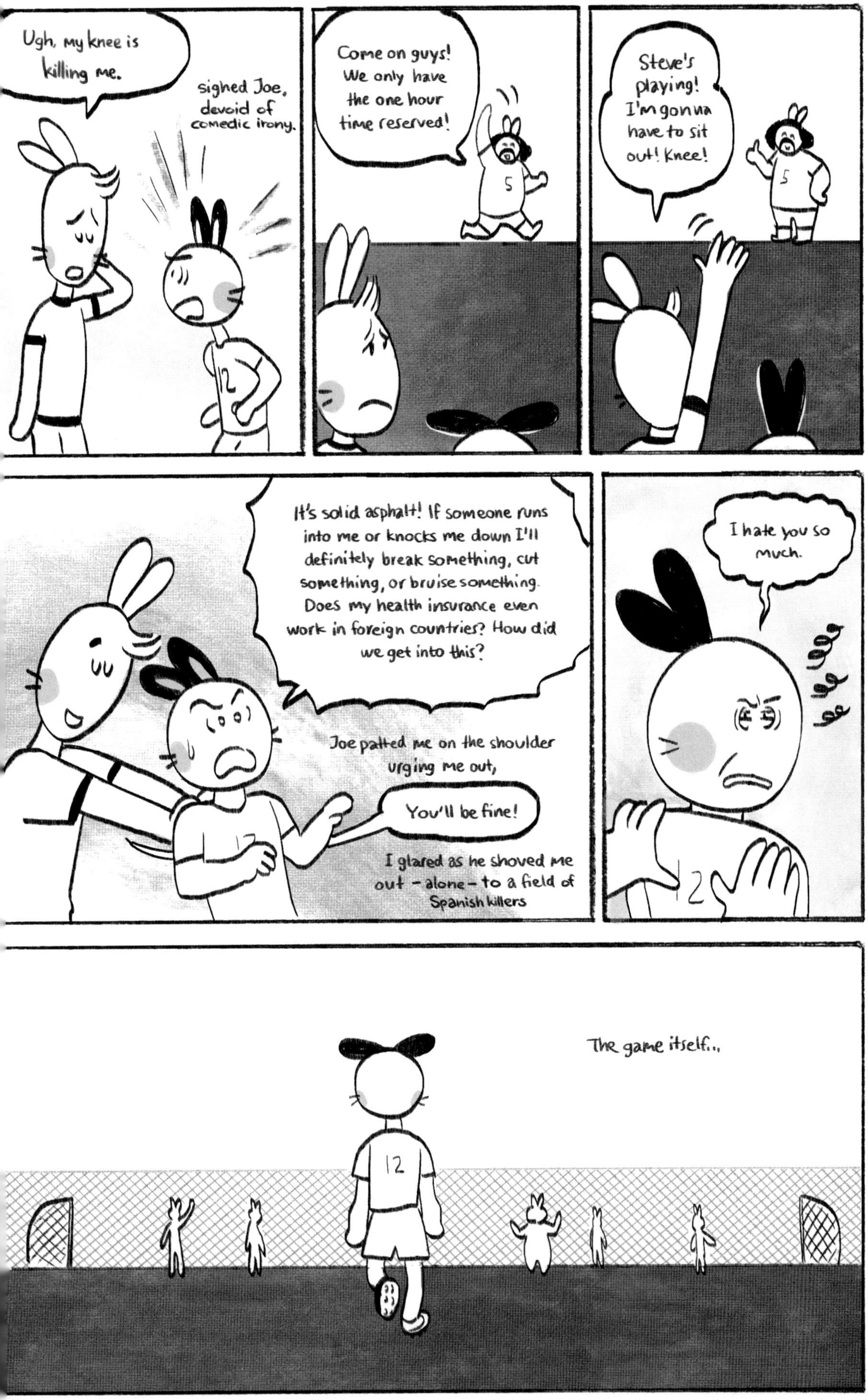
Ugh, my knee is killing me.
sighed Joe, devoid of comedic irony.
Come on guys! We only have the one hour time reserved!
Steve's playing! I'm gonna have to sit out! Knee!
It's solid asphalt! If someone runs into me or knocks me down I'll definitely break something, cut something, or bruise something. Does my health insurance even work in foreign countries? How did we get into this?
Joe patted me on the shoulder urging me out,
You'll be fine!
I glared as he shoved me out - alone - to a field of Spanish killers
I hate you so much.
The game itself...

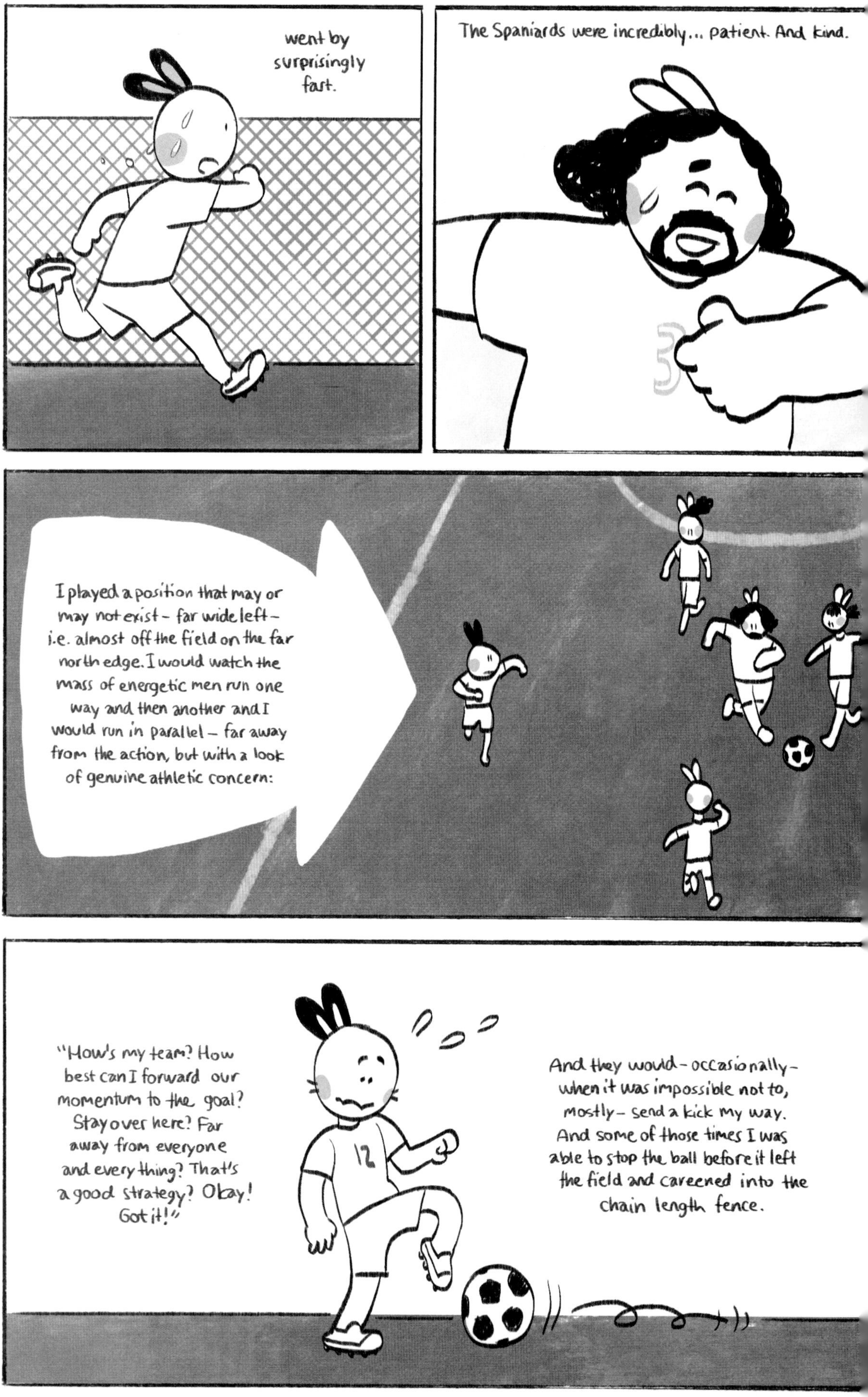
went by surprisingly fast.
The Spaniards were incredibly... patient. And kind.
I played a position that may or may not exist – far wide left – i.e. almost off the field on the far north edge. I would watch the mass of energetic men run one way and then another and I would run in parallel – far away from the action, but with a look of genuine athletic concern:
"How's my team? How best can I forward our momentum to the goal? Stay over here? Far away from everyone and everything? That's a good strategy? Okay! Got it!"
12
And they would – occasionally – when it was impossible not to, mostly – send a kick my way. And some of those times I was able to stop the ball before it left the field and careened into the chain length fence.

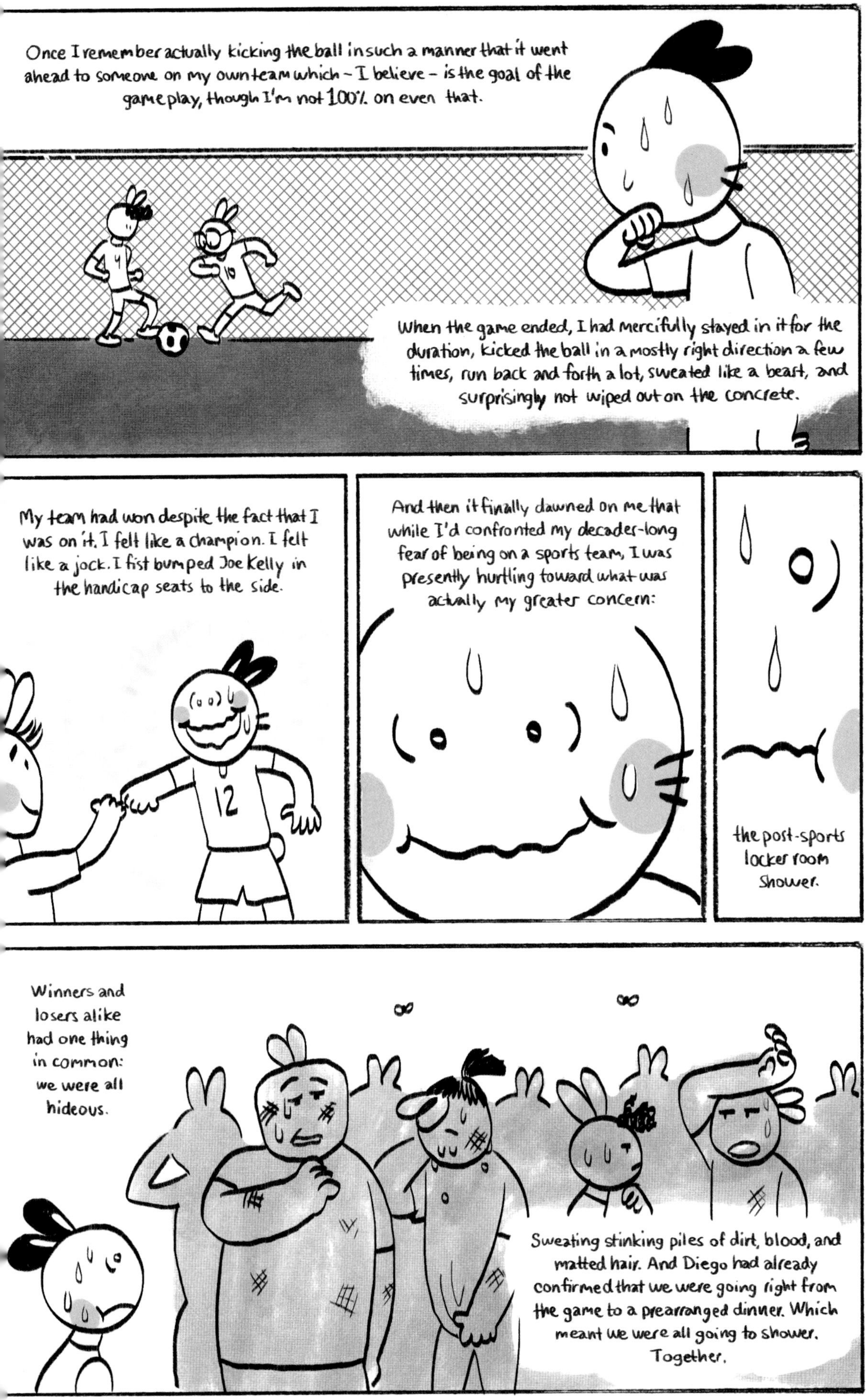
Once I remember actually kicking the ball in such a manner that it went ahead to someone on my own team which - I believe - is the goal of the gameplay, though I'm not 100% on even that.
4
10
When the game ended, I had mercifully stayed in it for the duration, kicked the ball in a mostly right direction a few times, run back and forth a lot, sweated like a beast, and surprisingly not wiped out on the concrete.
My team had won despite the fact that I was on it. I felt like a champion. I felt like a jock. I fist bumped Joe Kelly in the handicap seats to the side.
12
And then it finally dawned on me that while I'd confronted my decades-long fear of being on a sports team, I was presently hurtling toward what was actually my greater concern:
the post-sports locker room shower.
Winners and losers alike had one thing in common: we were all hideous.
Sweating stinking piles of dirt, blood, and matted hair. And Diego had already confirmed that we were going right from the game to a prearranged dinner. Which meant we were all going to shower. Together.

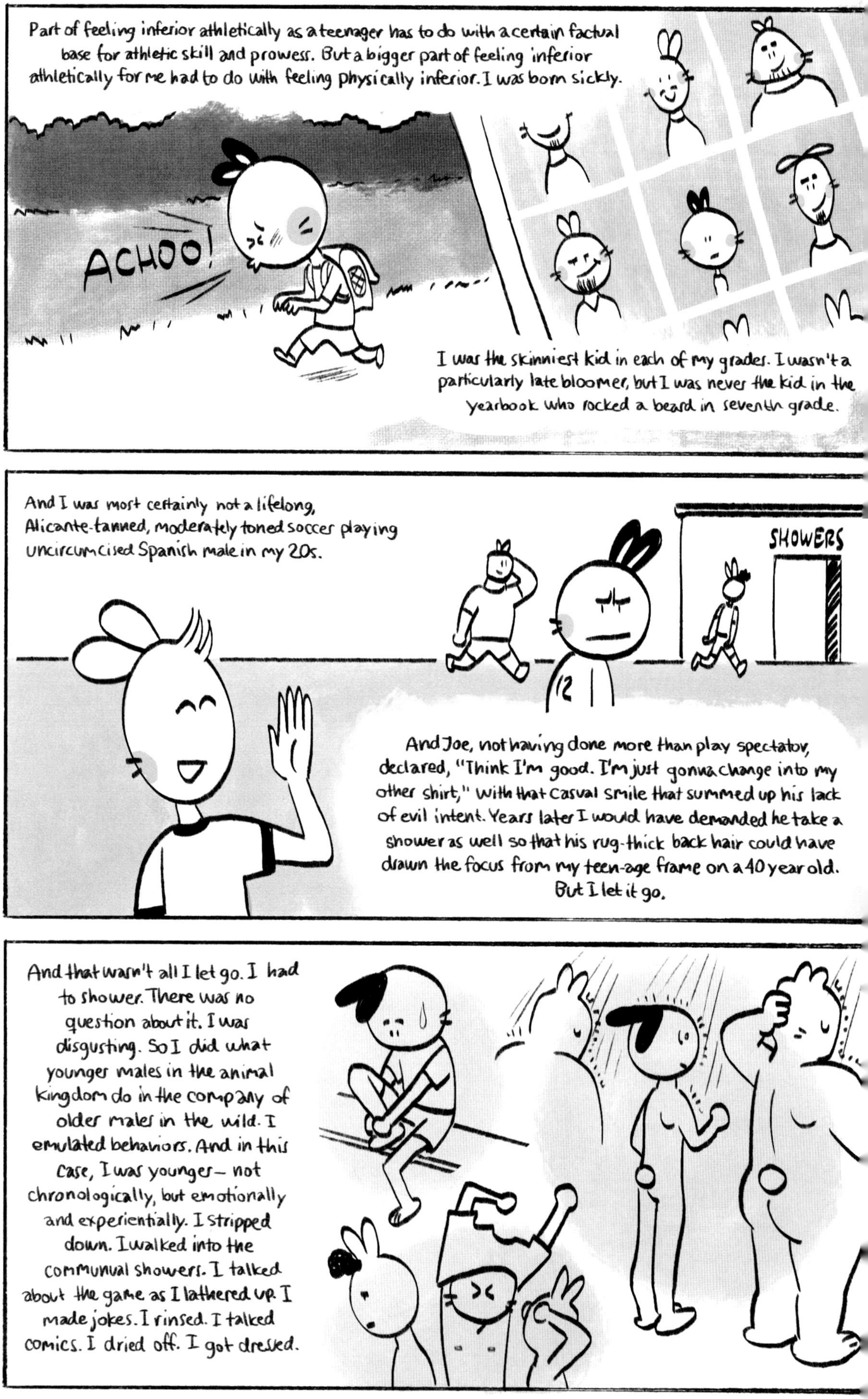
Part of feeling inferior athletically as a teenager has to do with a certain factual base for athletic skill and prowess. But a bigger part of feeling inferior athletically for me had to do with feeling physically inferior. I was born sickly.
ACHOO!
I was the skinniest kid in each of my grades. I wasn't a particularly late bloomer, but I was never the kid in the yearbook who rocked a beard in seventh grade.
And I was most certainly not a lifelong, Alicante-tanned, moderately toned soccer playing uncircumcised Spanish male in my 20s.
SHOWERS
12
And Joe, not having done more than play spectator, declared, "Think I'm good. I'm just gonna change into my other shirt," with that casual smile that summed up his lack of evil intent. Years later I would have demanded he take a shower as well so that his rug-thick back hair could have drawn the focus from my teen-age frame on a 40 year old. But I let it go.
And that wasn't all I let go. I had to shower. There was no question about it. I was disgusting. So I did what younger males in the animal kingdom do in the company of older males in the wild. I emulated behaviors. And in this case, I was younger— not chronologically, but emotionally and experientially. I stripped down. I walked into the communual showers. I talked about the game as I lathered up. I made jokes. I rinsed. I talked comics. I dried off. I got dressed.

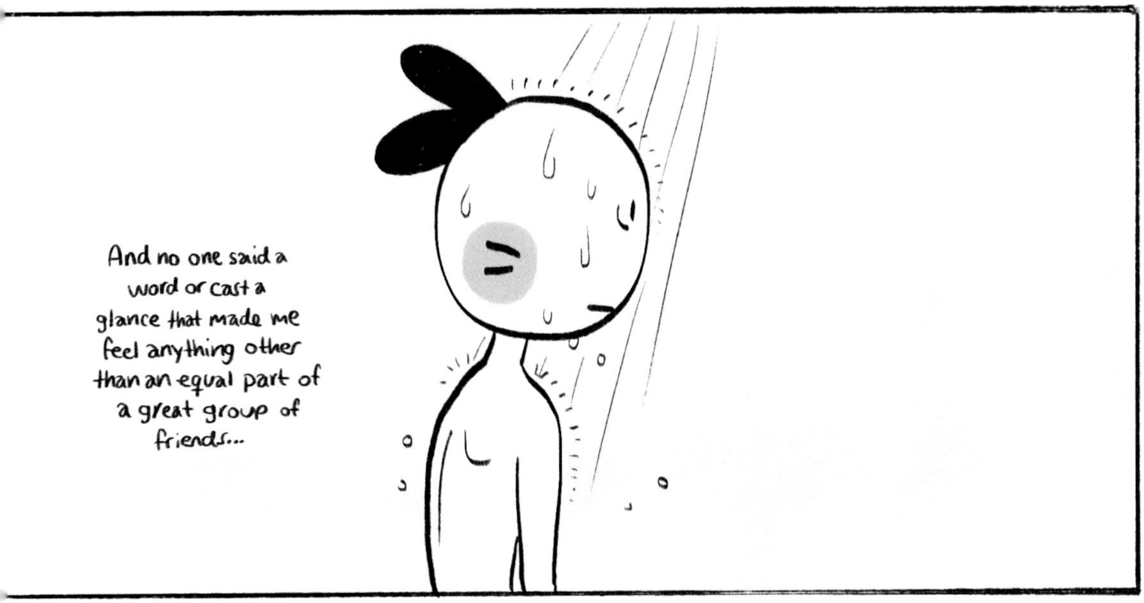
And no one said a word or cast a glance that made me feel anything other than an equal part of a great group of friends...

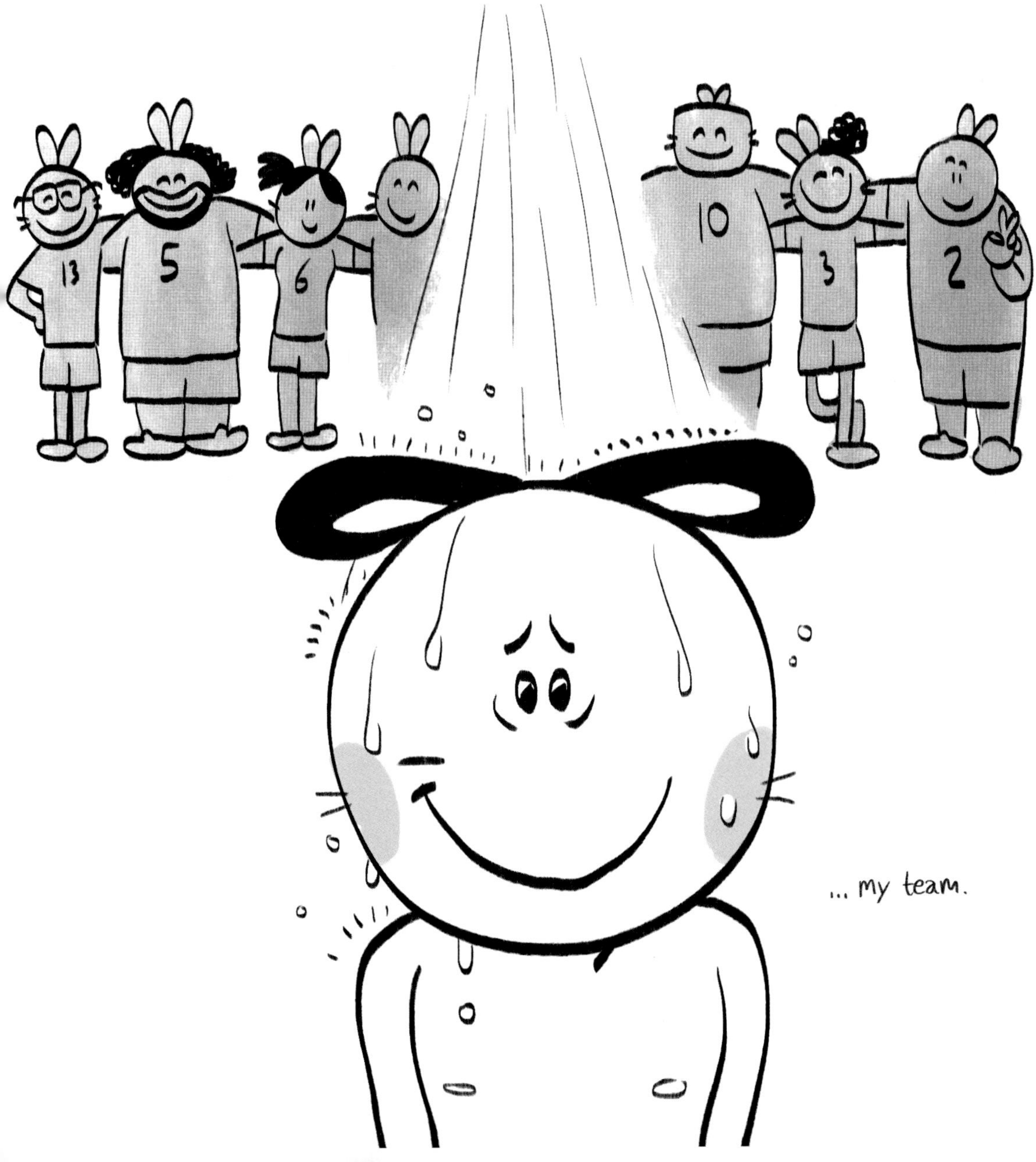
13
5
6
10
3
2
... my team.

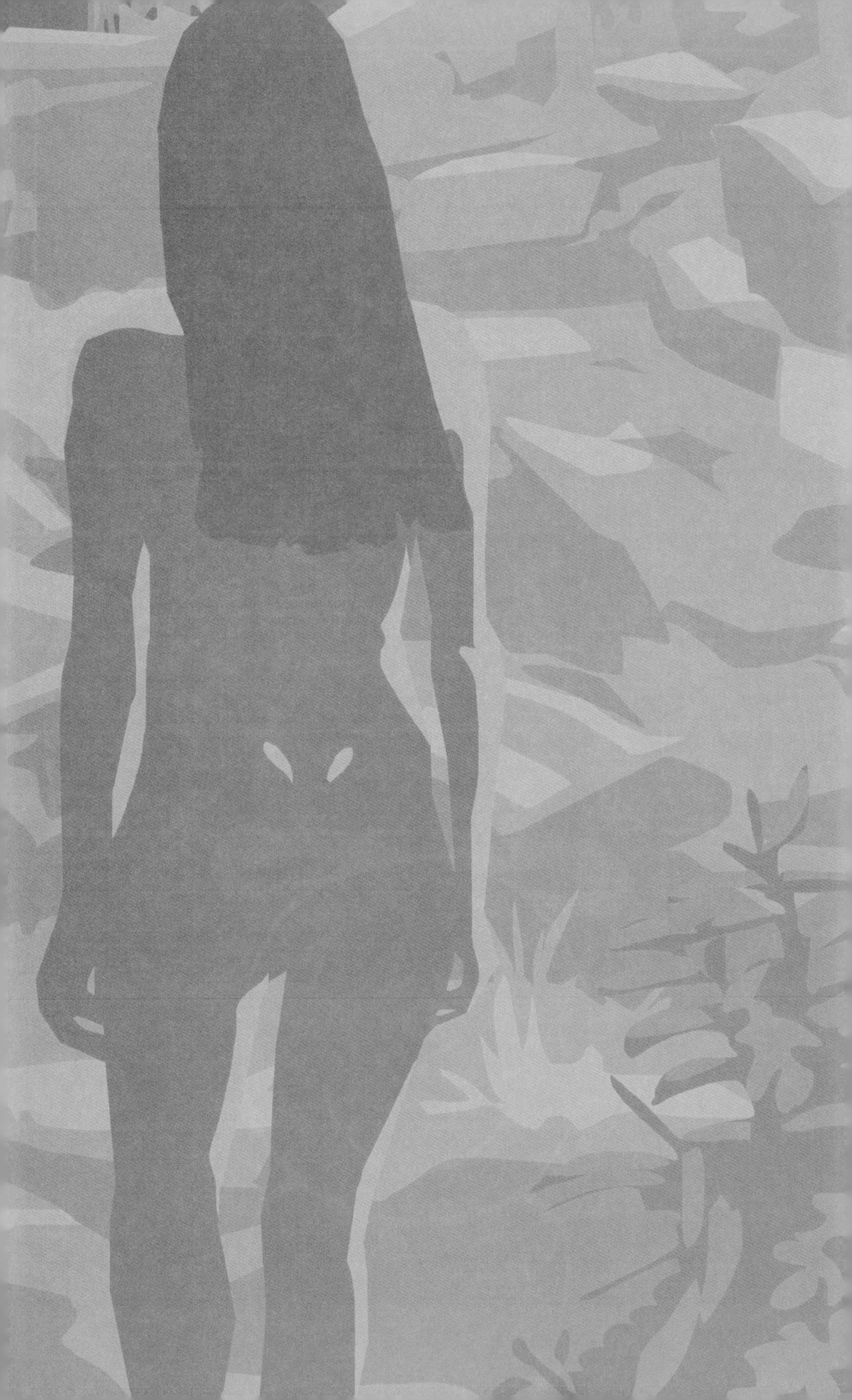

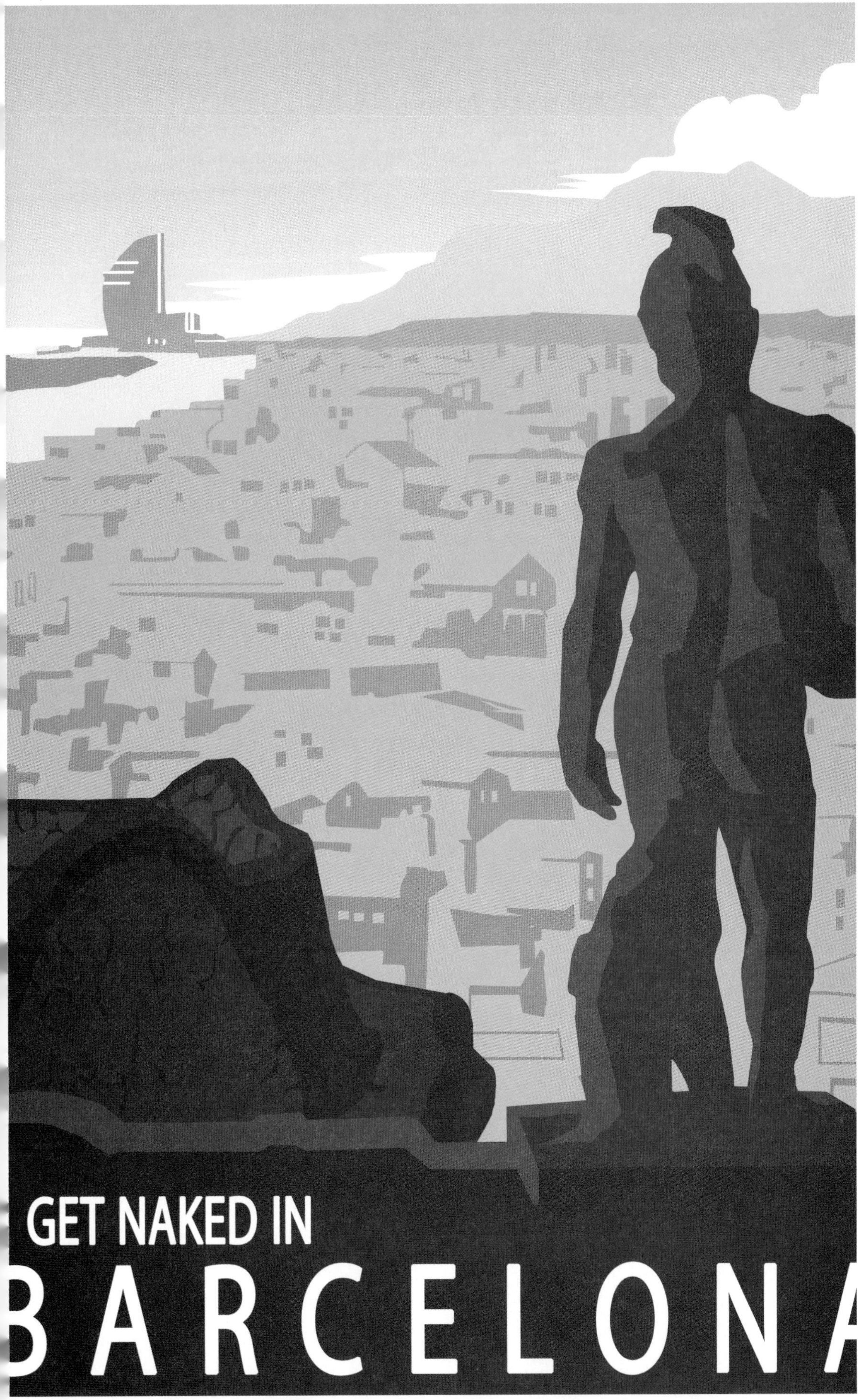
GET NAKED IN
BARCELONA

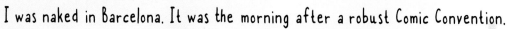

I was naked in Barcelona. It was the morning after a robust Comic Convention.

My collaborator, Teddy, had caught the night flight out the previous evening. My plane the next morning would chase him back to his home town of Copenhagen where we would plot out our next project together.

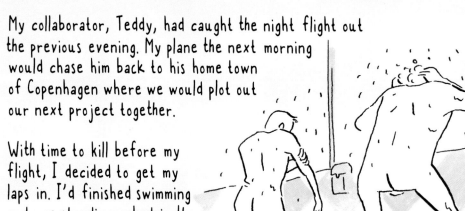

With time to kill before my flight, I decided to get my laps in. I'd finished swimming and was standing naked in the shower when I noticed that the clock on the wall was an hour later than I had been thinking.

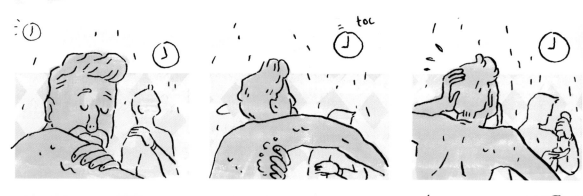

It's awkward to strike up a conversation with a naked Spanish guy in the showers, especially when you don't speak Spanish yourself, but he had a watch.

Is that the right time?

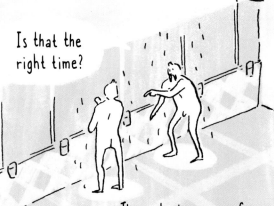

The naked guy confirmed for me that I was now naked and late — in danger of missing my flight altogether.

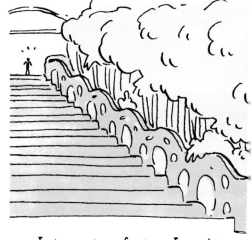

I dressed as fast as I could, ran down the endless stairs that separated the Bernat Picornell pool from my hotel at the bottom of a steep hill, grabbed my bags, and dashed for an airport bus.

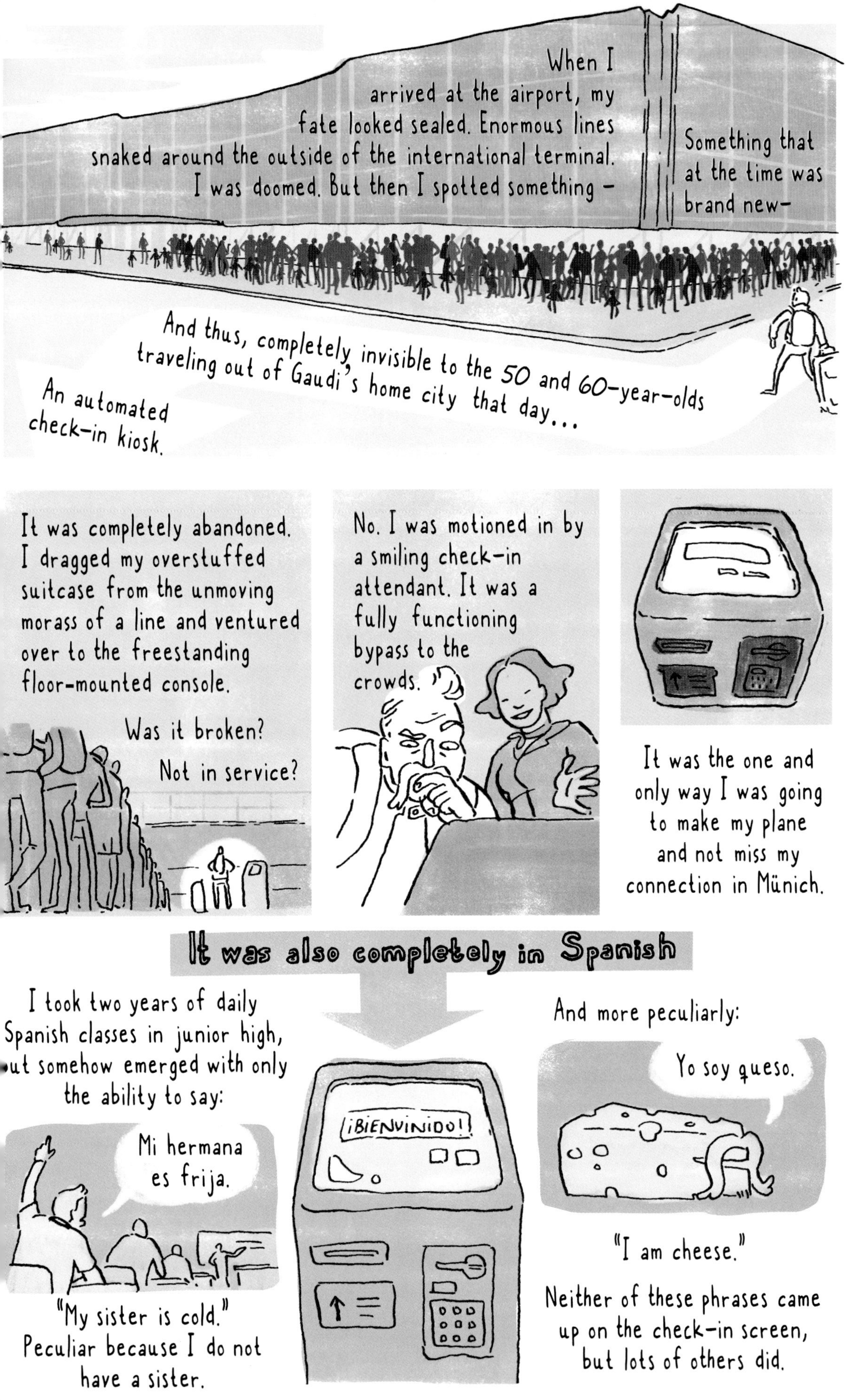
When I arrived at the airport, my fate looked sealed. Enormous lines snaked around the outside of the international terminal. I was doomed. But then I spotted something –
Something that at the time was brand new–
An automated check-in kiosk.
And thus, completely invisible to the 50 and 60-year-olds traveling out of Gaudi's home city that day...
It was completely abandoned. I dragged my overstuffed suitcase from the unmoving morass of a line and ventured over to the freestanding floor-mounted console.
Was it broken?
Not in service?
No. I was motioned in by a smiling check-in attendant. It was a fully functioning bypass to the crowds.
It was the one and only way I was going to make my plane and not miss my connection in Münich.
It was also completely in Spanish
I took two years of daily Spanish classes in junior high, but somehow emerged with only the ability to say:
Mi hermana es frija.
"My sister is cold." Peculiar because I do not have a sister.
¡BIENVINIDO!
And more peculiarly:
Yo soy queso.
"I am cheese."
Neither of these phrases came up on the check-in screen, but lots of others did.

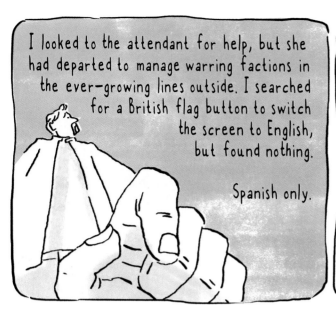

I looked to the attendant for help, but she had departed to manage warring factions in the ever-growing lines outside. I searched for a British flag button to switch the screen to English, but found nothing.

Spanish only.

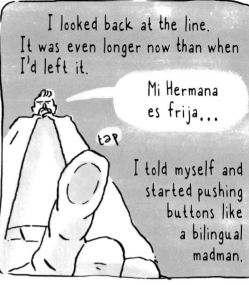

I looked back at the line. It was even longer now than when I'd left it.

Mi Hermana es frija...

I told myself and started pushing buttons like a bilingual madman.

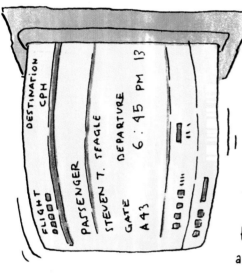

DESTINATION CPH

FLIGHT 00000

PASSENGER STEVEN T. SEAGLE

DEPARTURE 6:45 PM 13

GATE A43

After numerous screens came and went with me making various bi and tri-nary decisions, my boarding pass spat out at me.

- SUCCESS -

I took it over to the bag check counter looking wistfully back at the throngs of summer travelers certain to miss their connections for not having the brash willfulness to check themselves in at the automated kiosk using a language they do not speak.

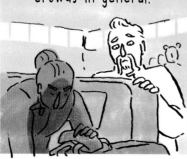

The woman behind the counter yelled something at me in Spanish and yanked my bag away. I couldn't tell if she was mad at me in particular or just frayed from the acidic crowds in general.

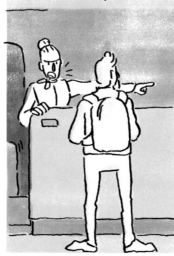

I smiled and she yelled again pointing this time— deadly serious.

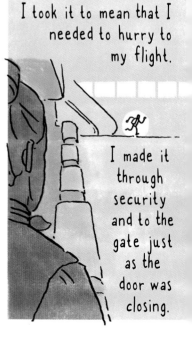

I took it to mean that I needed to hurry to my flight.

I made it through security and to the gate just as the door was closing.

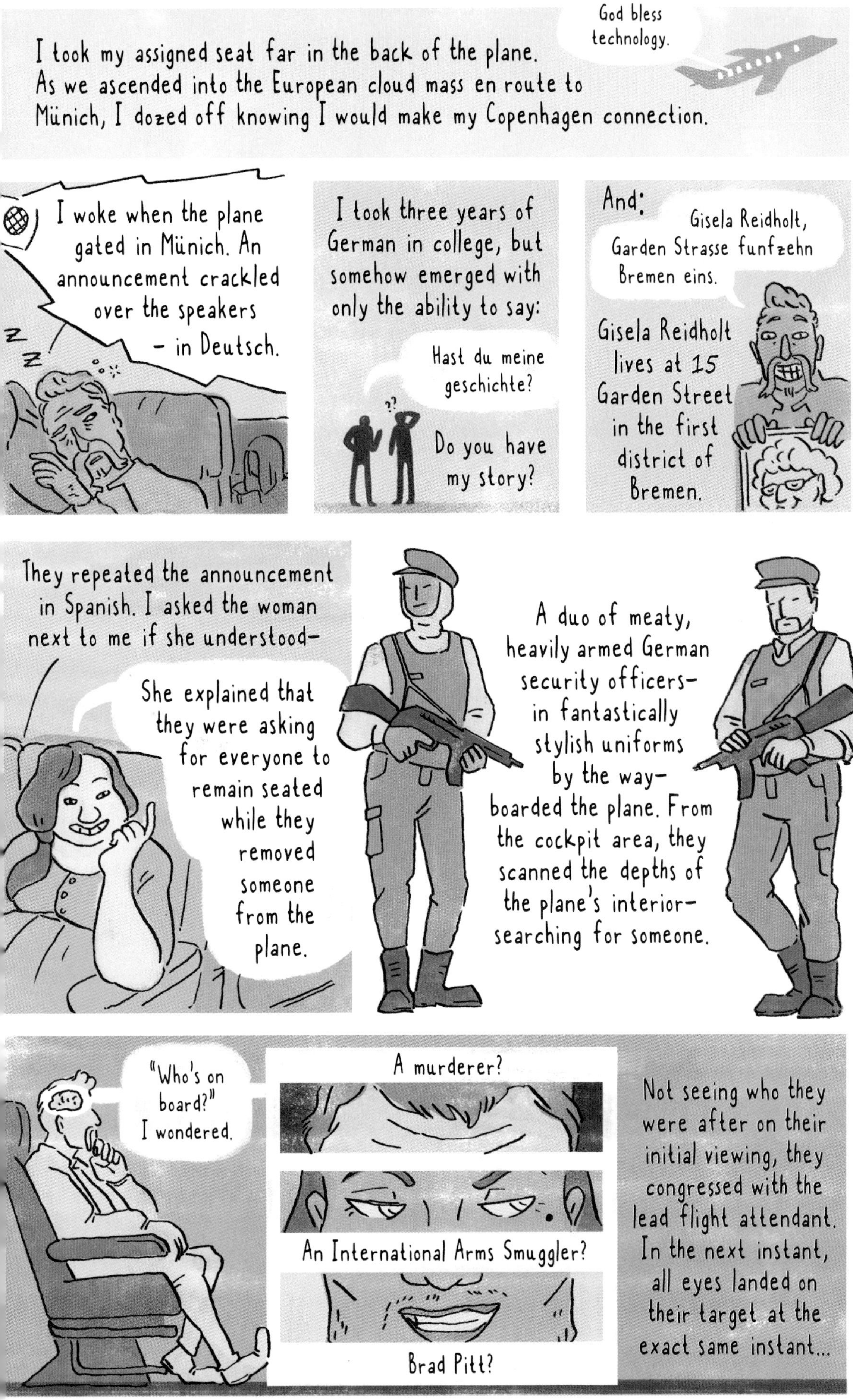
I took my assigned seat far in the back of the plane. As we ascended into the European cloud mass en route to Münich, I dozed off knowing I would make my Copenhagen connection.
God bless technology.
I woke when the plane gated in Münich. An announcement crackled over the speakers - in Deutsch.
Z Z
I took three years of German in college, but somehow emerged with only the ability to say:
Hast du meine geschichte?
??
Do you have my story?
And:
Gisela Reidholt, Garden Strasse funfzehn Bremen eins.
Gisela Reidholt lives at 15 Garden Street in the first district of Bremen.
They repeated the announcement in Spanish. I asked the woman next to me if she understood-
She explained that they were asking for everyone to remain seated while they removed someone from the plane.
A duo of meaty, heavily armed German security officers- in fantastically stylish uniforms by the way- boarded the plane. From the cockpit area, they scanned the depths of the plane's interior- searching for someone.
"Who's on board?" I wondered.
A murderer?
An International Arms Smuggler?
Brad Pitt?
Not seeing who they were after on their initial viewing, they congressed with the lead flight attendant. In the next instant, all eyes landed on their target at the exact same instant...

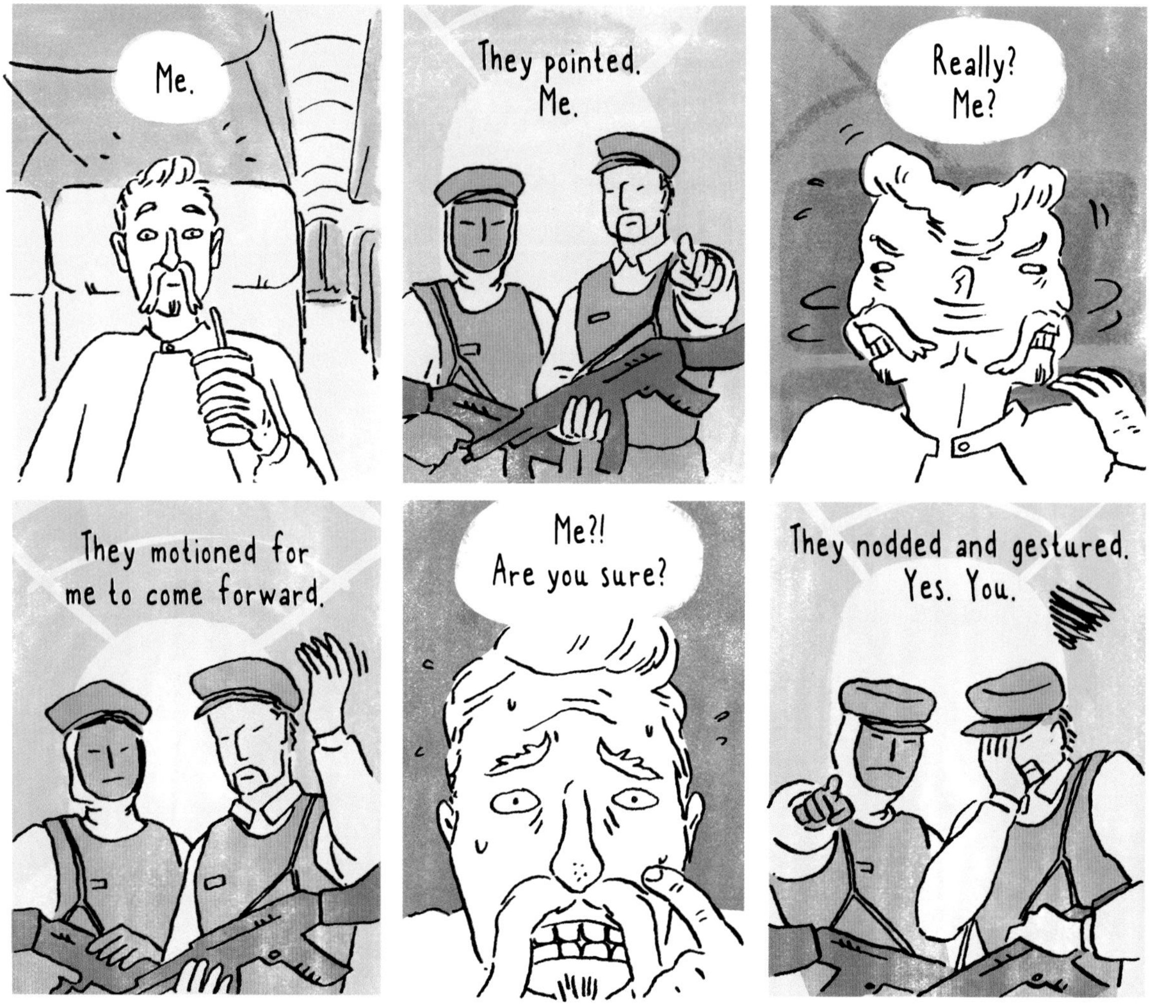
Me.
They pointed.
Me.
Really?
Me?
They motioned for
me to come forward.
Me?!
Are you sure?
They nodded and gestured.
Yes. You.

I studied nonverbal communication in grad school. I speak it fluently.
I think they wanted me to come forward.
FUCK.

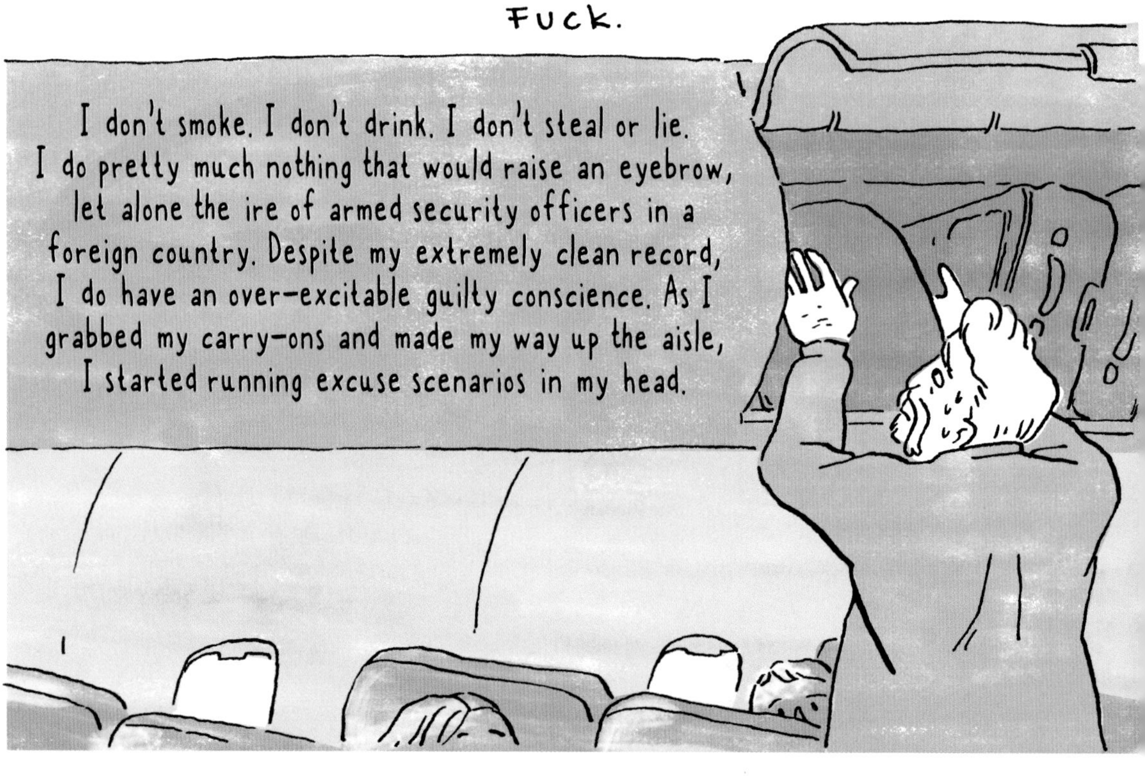
I don't smoke. I don't drink. I don't steal or lie. I do pretty much nothing that would raise an eyebrow, let alone the ire of armed security officers in a foreign country. Despite my extremely clean record, I do have an over-excitable guilty conscience. As I grabbed my carry-ons and made my way up the aisle, I started running excuse scenarios in my head.

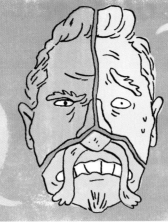

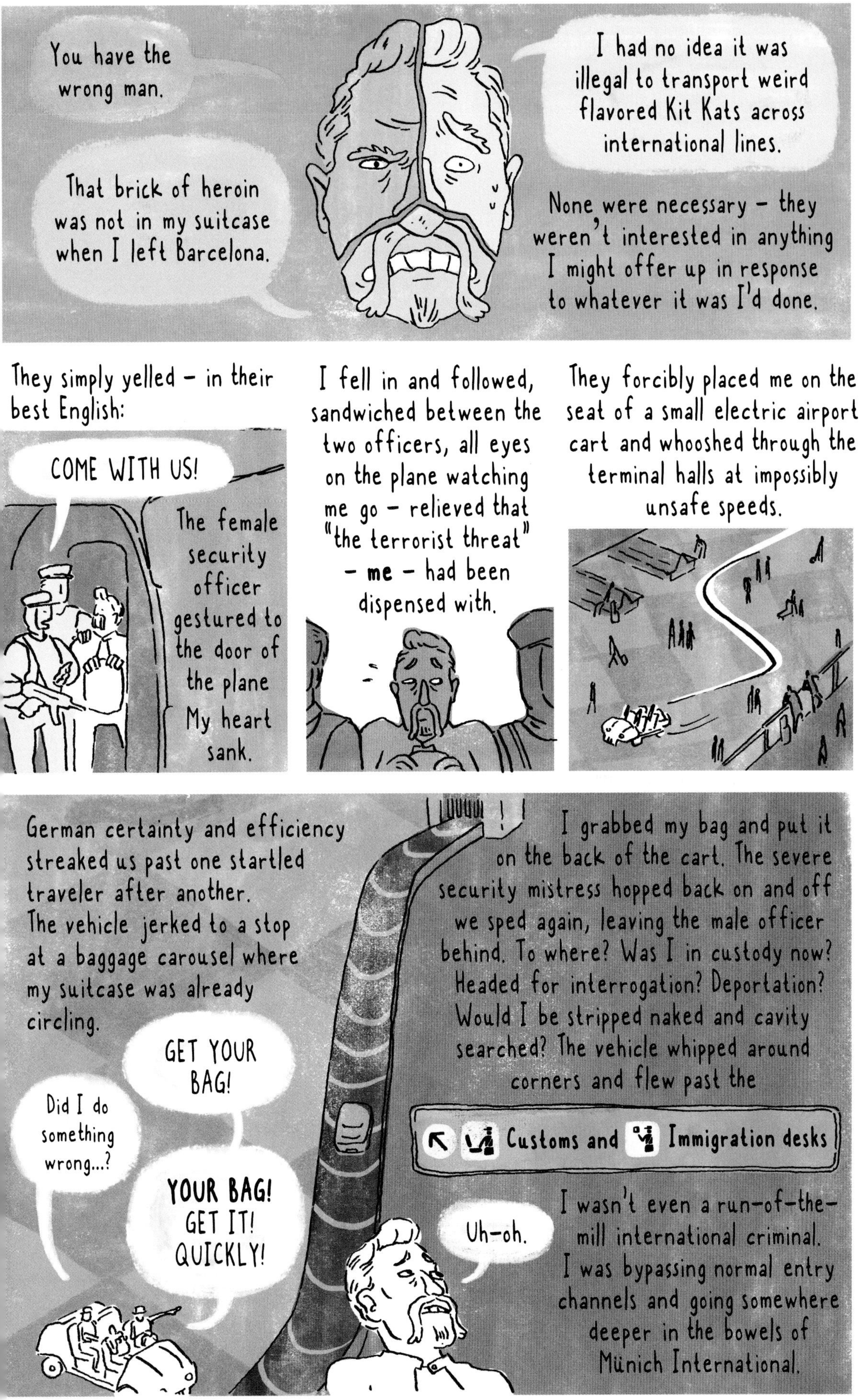

You have the wrong man.

That brick of heroin was not in my suitcase when I left Barcelona.

I had no idea it was illegal to transport weird flavored Kit Kats across international lines.

None were necessary — they weren't interested in anything I might offer up in response to whatever it was I'd done.

They simply yelled — in their best English:

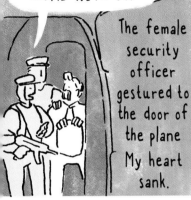

COME WITH US!

The female security officer gestured to the door of the plane My heart sank.

I fell in and followed, sandwiched between the two officers, all eyes on the plane watching me go — relieved that "the terrorist threat" — **me** — had been dispensed with.

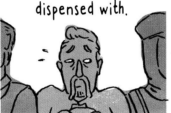

They forcibly placed me on the seat of a small electric airport cart and whooshed through the terminal halls at impossibly unsafe speeds.

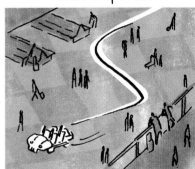

German certainty and efficiency streaked us past one startled traveler after another. The vehicle jerked to a stop at a baggage carousel where my suitcase was already circling.

GET YOUR BAG!

Did I do something wrong...?

YOUR BAG! GET IT! QUICKLY!

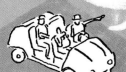

I grabbed my bag and put it on the back of the cart. The severe security mistress hopped back on and off we sped again, leaving the male officer behind. To where? Was I in custody now? Headed for interrogation? Deportation? Would I be stripped naked and cavity searched? The vehicle whipped around corners and flew past the

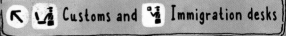

Customs and Immigration desks

Uh-oh.

I wasn't even a run-of-the-mill international criminal. I was bypassing normal entry channels and going somewhere deeper in the bowels of München International.

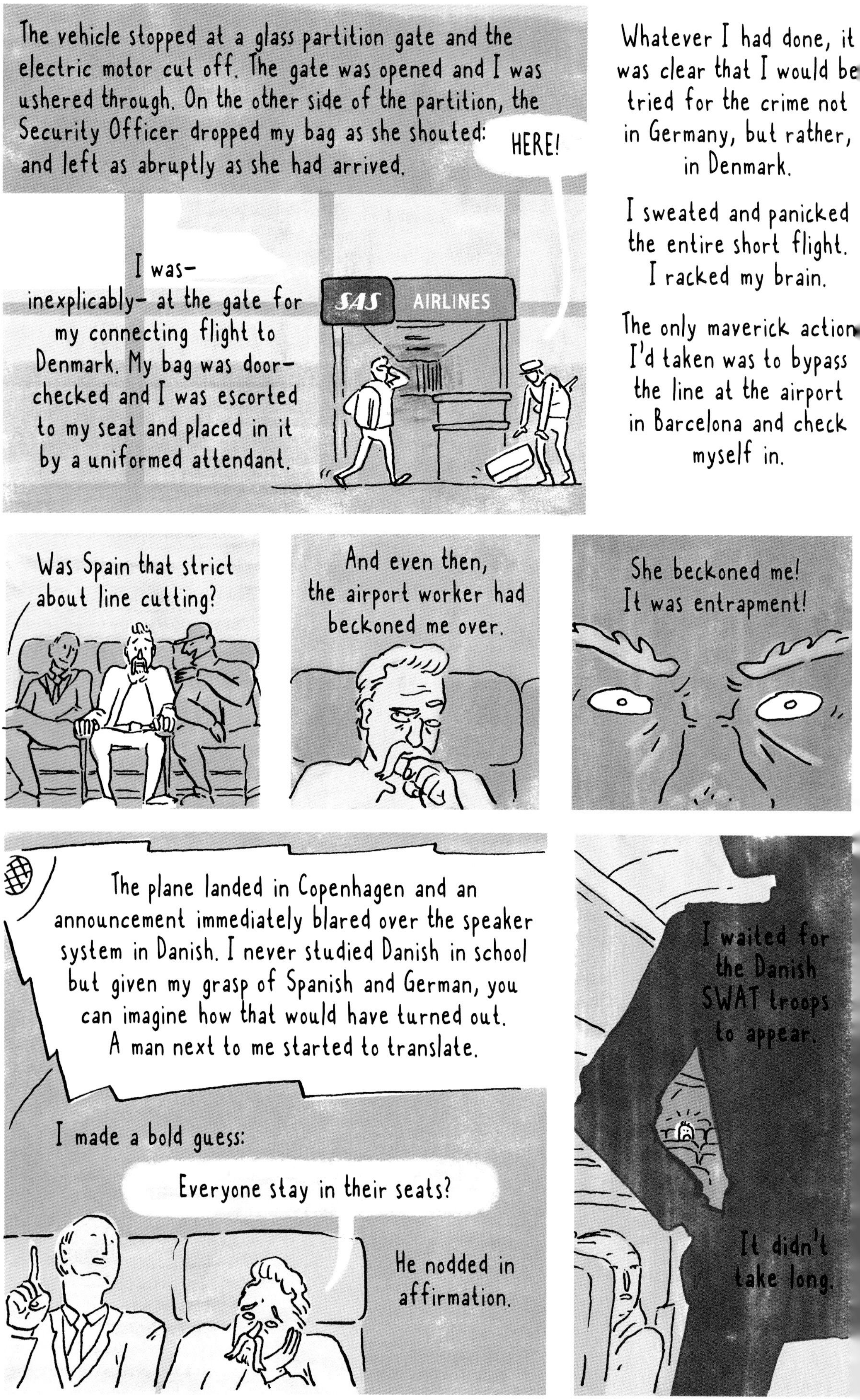

The vehicle stopped at a glass partition gate and the electric motor cut off. The gate was opened and I was ushered through. On the other side of the partition, the Security Officer dropped my bag as she shouted:
HERE!
and left as abruptly as she had arrived.
I was—inexplicably— at the gate for my connecting flight to Denmark. My bag was door-checked and I was escorted to my seat and placed in it by a uniformed attendant.
SAS
AIRLINES
Whatever I had done, it was clear that I would be tried for the crime not in Germany, but rather, in Denmark.
I sweated and panicked the entire short flight. I racked my brain.
The only maverick action I'd taken was to bypass the line at the airport in Barcelona and check myself in.
Was Spain that strict about line cutting?
And even then, the airport worker had beckoned me over.
She beckoned me! It was entrapment!
The plane landed in Copenhagen and an announcement immediately blared over the speaker system in Danish. I never studied Danish in school but given my grasp of Spanish and German, you can imagine how that would have turned out. A man next to me started to translate.
I made a bold guess:
Everyone stay in their seats?
He nodded in affirmation.
I waited for the Danish SWAT troops to appear.
It didn't take long.

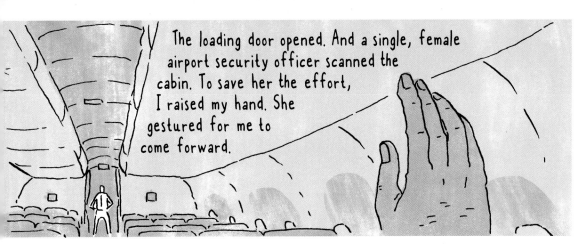

The loading door opened. And a single, female airport security officer scanned the cabin. To save her the effort, I raised my hand. She gestured for me to come forward.

Uh-oh, busted! What did you do?

A fellow traveling American I had chatted with during the flight asked as I crawled past him.

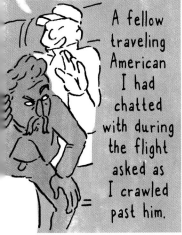

I checked myself in.

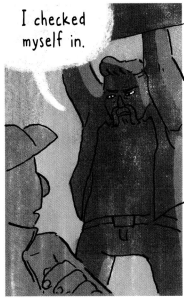

I made my way through all the other waiting passengers and met my new warden at the front of the plane.

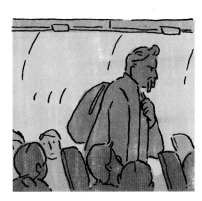

COME WITH ME! NOW!

She barked loudly in a pointed Danish-accented English. I followed her to a similar electric cart. I knew the drill. No need for instruction. I hopped in, sat down and remained silent. I'd been yelled at enough for one day. I started composing my single phone call to my parents:

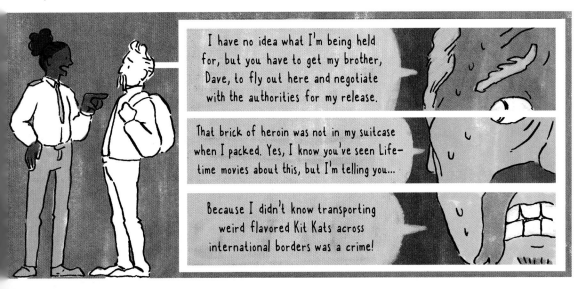

I have no idea what I'm being held for, but you have to get my brother, Dave, to fly out here and negotiate with the authorities for my release.

That brick of heroin was not in my suitcase when I packed. Yes, I know you've seen Life-time movies about this, but I'm telling you...

Because I didn't know transporting weird flavored Kit Kats across international borders was a crime!

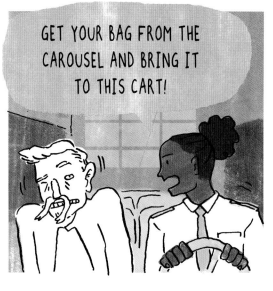

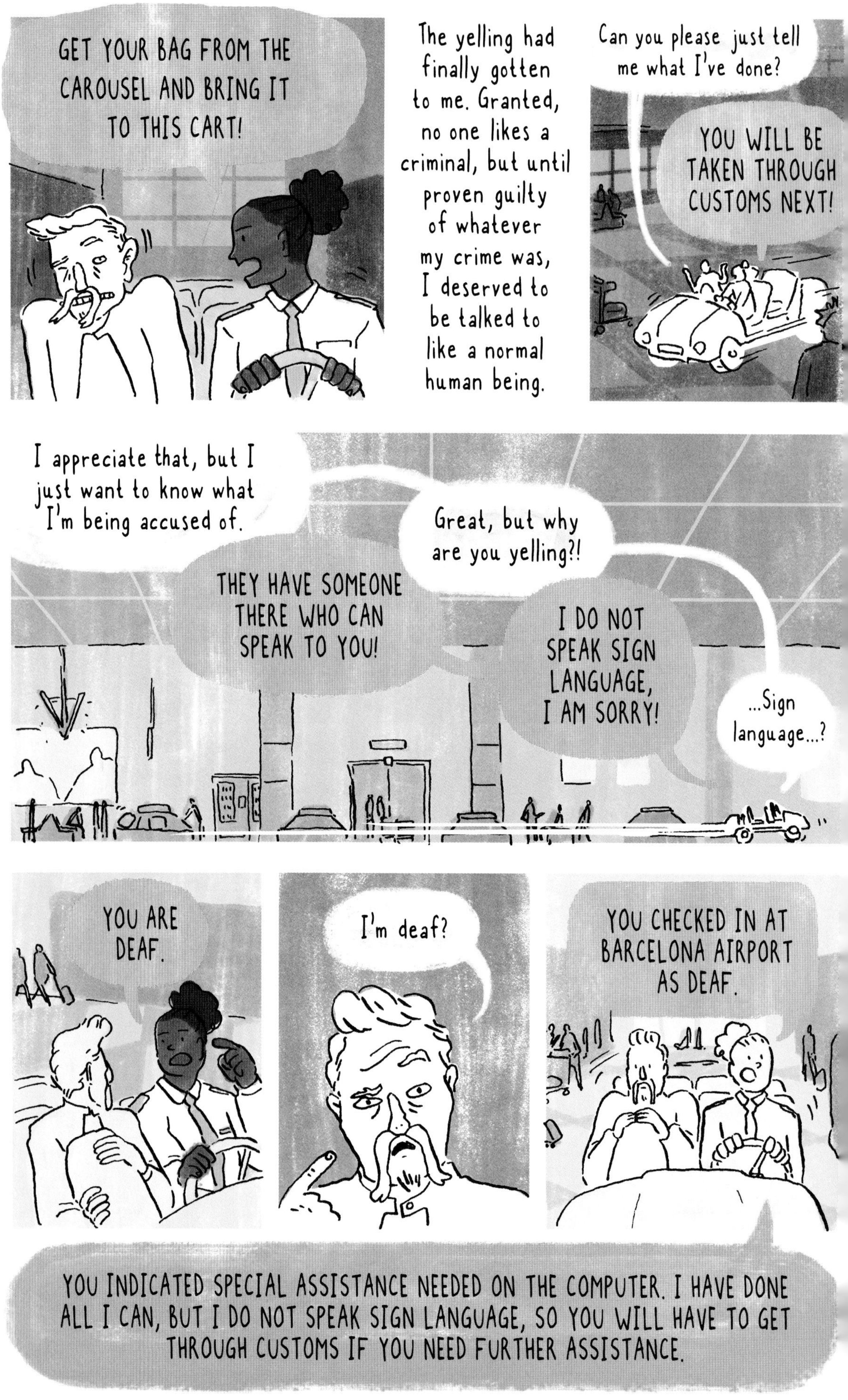

GET YOUR BAG FROM THE CAROUSEL AND BRING IT TO THIS CART!

The yelling had finally gotten to me. Granted, no one likes a criminal, but until proven guilty of whatever my crime was, I deserved to be talked to like a normal human being.

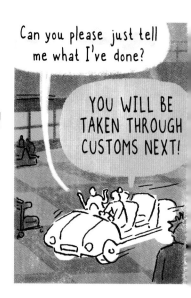

Can you please just tell me what I've done?

YOU WILL BE TAKEN THROUGH CUSTOMS NEXT!

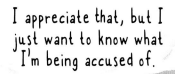

I appreciate that, but I just want to know what I'm being accused of.

THEY HAVE SOMEONE THERE WHO CAN SPEAK TO YOU!

Great, but why are you yelling?!

I DO NOT SPEAK SIGN LANGUAGE, I AM SORRY!

...Sign language...?

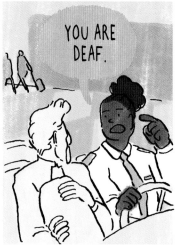

YOU ARE DEAF.

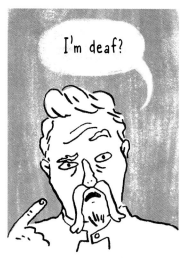

I'm deaf?

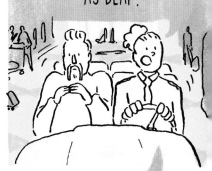

YOU CHECKED IN AT BARCELONA AIRPORT AS DEAF.

YOU INDICATED SPECIAL ASSISTANCE NEEDED ON THE COMPUTER. I HAVE DONE ALL I CAN, BUT I DO NOT SPEAK SIGN LANGUAGE, SO YOU WILL HAVE TO GET THROUGH CUSTOMS IF YOU NEED FURTHER ASSISTANCE.

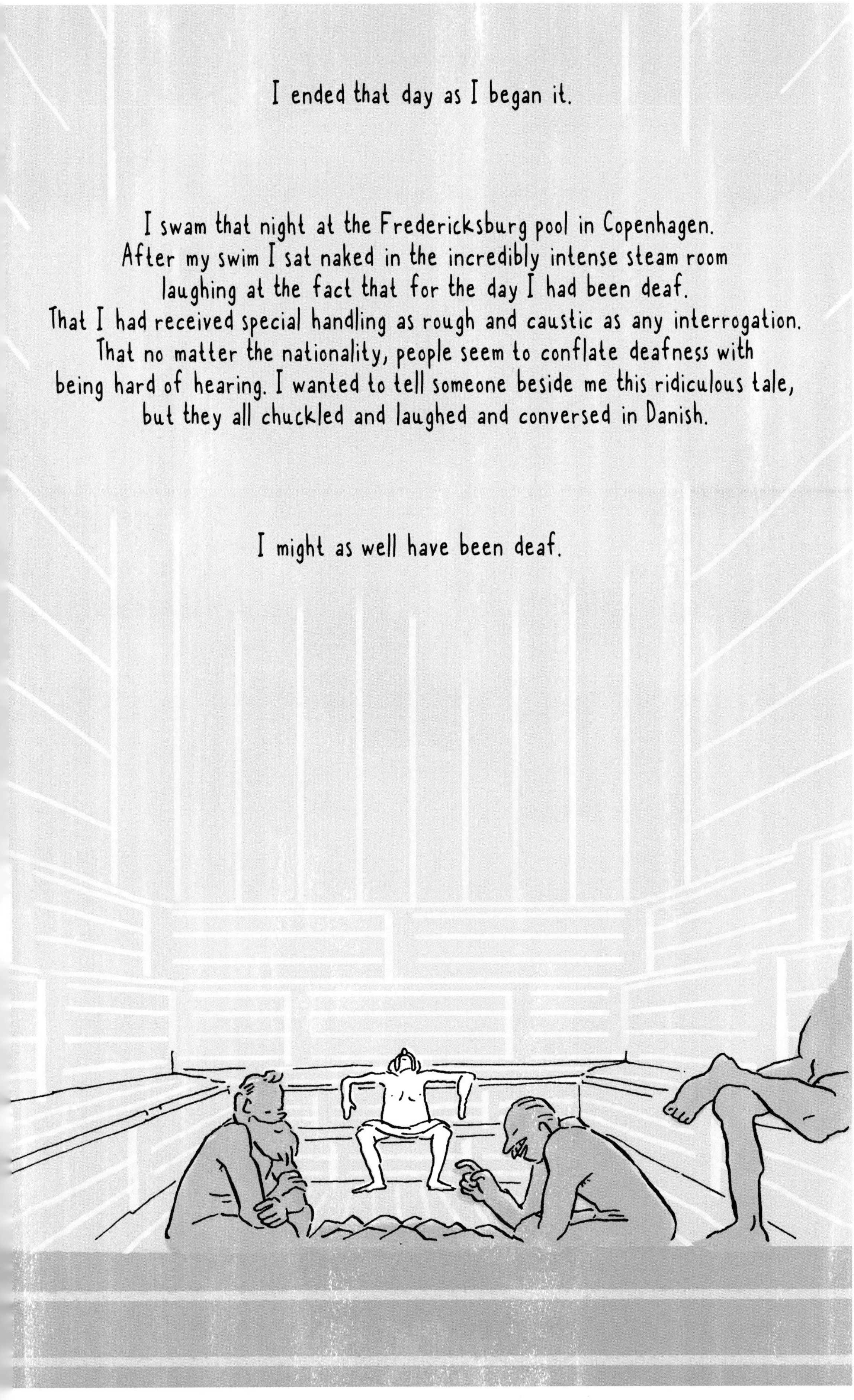
I ended that day as I began it.
I swam that night at the Fredericksburg pool in Copenhagen. After my swim I sat naked in the incredibly intense steam room laughing at the fact that for the day I had been deaf. That I had received special handling as rough and caustic as any interrogation. That no matter the nationality, people seem to conflate deafness with being hard of hearing. I wanted to tell someone beside me this ridiculous tale, but they all chuckled and laughed and conversed in Danish.
I might as well have been deaf.

Footnote: When I left Denmark about a week later,
I had forgotten all about my special status – I'd also forgotten to change it.
I checked in and boarded my flight. When it landed in Münich for the transfer,
the order for everyone to remain seated erupted through the speakers and I knew
what was to follow. As the security officers boarded the plane,
I simply stood and walked to the front.

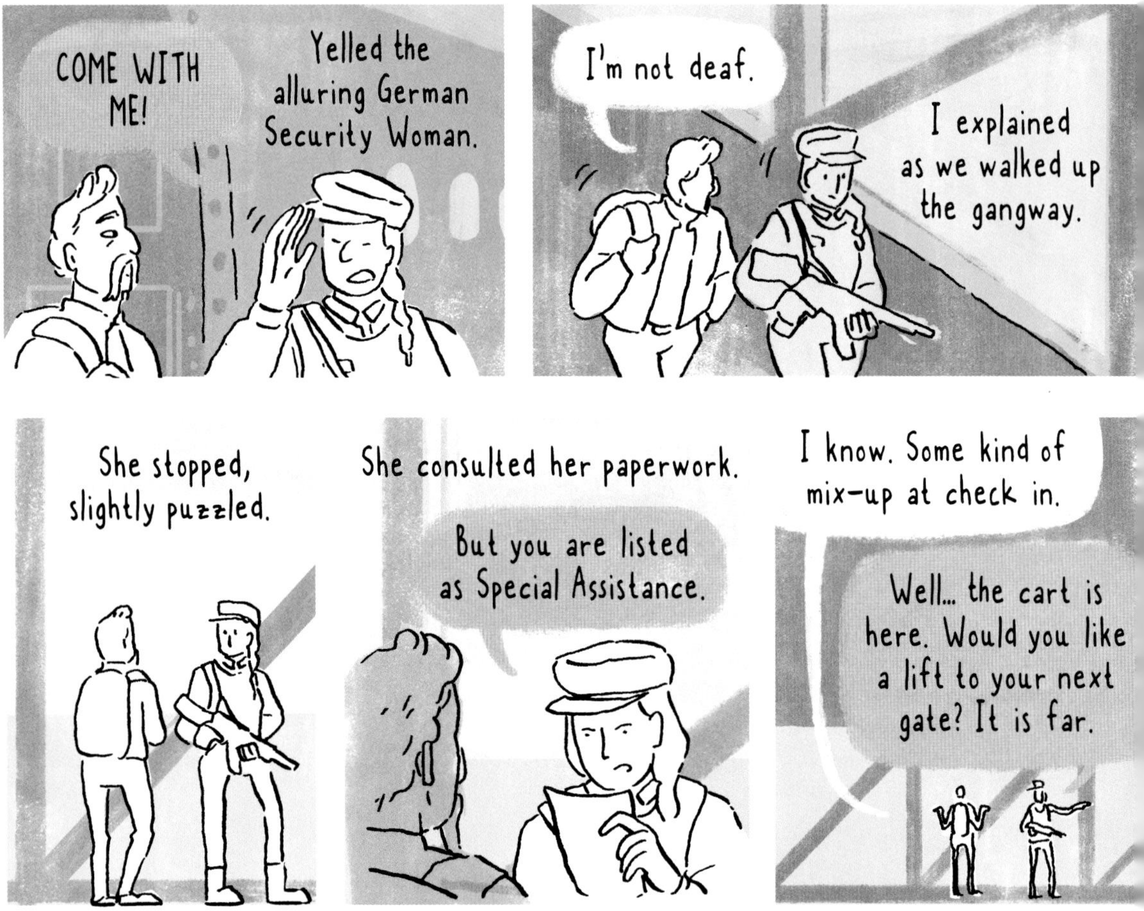
COME WITH ME!
Yelled the alluring German Security Woman.
I'm not deaf.
I explained as we walked up the gangway.
She stopped, slightly puzzled.
She consulted her paperwork.
But you are listed as Special Assistance.
I know. Some kind of mix-up at check in.
Well... the cart is here. Would you like a lift to your next gate? It is far.

I hopped in.
Traveling deaf is the only way to fly.
We sped off for parts unknown.

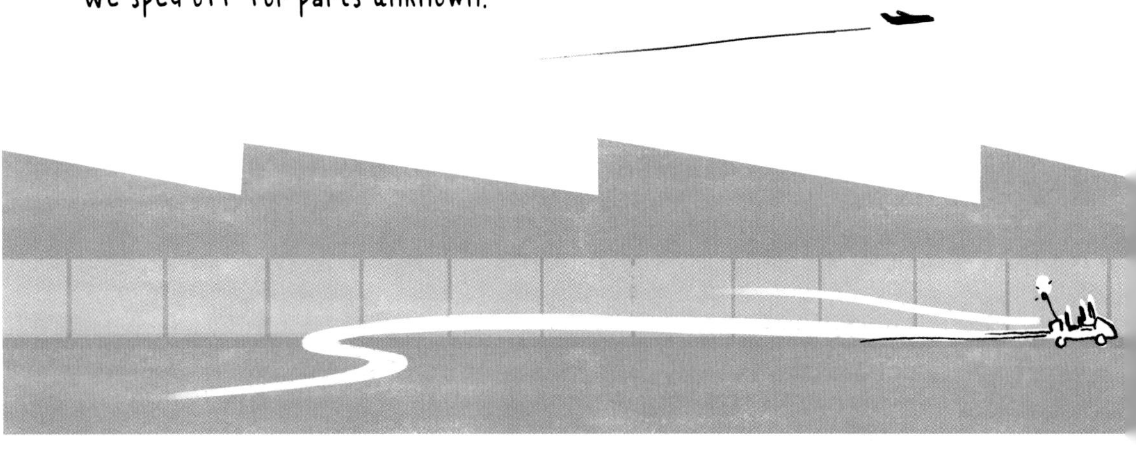

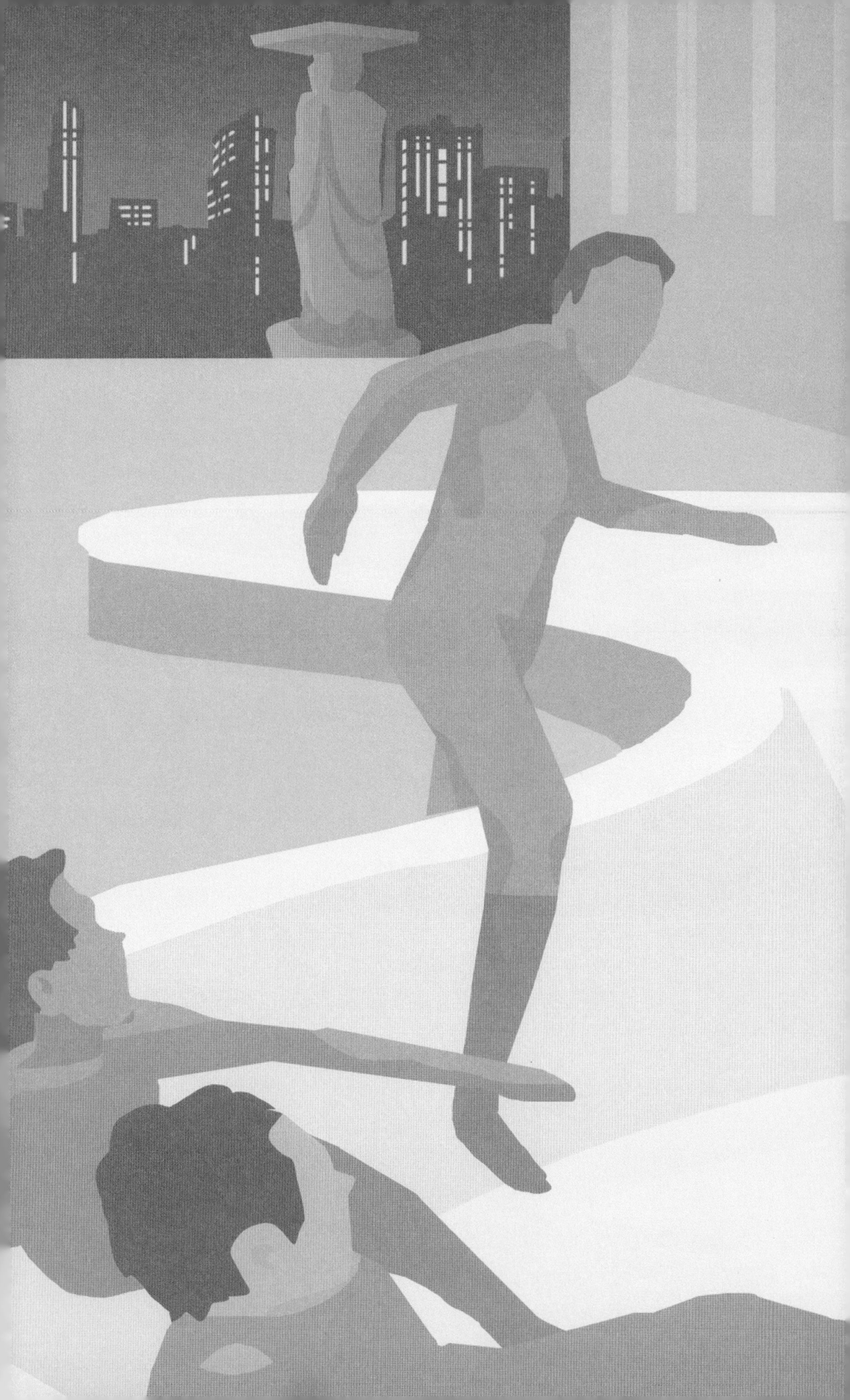

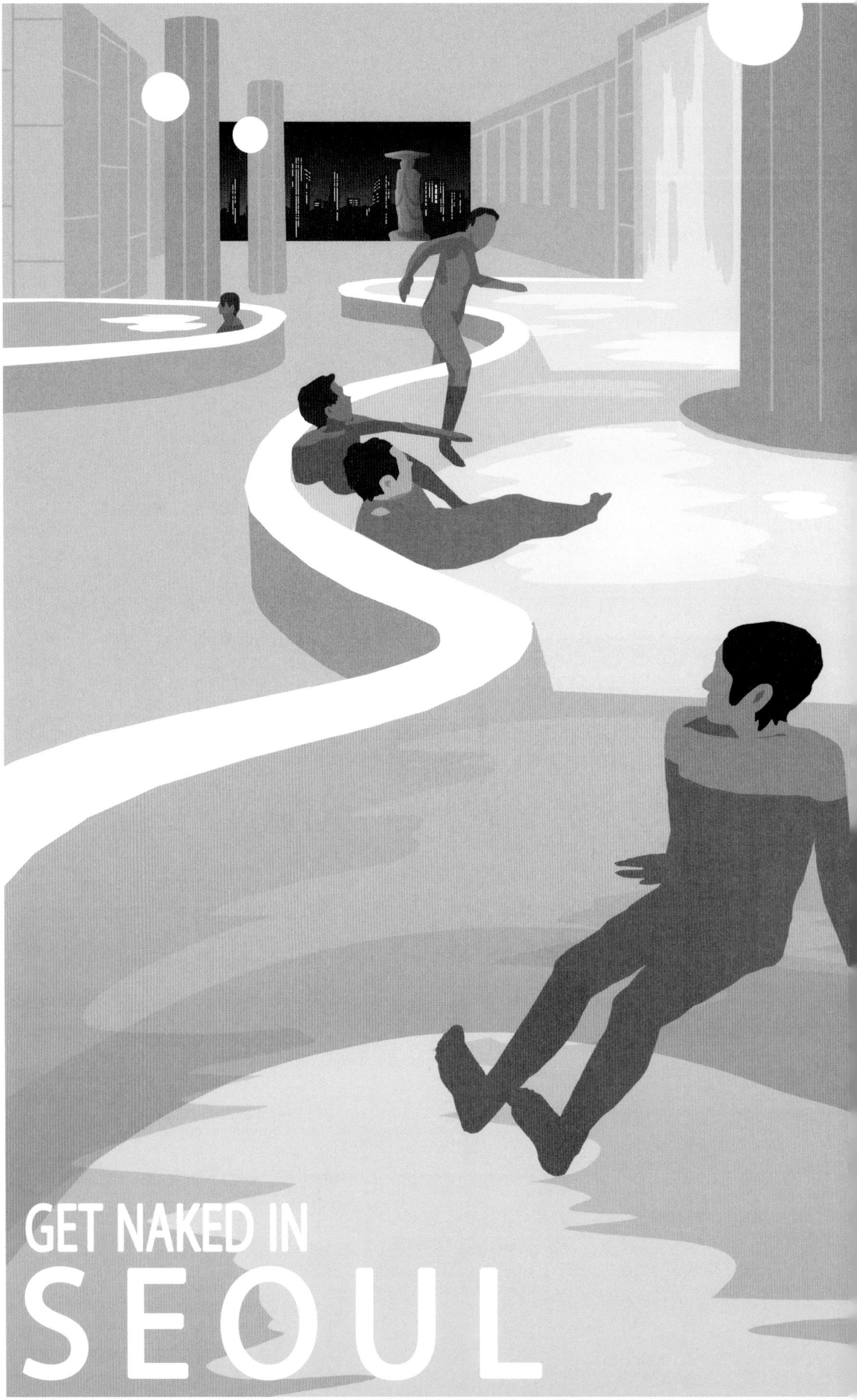
GET NAKED IN
SEOUL

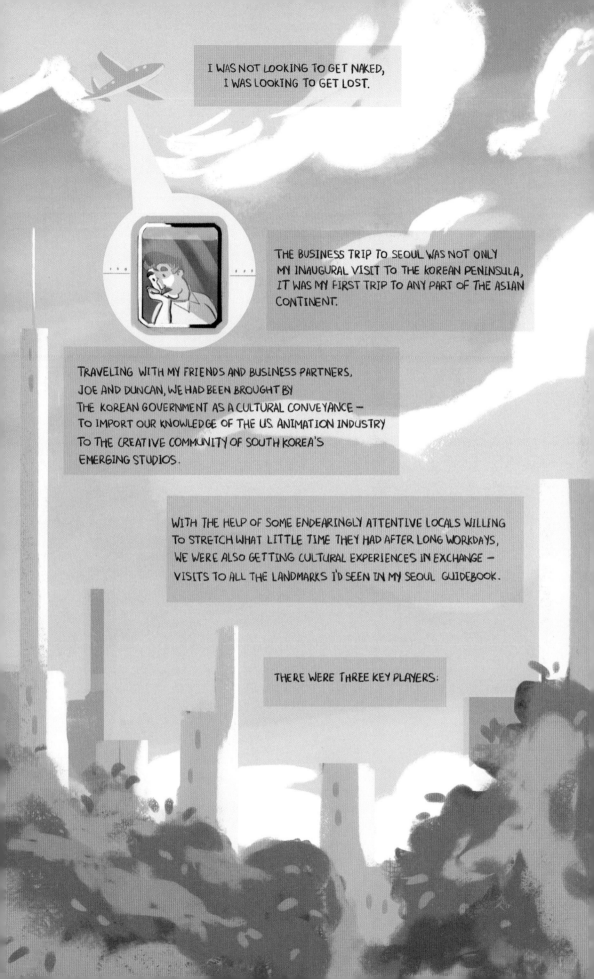

I WAS NOT LOOKING TO GET NAKED,
I WAS LOOKING TO GET LOST.

THE BUSINESS TRIP TO SEOUL WAS NOT ONLY
MY INAUGURAL VISIT TO THE KOREAN PENINSULA,
IT WAS MY FIRST TRIP TO ANY PART OF THE ASIAN
CONTINENT.

TRAVELING WITH MY FRIENDS AND BUSINESS PARTNERS,
JOE AND DUNCAN, WE HAD BEEN BROUGHT BY
THE KOREAN GOVERNMENT AS A CULTURAL CONVEYANCE —
TO IMPORT OUR KNOWLEDGE OF THE U.S. ANIMATION INDUSTRY
TO THE CREATIVE COMMUNITY OF SOUTH KOREA'S
EMERGING STUDIOS.

WITH THE HELP OF SOME ENDEARINGLY ATTENTIVE LOCALS WILLING
TO STRETCH WHAT LITTLE TIME THEY HAD AFTER LONG WORKDAYS,
WE WERE ALSO GETTING CULTURAL EXPERIENCES IN EXCHANGE —
VISITS TO ALL THE LANDMARKS I'D SEEN IN MY SEOUL GUIDEBOOK.

THERE WERE THREE KEY PLAYERS:

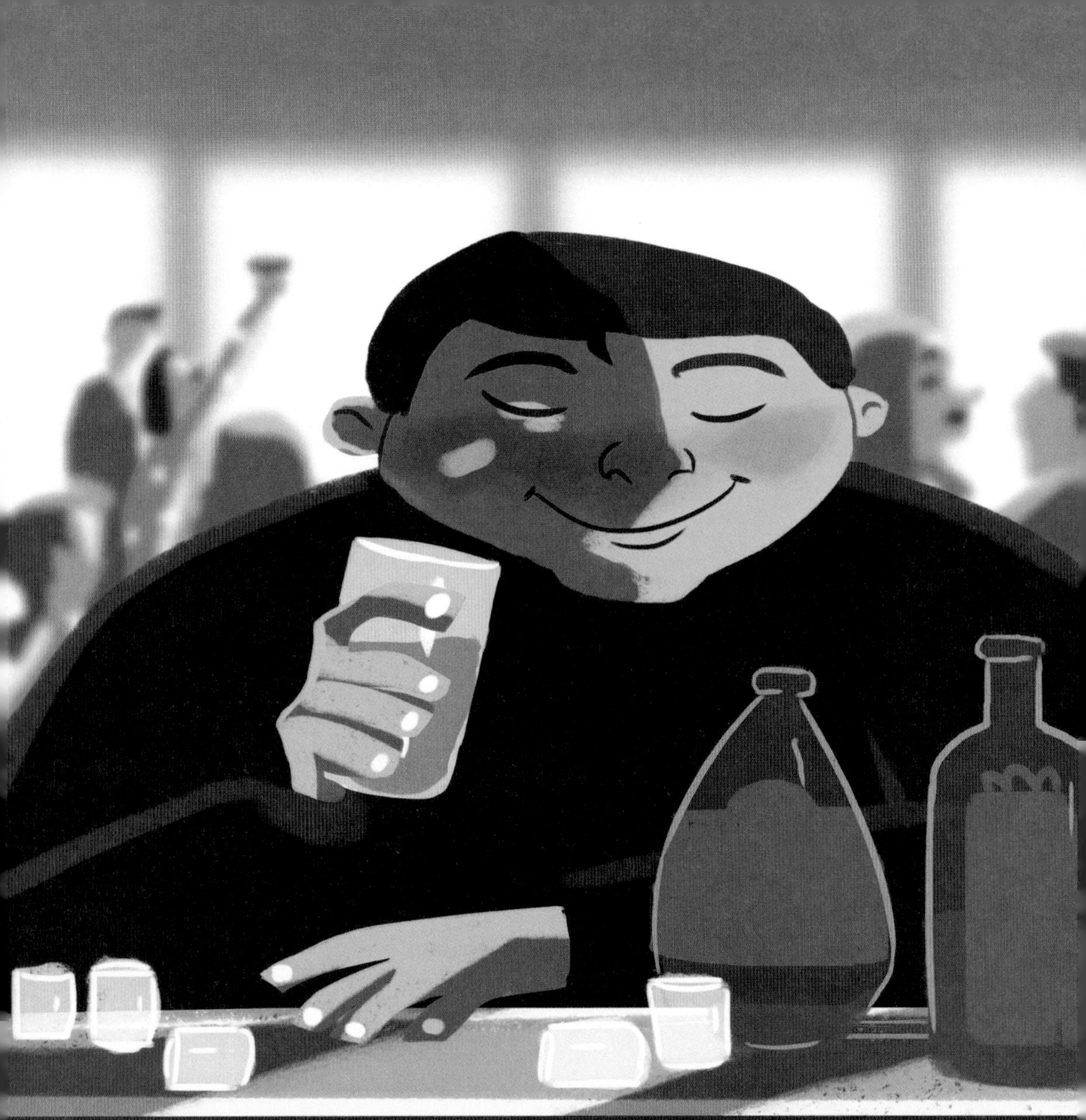

MR. KIM — HEAD OF THE ANIMATION STUDIO WE WERE DEVELOPING A PROJECT WITH — WAS OUR CONDUIT TO THE POST-WORKDAY UNDERGROUND OF LOCAL RESTAURANTS. MANY A NIGHT WAS SPENT WITH KOREAN BBQ COOKED AT THE TABLE WHILE MASSIVE INDUSTRIAL EXHAUST FANS SUCKED THE KIMCHI-SCENTED MEAT SMOKE OUT THROUGH THE ROOF.

DINNER WAS ONLY A STARTING POINT FOR A MR. KIM-HOSTED NIGHT OUT. THOUGH QUIET AND RESERVED DURING THE DAY, HE COULD EASILY PARTY UNTIL 2...3...4 IN THE MORNING - BUYING ROUNDS AT LOCAL BARS.

HE TOOK ON ALL CHALLENGERS WHEN IT CAME TO SOJU BOMBS — A WIDE POUR OF THE STURDY KOREAN ETHANOL DRINK WITH A SHOT-GLASSED BEER CHASER DROPPED DOWN INTO THE CENTER OF IT — BOTH DRINKS SLAMMED BACK SIMULTANEOUSLY TO A CHANT OF "BONGA BONGA!"

IF THE CHANT PHRASE IS DIRTY, RACIST, INSENSITIVE, OR ALL OF THE ABOVE, I APOLOGIZE. I STILL HAVE NO IDEA WHAT IT MEANS TO THIS DAY.

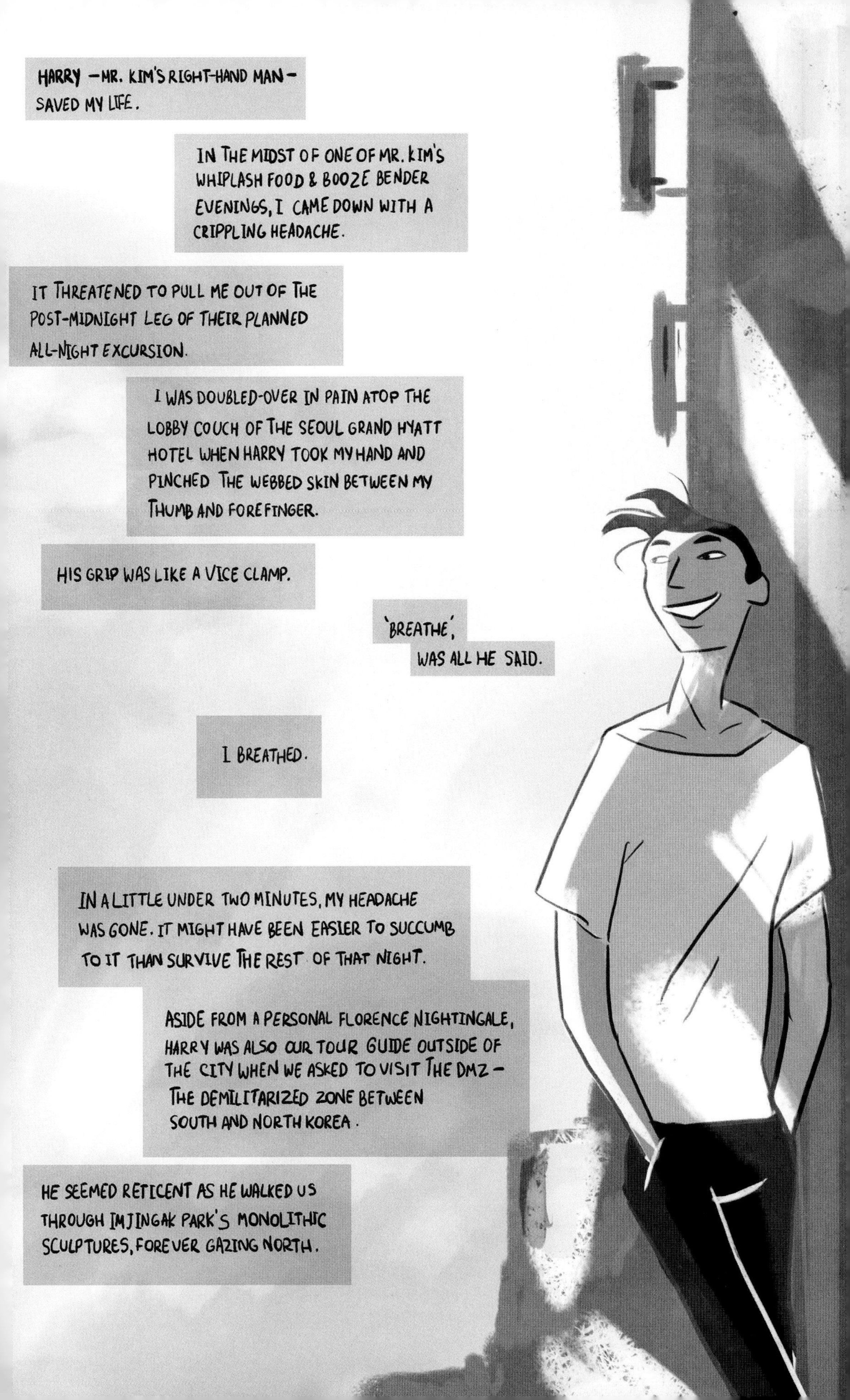
HARRY —MR. KIM'S RIGHT-HAND MAN— SAVED MY LIFE.
IN THE MIDST OF ONE OF MR. KIM'S WHIPLASH FOOD & BOOZE BENDER EVENINGS, I CAME DOWN WITH A CRIPPLING HEADACHE.
IT THREATENED TO PULL ME OUT OF THE POST-MIDNIGHT LEG OF THEIR PLANNED ALL-NIGHT EXCURSION.
I WAS DOUBLED-OVER IN PAIN ATOP THE LOBBY COUCH OF THE SEOUL GRAND HYATT HOTEL WHEN HARRY TOOK MY HAND AND PINCHED THE WEBBED SKIN BETWEEN MY THUMB AND FOREFINGER.
HIS GRIP WAS LIKE A VICE CLAMP.
'BREATHE',
WAS ALL HE SAID.
I BREATHED.
IN A LITTLE UNDER TWO MINUTES, MY HEADACHE WAS GONE. IT MIGHT HAVE BEEN EASIER TO SUCCUMB TO IT THAN SURVIVE THE REST OF THAT NIGHT.
ASIDE FROM A PERSONAL FLORENCE NIGHTINGALE, HARRY WAS ALSO OUR TOUR GUIDE OUTSIDE OF THE CITY WHEN WE ASKED TO VISIT THE DMZ — THE DEMILITARIZED ZONE BETWEEN SOUTH AND NORTH KOREA.
HE SEEMED RETICENT AS HE WALKED US THROUGH IMJINGAK PARK'S MONOLITHIC SCULPTURES, FOREVER GAZING NORTH.

HARRY WAS NOTICEABLY MORE UPBEAT ABOUT DORASAN, THE SPARKLING NEW TRAIN STATION AT THE DMZ.

HE SAID IT WAS BUILT TO WELCOME NORTH KOREANS ON THE DAY OF REUNIFICATION.

IT WAS A TOUCHING THOUGHT, BUT WHAT WAS A GHOST STATION THEN REMAINS SO A DECADE LATER — WITH NO HINT OF ARRIVING PASSENGERS FROM THE NORTH ANYWHERE ON THE HORIZON.

HARRY RELUCTANTLY ACCOMPANIED US DOWN A PLUNGING MINE SHAFT THAT INTERCEPTED A TUNNEL NORTH KOREA SECRETLY DUG INTO SOUTH KOREA IN THE LATE 1970s.

ONLY AFTER EXPLAINING ALL HE KNEW ABOUT THE CULTURE OF THIS CHARGED PLACE DID HARRY REVEAL THAT HE HAD NEVER PREVIOUSLY BEEN TO THE DMZ, EVEN THOUGH HE'D LIVED IN SEOUL HIS ENTIRE LIFE.

HE WAS FEARFUL OF IT—

BUT HAD EXPOSED HIMSELF TO THIS PAINFUL PLACE BECAUSE WE'D ASKED.

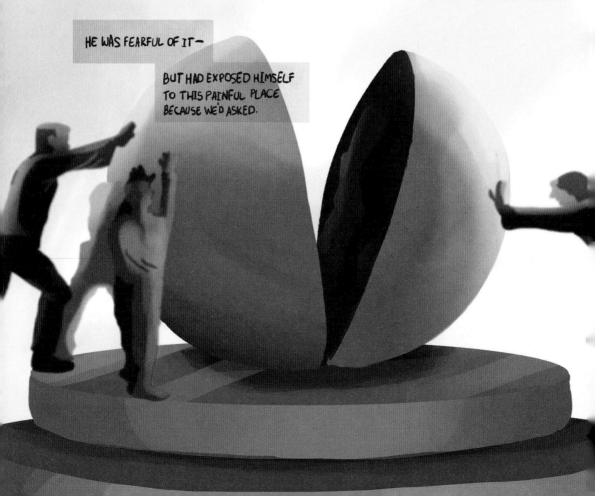

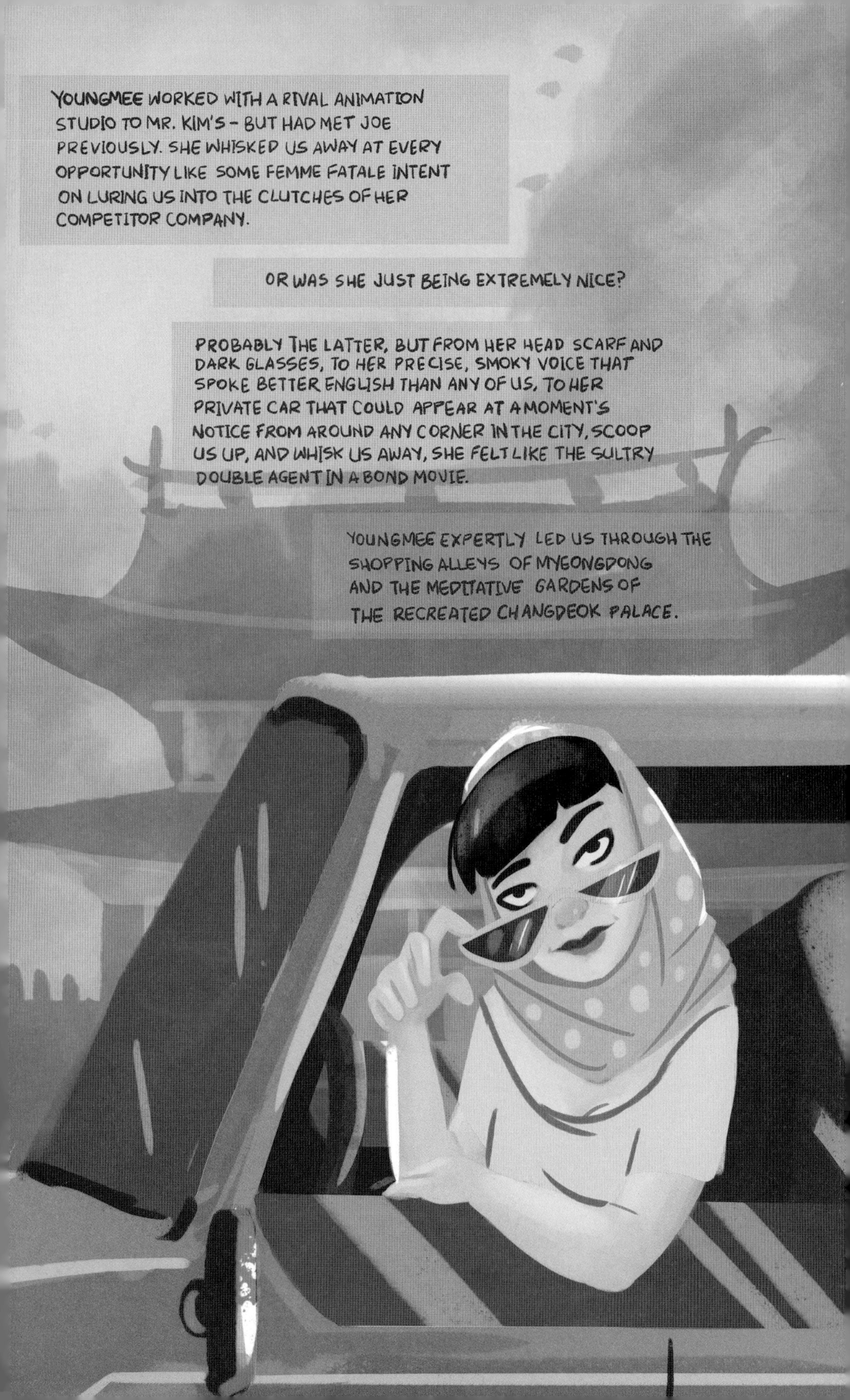
YOUNGMEE WORKED WITH A RIVAL ANIMATION STUDIO TO MR. KIM'S – BUT HAD MET JOE PREVIOUSLY. SHE WHISKED US AWAY AT EVERY OPPORTUNITY LIKE SOME FEMME FATALE INTENT ON LURING US INTO THE CLUTCHES OF HER COMPETITOR COMPANY.
OR WAS SHE JUST BEING EXTREMELY NICE?
PROBABLY THE LATTER, BUT FROM HER HEAD SCARF AND DARK GLASSES, TO HER PRECISE, SMOKY VOICE THAT SPOKE BETTER ENGLISH THAN ANY OF US, TO HER PRIVATE CAR THAT COULD APPEAR AT A MOMENT'S NOTICE FROM AROUND ANY CORNER IN THE CITY, SCOOP US UP, AND WHISK US AWAY, SHE FELT LIKE THE SULTRY DOUBLE AGENT IN A BOND MOVIE.
YOUNGMEE EXPERTLY LED US THROUGH THE SHOPPING ALLEYS OF MYEONGDONG AND THE MEDITATIVE GARDENS OF THE RECREATED CHANGDEOK PALACE.

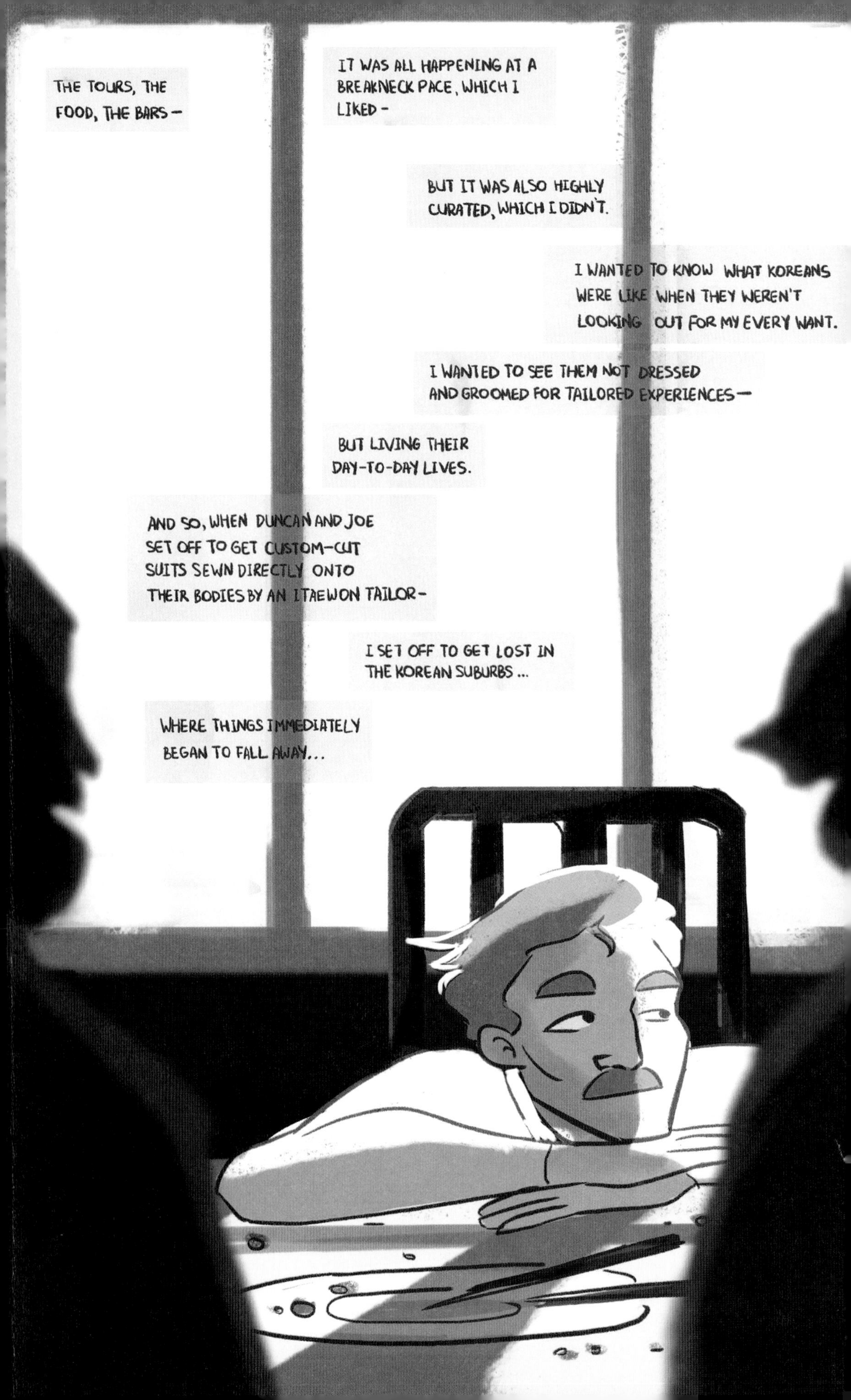
THE TOURS, THE FOOD, THE BARS –
IT WAS ALL HAPPENING AT A BREAKNECK PACE, WHICH I LIKED –
BUT IT WAS ALSO HIGHLY CURATED, WHICH I DIDN'T.
I WANTED TO KNOW WHAT KOREANS WERE LIKE WHEN THEY WEREN'T LOOKING OUT FOR MY EVERY WANT.
I WANTED TO SEE THEM NOT DRESSED AND GROOMED FOR TAILORED EXPERIENCES –
BUT LIVING THEIR DAY-TO-DAY LIVES.
AND SO, WHEN DUNCAN AND JOE SET OFF TO GET CUSTOM-CUT SUITS SEWN DIRECTLY ONTO THEIR BODIES BY AN ITAEWON TAILOR –
I SET OFF TO GET LOST IN THE KOREAN SUBURBS ...
WHERE THINGS IMMEDIATELY BEGAN TO FALL AWAY...

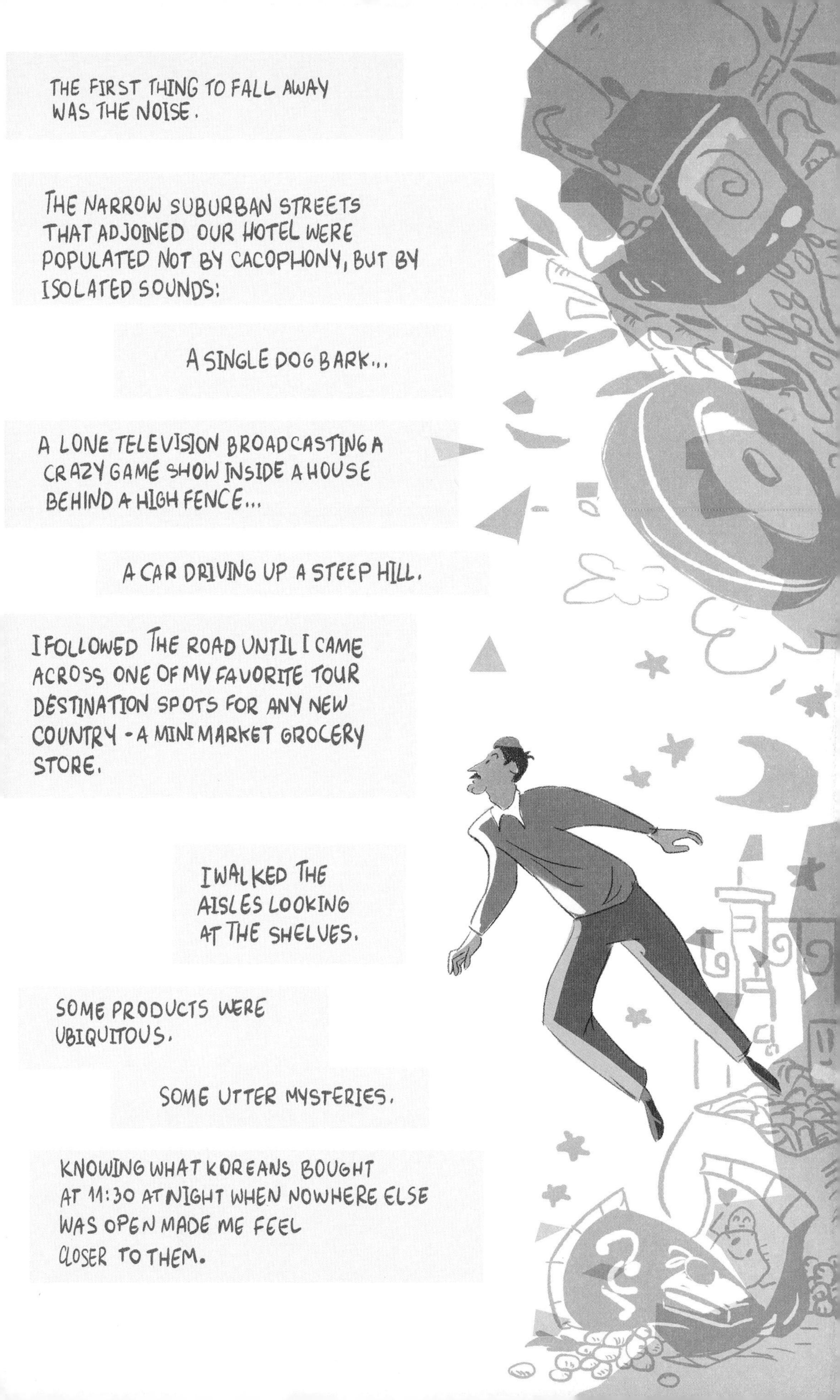
THE FIRST THING TO FALL AWAY WAS THE NOISE.
THE NARROW SUBURBAN STREETS THAT ADJOINED OUR HOTEL WERE POPULATED NOT BY CACOPHONY, BUT BY ISOLATED SOUNDS:
A SINGLE DOG BARK...
A LONE TELEVISION BROADCASTING A CRAZY GAME SHOW INSIDE A HOUSE BEHIND A HIGH FENCE...
A CAR DRIVING UP A STEEP HILL.
I FOLLOWED THE ROAD UNTIL I CAME ACROSS ONE OF MY FAVORITE TOUR DESTINATION SPOTS FOR ANY NEW COUNTRY - A MINI MARKET GROCERY STORE.
I WALKED THE AISLES LOOKING AT THE SHELVES.
SOME PRODUCTS WERE UBIQUITOUS.
SOME UTTER MYSTERIES.
KNOWING WHAT KOREANS BOUGHT AT 11:30 AT NIGHT WHEN NOWHERE ELSE WAS OPEN MADE ME FEEL CLOSER TO THEM.

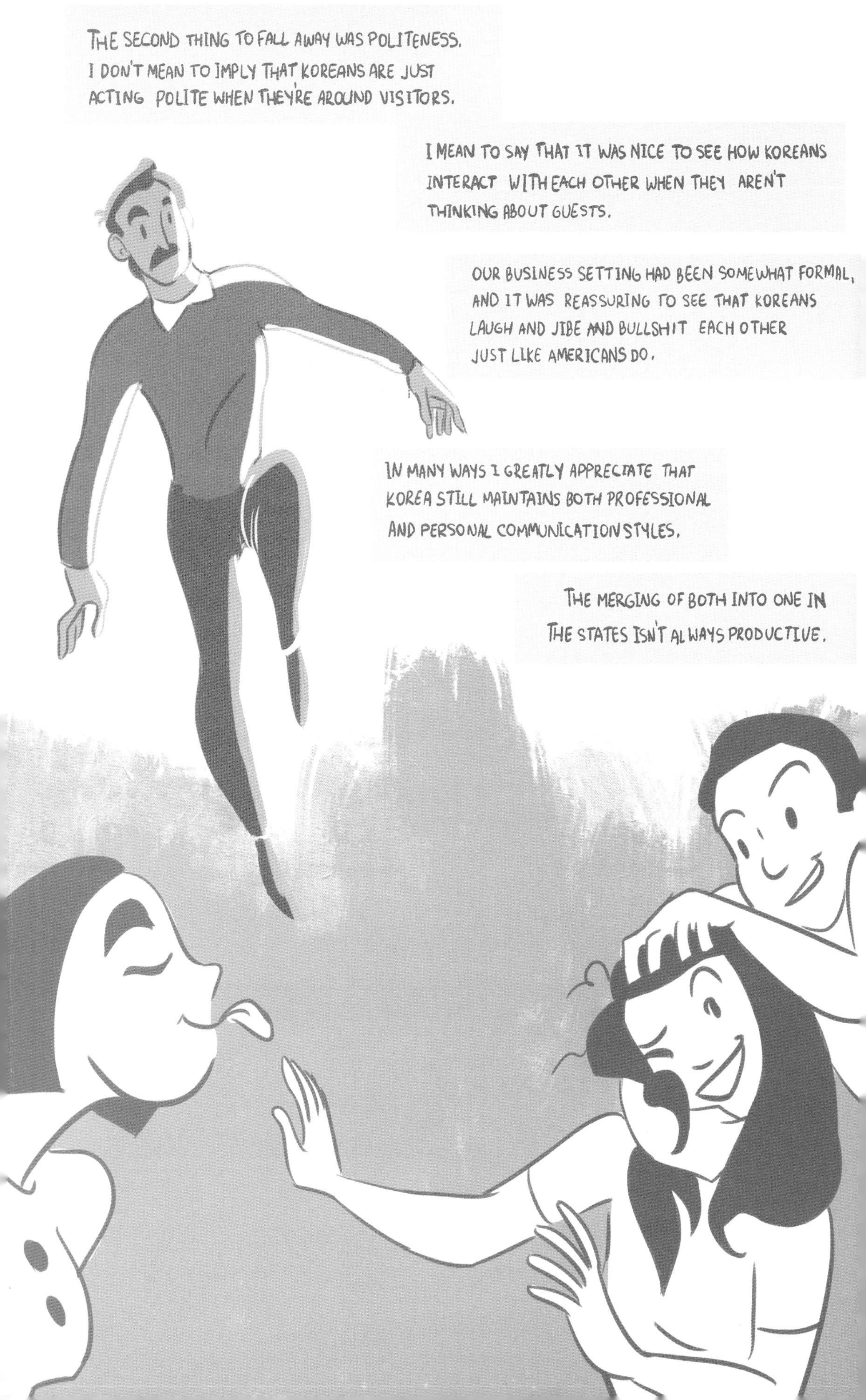
THE SECOND THING TO FALL AWAY WAS POLITENESS. I DON'T MEAN TO IMPLY THAT KOREANS ARE JUST ACTING POLITE WHEN THEY'RE AROUND VISITORS.
I MEAN TO SAY THAT IT WAS NICE TO SEE HOW KOREANS INTERACT WITH EACH OTHER WHEN THEY AREN'T THINKING ABOUT GUESTS.
OUR BUSINESS SETTING HAD BEEN SOMEWHAT FORMAL, AND IT WAS REASSURING TO SEE THAT KOREANS LAUGH AND JIBE AND BULLSHIT EACH OTHER JUST LIKE AMERICANS DO.
IN MANY WAYS I GREATLY APPRECIATE THAT KOREA STILL MAINTAINS BOTH PROFESSIONAL AND PERSONAL COMMUNICATION STYLES.
THE MERGING OF BOTH INTO ONE IN THE STATES ISN'T ALWAYS PRODUCTIVE.

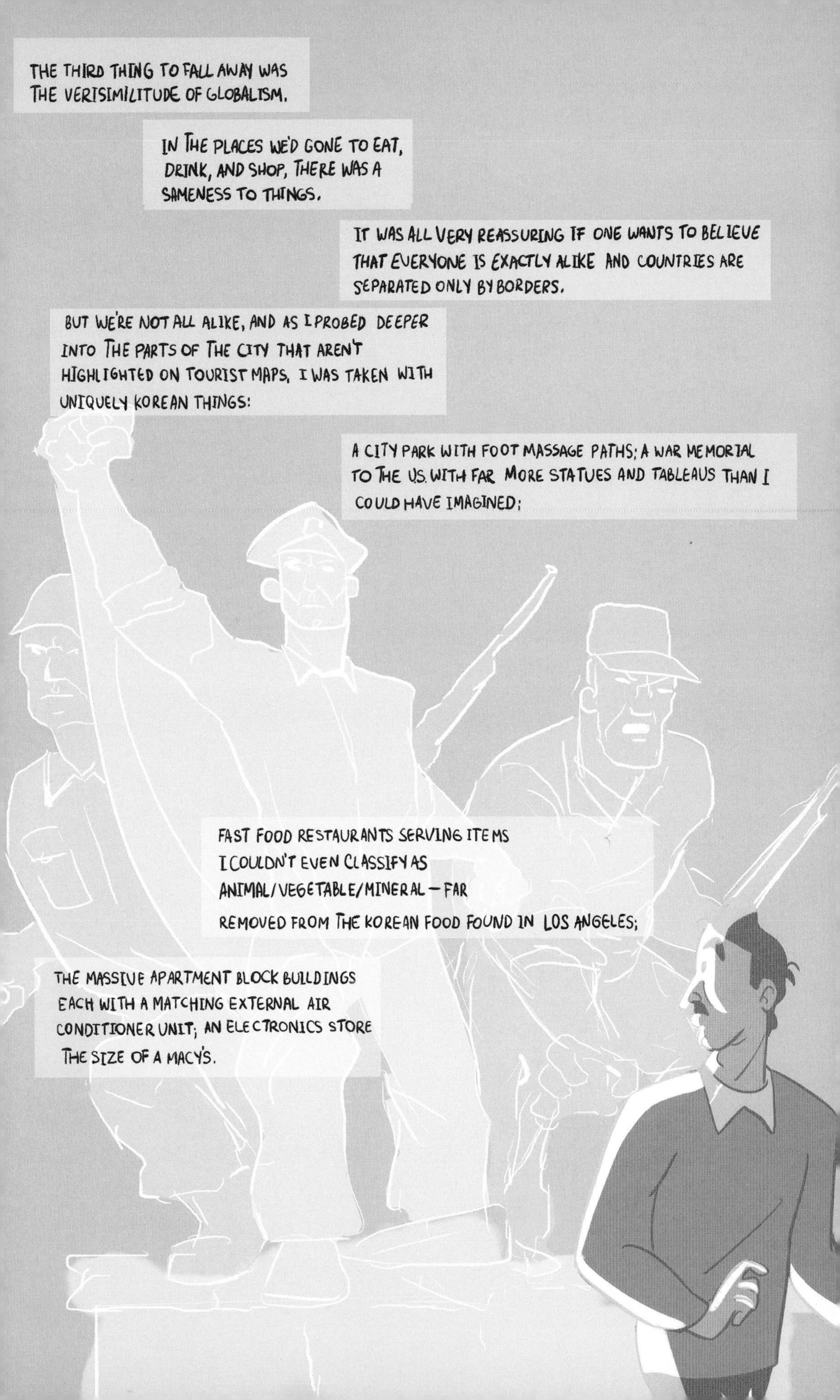
THE THIRD THING TO FALL AWAY WAS THE VERISIMILITUDE OF GLOBALISM.
IN THE PLACES WE'D GONE TO EAT, DRINK, AND SHOP, THERE WAS A SAMENESS TO THINGS.
IT WAS ALL VERY REASSURING IF ONE WANTS TO BELIEVE THAT EVERYONE IS EXACTLY ALIKE AND COUNTRIES ARE SEPARATED ONLY BY BORDERS.
BUT WE'RE NOT ALL ALIKE, AND AS I PROBED DEEPER INTO THE PARTS OF THE CITY THAT AREN'T HIGHLIGHTED ON TOURIST MAPS, I WAS TAKEN WITH UNIQUELY KOREAN THINGS:
A CITY PARK WITH FOOT MASSAGE PATHS; A WAR MEMORIAL TO THE U.S. WITH FAR MORE STATUES AND TABLEAUS THAN I COULD HAVE IMAGINED;
FAST FOOD RESTAURANTS SERVING ITEMS I COULDN'T EVEN CLASSIFY AS ANIMAL/VEGETABLE/MINERAL — FAR REMOVED FROM THE KOREAN FOOD FOUND IN LOS ANGELES;
THE MASSIVE APARTMENT BLOCK BUILDINGS EACH WITH A MATCHING EXTERNAL AIR CONDITIONER UNIT; AN ELECTRONICS STORE THE SIZE OF A MACY'S.

THE NEXT THING TO FALL AWAY WAS MY FEAR OF STANDING OUT.

THERE WAS A VERY SMALL, PEACEFUL KOREAN SPA IN THE BASEMENT OF THE HYATT.

AND I'D ALREADY PUT A FOOT IN THE WATER AND A BUTT ON THE SEAT OF THE HOT SAUNA THERE.

IT WAS ONE THING TO GET NAKED IN A SMALL FACILITY WITH A SMATTERING OF INTERNATIONAL TOURISTS.

YES, THE HUGE PICTURE WINDOW ADJACENT TO THE HOT TUBS WAS A BIT OFF-PUTTING AT FIRST, BUT EVEN THAT WAS PROTECTED – IT LOOKED ON TO A PRIVATE GARDEN, SO THERE WAS LITTLE RISK OF PAPARAZZI.

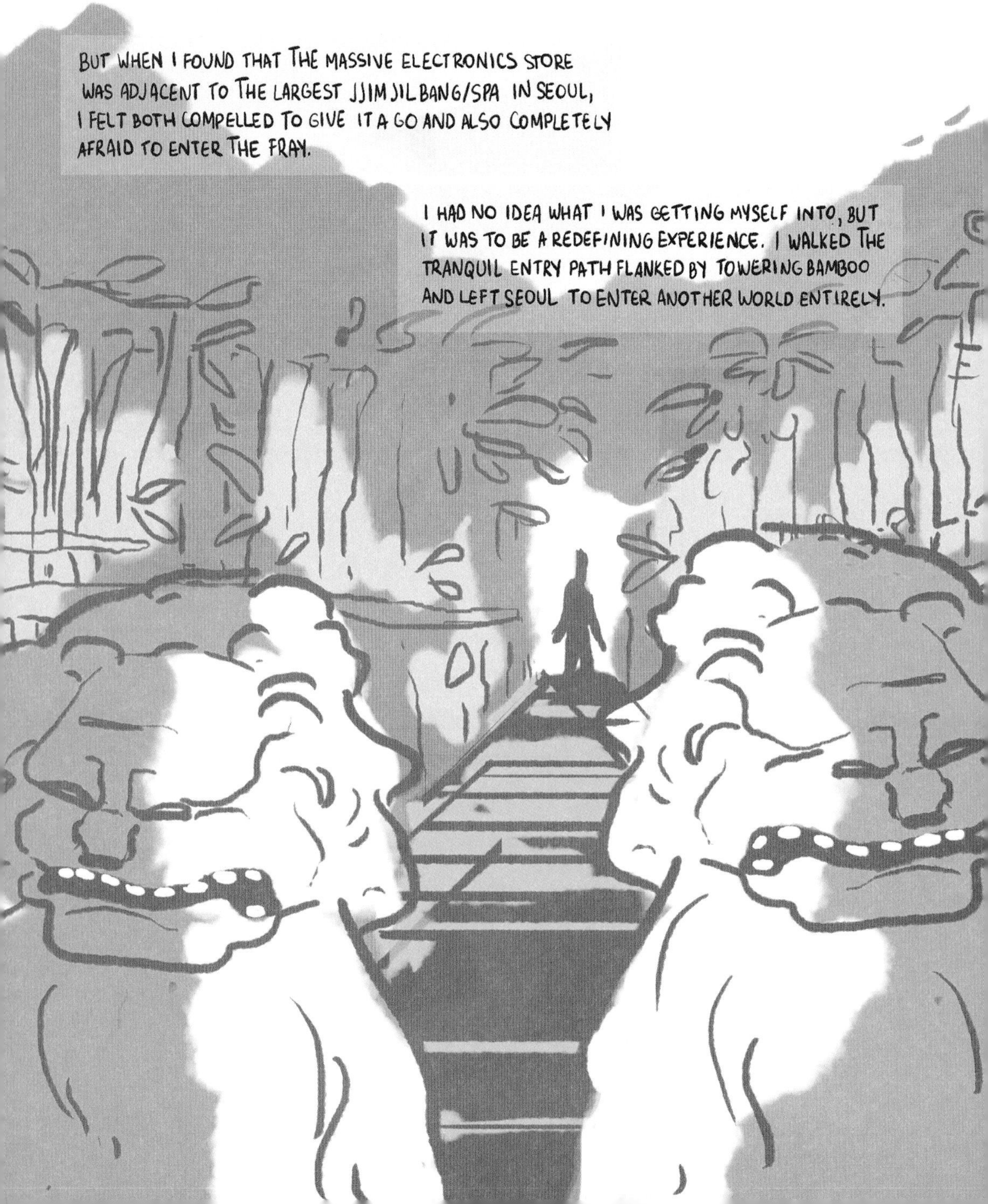
BUT WHEN I FOUND THAT THE MASSIVE ELECTRONICS STORE WAS ADJACENT TO THE LARGEST JJIMJILBANG/SPA IN SEOUL, I FELT BOTH COMPELLED TO GIVE IT A GO AND ALSO COMPLETELY AFRAID TO ENTER THE FRAY.
I HAD NO IDEA WHAT I WAS GETTING MYSELF INTO, BUT IT WAS TO BE A REDEFINING EXPERIENCE. I WALKED THE TRANQUIL ENTRY PATH FLANKED BY TOWERING BAMBOO AND LEFT SEOUL TO ENTER ANOTHER WORLD ENTIRELY.

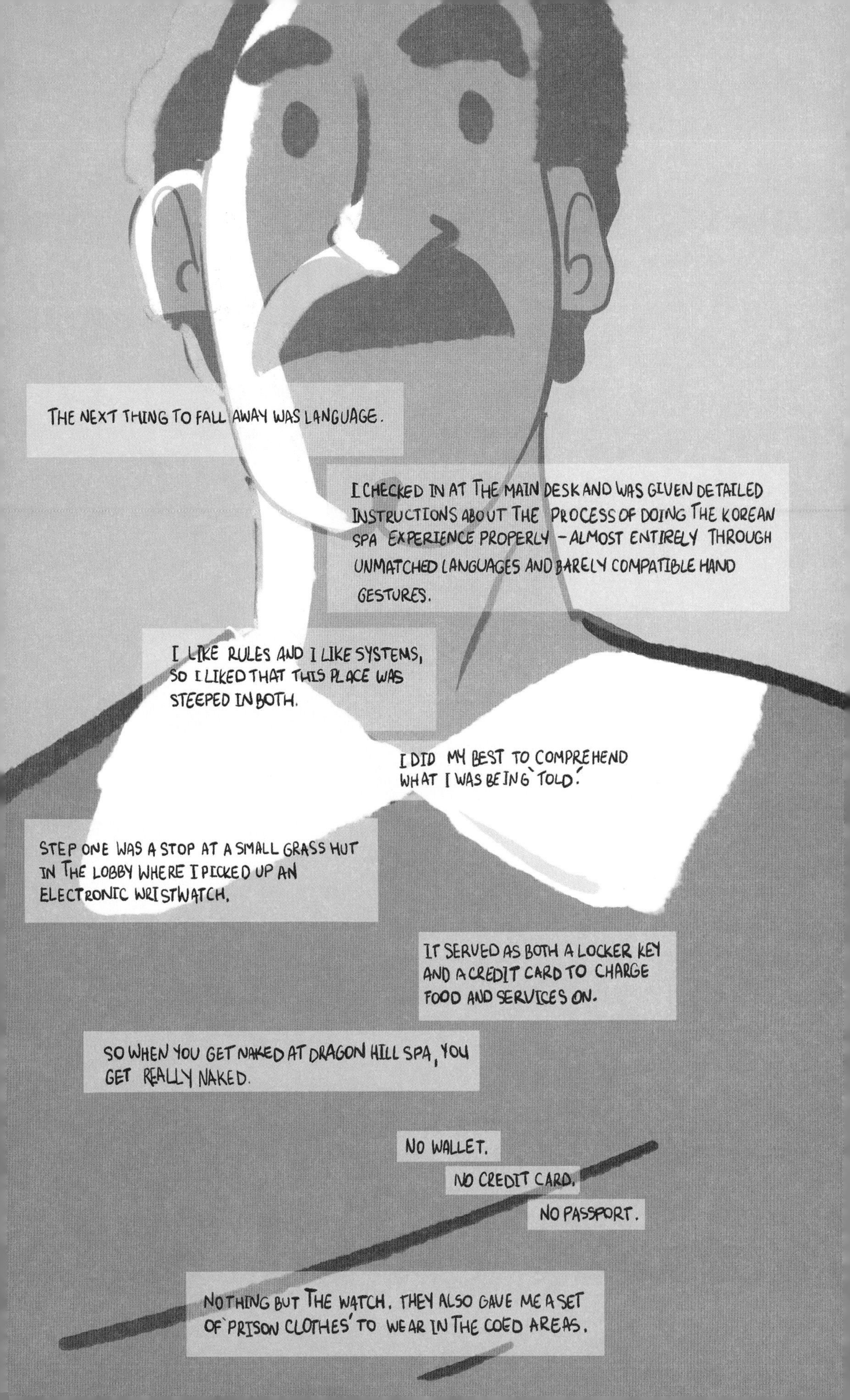
THE NEXT THING TO FALL AWAY WAS LANGUAGE.
I CHECKED IN AT THE MAIN DESK AND WAS GIVEN DETAILED INSTRUCTIONS ABOUT THE PROCESS OF DOING THE KOREAN SPA EXPERIENCE PROPERLY - ALMOST ENTIRELY THROUGH UNMATCHED LANGUAGES AND BARELY COMPATIBLE HAND GESTURES.
I LIKE RULES AND I LIKE SYSTEMS, SO I LIKED THAT THIS PLACE WAS STEEPED IN BOTH.
I DID MY BEST TO COMPREHEND WHAT I WAS BEING 'TOLD.'
STEP ONE WAS A STOP AT A SMALL GRASS HUT IN THE LOBBY WHERE I PICKED UP AN ELECTRONIC WRISTWATCH.
IT SERVED AS BOTH A LOCKER KEY AND A CREDIT CARD TO CHARGE FOOD AND SERVICES ON.
SO WHEN YOU GET NAKED AT DRAGON HILL SPA, YOU GET REALLY NAKED.
NO WALLET.
NO CREDIT CARD.
NO PASSPORT.
NOTHING BUT THE WATCH. THEY ALSO GAVE ME A SET OF 'PRISON CLOTHES' TO WEAR IN THE COED AREAS.

THE NEXT THING TO FALL AWAY WAS MY SHOES.

THE WATCH OPENED A TURNSTILE THAT ADMITTED ME TO THE SHOE LOCKER AREA.

I WAS GLAD SOMEONE HAD EXPLAINED THAT THESE WERE JUST SHOE LOCKERS AS I SAW A GERMAN COUPLE TRYING TO CRAM ALL OF THEIR BELONGINGS INTO THE MINIMAL SPACE.

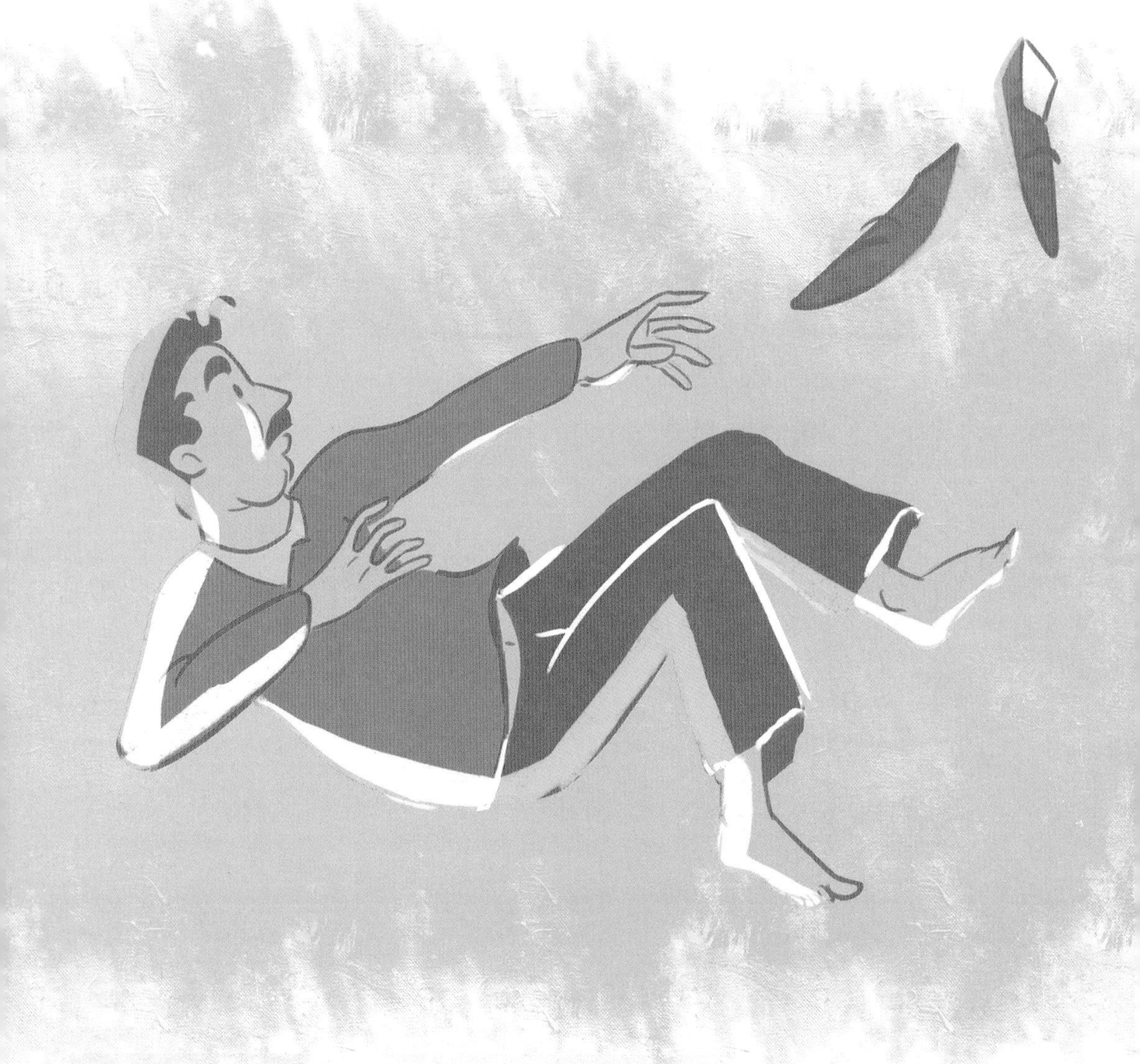

BECAUSE THEY WERE GERMANS, I HALF BELIEVED THEY WOULD FIND A PRECISE, EFFICIENT MEANS OF FITTING THEIR MASSIVE BACKPACKS IN THE TINY CUBBIES.

AFTER A MOMENT, AS IF I WERE A PRO, I LET THEM IN ON THE SECRET THAT THERE WERE OTHER LOCKERS AHEAD AND THIS WAS ONLY WHERE WE HAD TO SAY GOOD BYE TO OUR FOOTWEAR FOR THE DURATION OF THE VISIT.

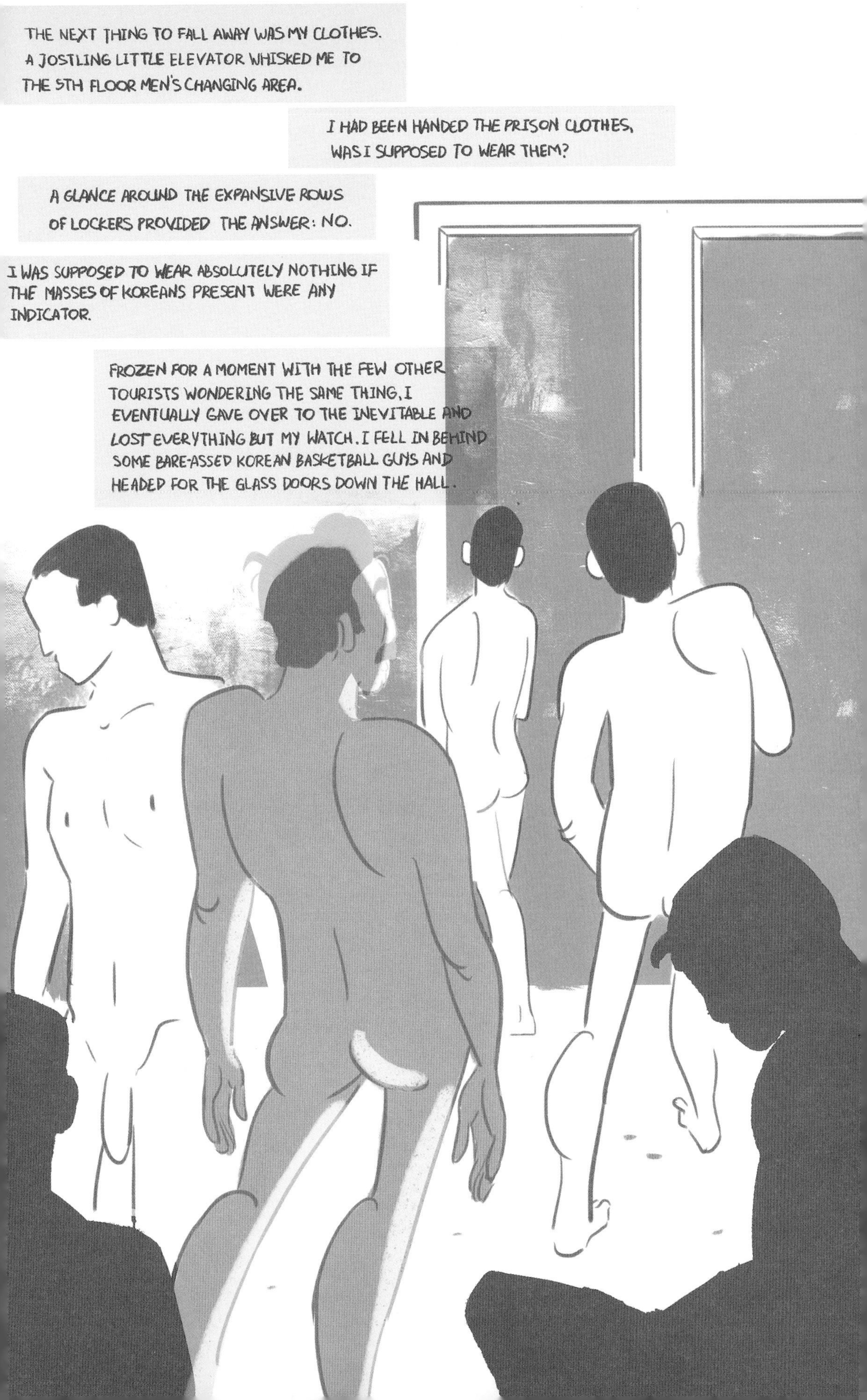
THE NEXT THING TO FALL AWAY WAS MY CLOTHES. A JOSTLING LITTLE ELEVATOR WHISKED ME TO THE 5TH FLOOR MEN'S CHANGING AREA.
I HAD BEEN HANDED THE PRISON CLOTHES, WAS I SUPPOSED TO WEAR THEM?
A GLANCE AROUND THE EXPANSIVE ROWS OF LOCKERS PROVIDED THE ANSWER: NO.
I WAS SUPPOSED TO WEAR ABSOLUTELY NOTHING IF THE MASSES OF KOREANS PRESENT WERE ANY INDICATOR.
FROZEN FOR A MOMENT WITH THE FEW OTHER TOURISTS WONDERING THE SAME THING, I EVENTUALLY GAVE OVER TO THE INEVITABLE AND LOST EVERYTHING BUT MY WATCH. I FELL IN BEHIND SOME BARE-ASSED KOREAN BASKETBALL GUYS AND HEADED FOR THE GLASS DOORS DOWN THE HALL.

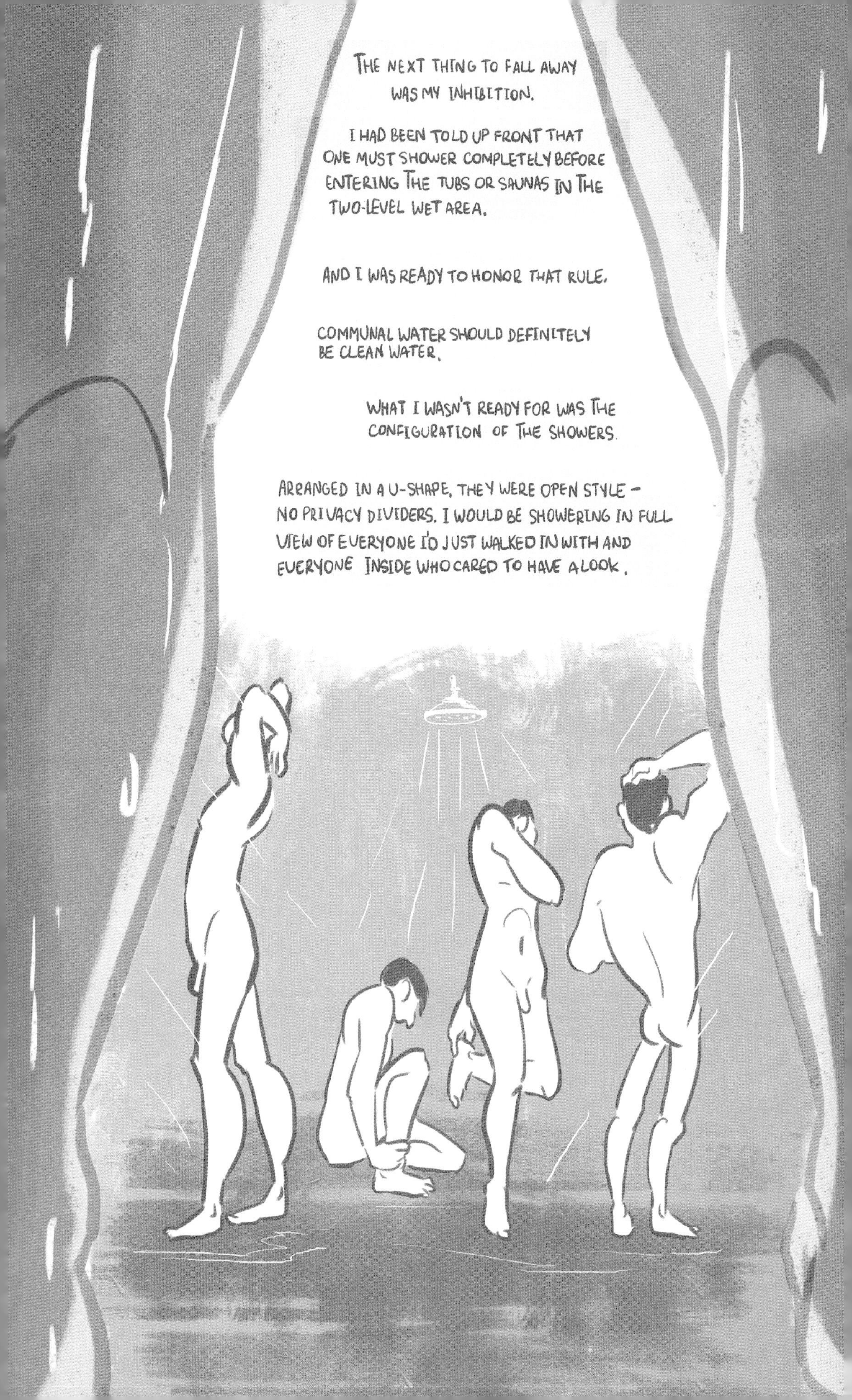
THE NEXT THING TO FALL AWAY WAS MY INHIBITION.
I HAD BEEN TOLD UP FRONT THAT ONE MUST SHOWER COMPLETELY BEFORE ENTERING THE TUBS OR SAUNAS IN THE TWO-LEVEL WET AREA.
AND I WAS READY TO HONOR THAT RULE.
COMMUNAL WATER SHOULD DEFINITELY BE CLEAN WATER.
WHAT I WASN'T READY FOR WAS THE CONFIGURATION OF THE SHOWERS.
ARRANGED IN A U-SHAPE, THEY WERE OPEN STYLE - NO PRIVACY DIVIDERS. I WOULD BE SHOWERING IN FULL VIEW OF EVERYONE I'D JUST WALKED IN WITH AND EVERYONE INSIDE WHO CARED TO HAVE A LOOK.

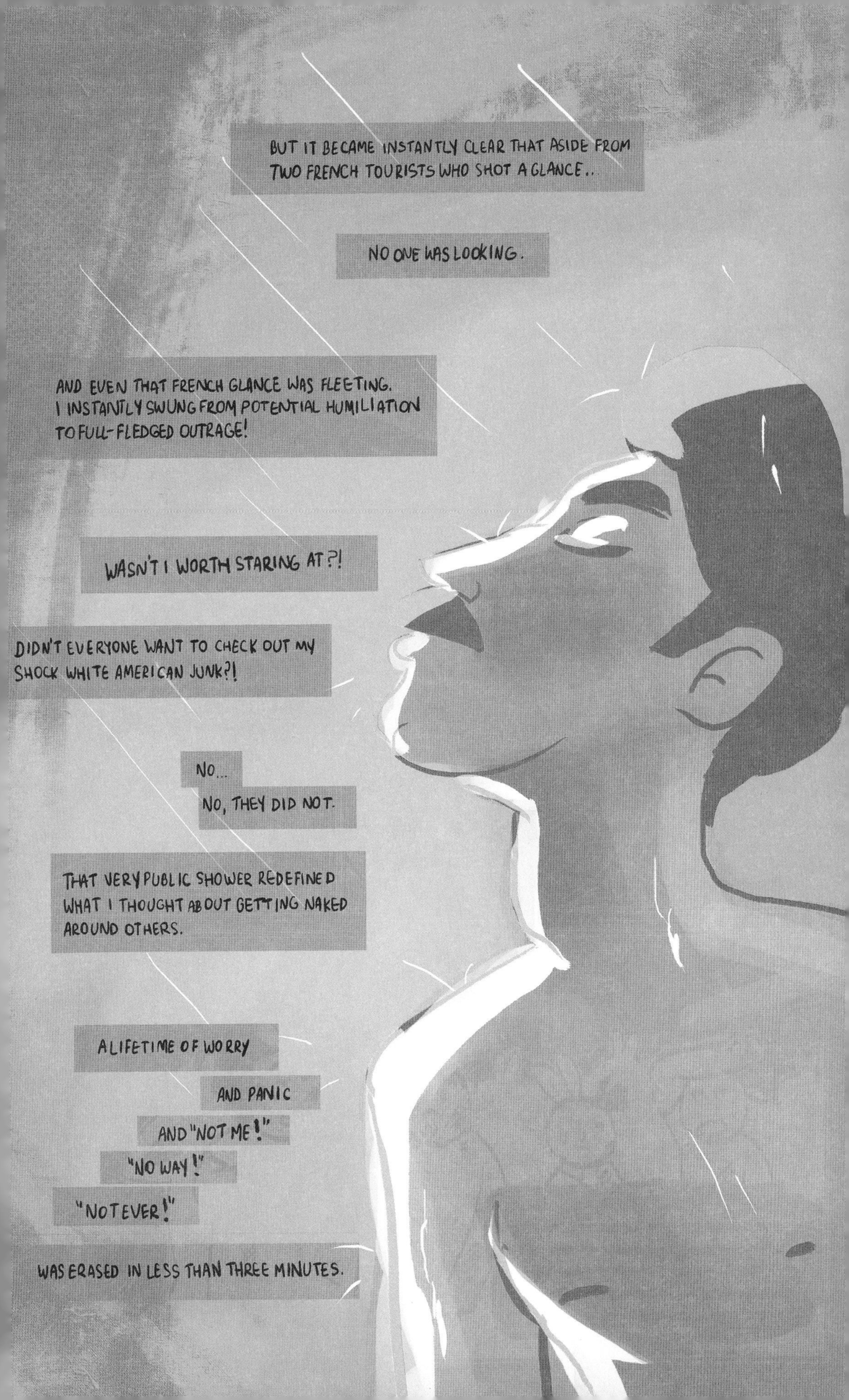
BUT IT BECAME INSTANTLY CLEAR THAT ASIDE FROM TWO FRENCH TOURISTS WHO SHOT A GLANCE..
NO ONE WAS LOOKING.
AND EVEN THAT FRENCH GLANCE WAS FLEETING. I INSTANTLY SWUNG FROM POTENTIAL HUMILIATION TO FULL-FLEDGED OUTRAGE!
WASN'T I WORTH STARING AT?!
DIDN'T EVERYONE WANT TO CHECK OUT MY SHOCK WHITE AMERICAN JUNK?!
NO...
NO, THEY DID NOT.
THAT VERY PUBLIC SHOWER REDEFINED WHAT I THOUGHT ABOUT GETTING NAKED AROUND OTHERS.
A LIFETIME OF WORRY
AND PANIC
AND "NOT ME!"
"NO WAY!"
"NOT EVER!"
WAS ERASED IN LESS THAN THREE MINUTES.

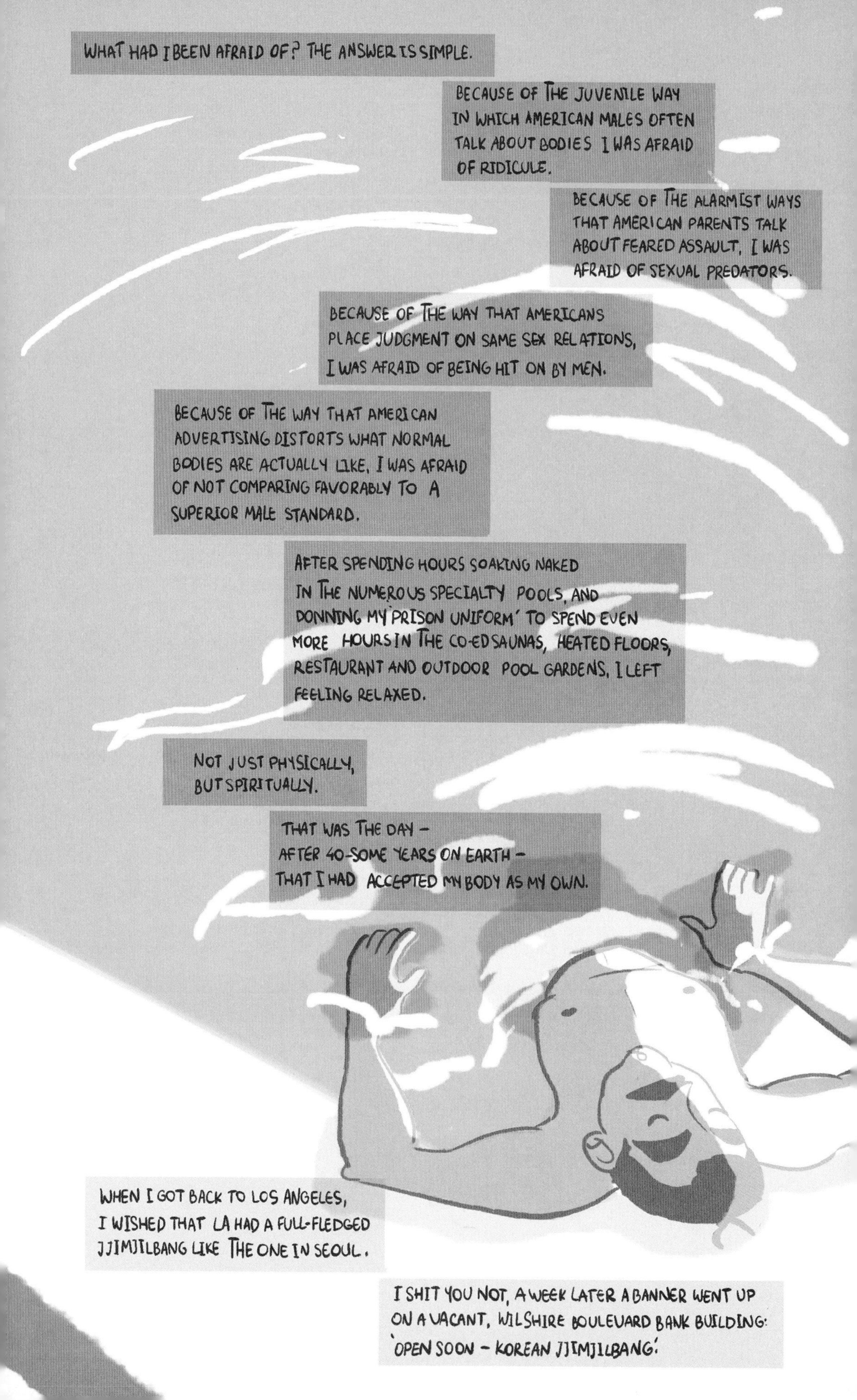
WHAT HAD I BEEN AFRAID OF? THE ANSWER IS SIMPLE.
BECAUSE OF THE JUVENILE WAY IN WHICH AMERICAN MALES OFTEN TALK ABOUT BODIES I WAS AFRAID OF RIDICULE.
BECAUSE OF THE ALARMIST WAYS THAT AMERICAN PARENTS TALK ABOUT FEARED ASSAULT, I WAS AFRAID OF SEXUAL PREDATORS.
BECAUSE OF THE WAY THAT AMERICANS PLACE JUDGMENT ON SAME SEX RELATIONS, I WAS AFRAID OF BEING HIT ON BY MEN.
BECAUSE OF THE WAY THAT AMERICAN ADVERTISING DISTORTS WHAT NORMAL BODIES ARE ACTUALLY LIKE, I WAS AFRAID OF NOT COMPARING FAVORABLY TO A SUPERIOR MALE STANDARD.
AFTER SPENDING HOURS SOAKING NAKED IN THE NUMEROUS SPECIALTY POOLS, AND DONNING MY 'PRISON UNIFORM' TO SPEND EVEN MORE HOURS IN THE CO-ED SAUNAS, HEATED FLOORS, RESTAURANT AND OUTDOOR POOL GARDENS, I LEFT FEELING RELAXED.
NOT JUST PHYSICALLY, BUT SPIRITUALLY.
THAT WAS THE DAY – AFTER 40-SOME YEARS ON EARTH – THAT I HAD ACCEPTED MY BODY AS MY OWN.
WHEN I GOT BACK TO LOS ANGELES, I WISHED THAT LA HAD A FULL-FLEDGED JJIMJILBANG LIKE THE ONE IN SEOUL.
I SHIT YOU NOT, A WEEK LATER A BANNER WENT UP ON A VACANT, WILSHIRE BOULEVARD BANK BUILDING: 'OPEN SOON – KOREAN JJIMJILBANG.'

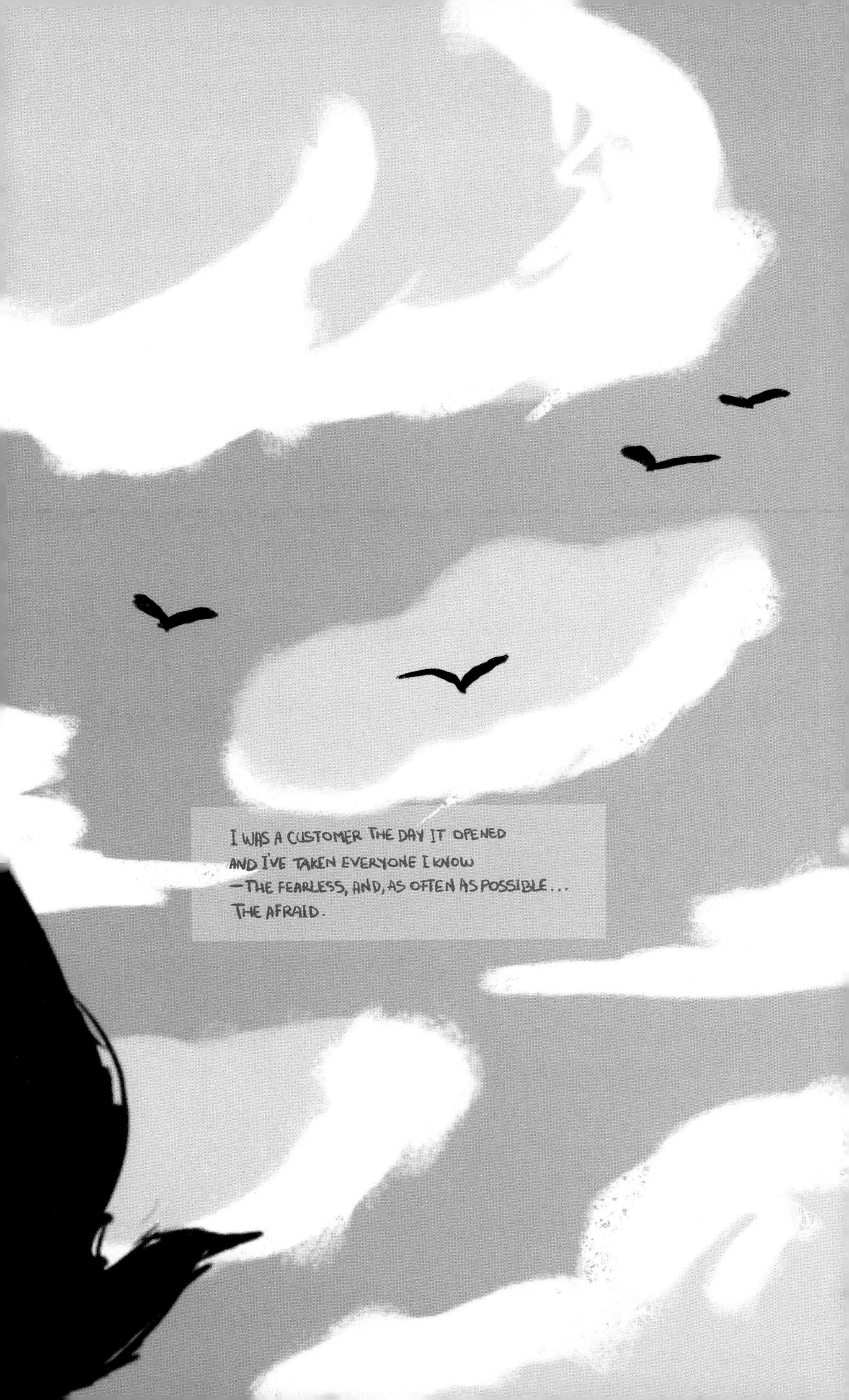
I WAS A CUSTOMER THE DAY IT OPENED
AND I'VE TAKEN EVERYONE I KNOW
—THE FEARLESS, AND, AS OFTEN AS POSSIBLE...
THE AFRAID.

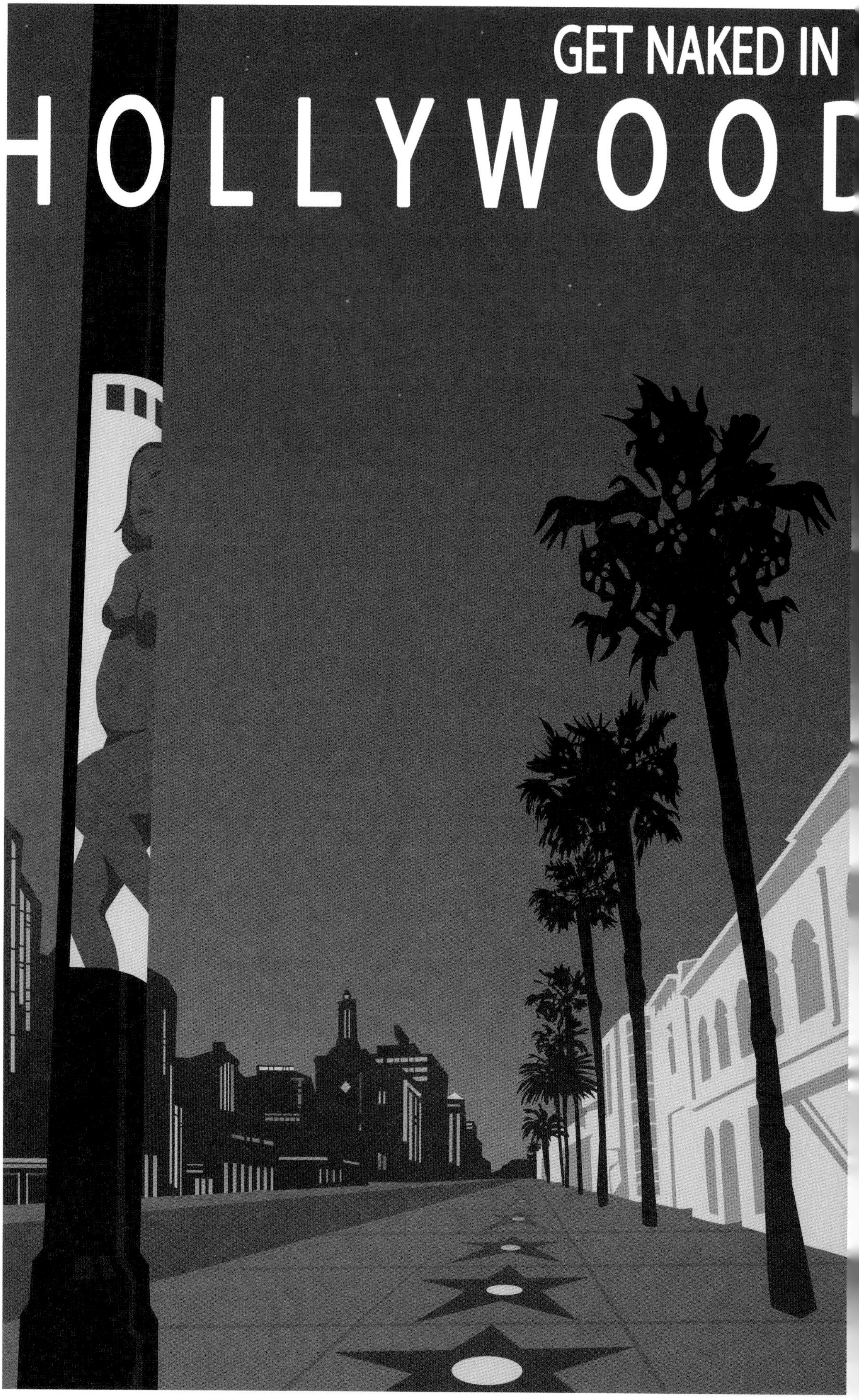
GET NAKED IN
HOLLYWOOD

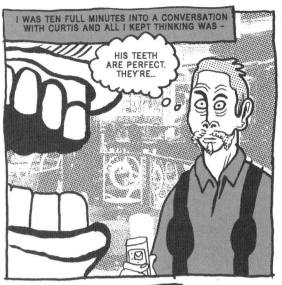

I WAS TEN FULL MINUTES INTO A CONVERSATION WITH CURTIS AND ALL I KEPT THINKING WAS -
HIS TEETH ARE PERFECT. THEY'RE...
ALIGNED
WHITE
RADIANT
MY OWN TEETH ARE A JUMBLED MESS SO BAD THAT MY CHILDHOOD DENTIST EXPRESSED TO MY MOTHER ABOUT THE POSSIBILITY OF BRACES-
I DON'T THINK I'D BOTHER.
Article Talk Read View source View history
WIKIPEDIA The Free Encyclopedia
BUT CURTIS'S WERE MARVELOUS - THE PERFECT CANDIDATES FOR THE PHOTOGRAPH OF THE WIKIPEDIA ENTRY ENTITLED:
Teeth
From Wikipedia, the free encyclopedia
Main page
Contents
Featured content
Current events
Random article
Donate to Wikipedia
Wikipedia store
Interaction
Help
About Wikipedia
Community portal
Recent changes
Contact page
Tools
What links here
Related changes
Upload file
Special pages
Permanent link
Page information
Wikidata item
Cite this page
HE HAD ASKED ABOUT THE "WHOLESTERS" I WEAR--
A WALLET/PHONE HOLSTER SYSTEM DESIGNED BY ONE OF THE VOICE ACTORS I WORK WITH - GREG CIPES. I EXPLAINED THE USUAL THINGS STRANGERS ASK ABOUT:
NO, THEY AREN'T CONFINING;
YES, BOTH POCKETS (GREG CALLS THEM BAGS) ARE ADJUSTABLE;
YES, THEY COME IN NYLON, LEATHER, AND FABRIC;
NO, THEY DON'T DRAW THAT MUCH ATTENTION AT AIRPORTS;
AND YES, YOU DO GET BETTER SEATS AT RESTAURANTS.
TO WHICH CURTIS CHUCKLED KNOWINGLY. TOO KNOWINGLY. DID HE SECRETLY OWN WHOLESTERS HIMSELF...?
WE PARTED WAYS WITH A FIST BUMP.

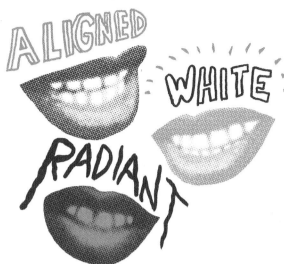

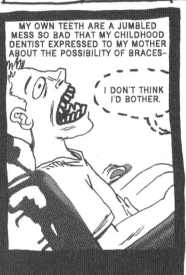

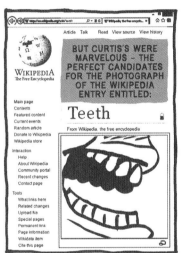

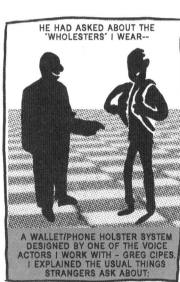

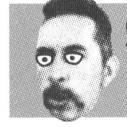

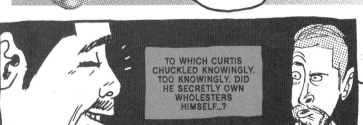

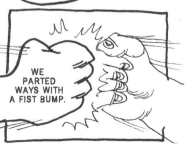

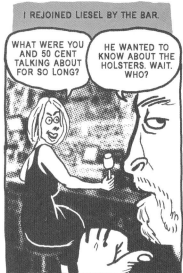

I REJOINED LIESEL BY THE BAR.

WHAT WERE YOU AND 50 CENT TALKING ABOUT FOR SO LONG?

HE WANTED TO KNOW ABOUT THE HOLSTERS. WAIT. WHO?

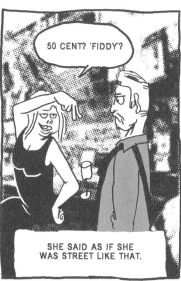

50 CENT? 'FIDDY'?

SHE SAID AS IF SHE WAS STREET LIKE THAT.

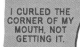

I CURLED THE CORNER OF MY MOUTH, NOT GETTING IT.

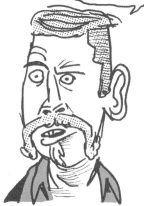

I THINK YOU'RE THINKING OF THE WRONG GUY. THAT GUY'S NAME IS CURTIS.

CURTIS JACKSON. FIDDY CENT? THE RAPPER. YOU HONESTLY DIDN'T KNOW?

I HONESTLY DIDN'T.

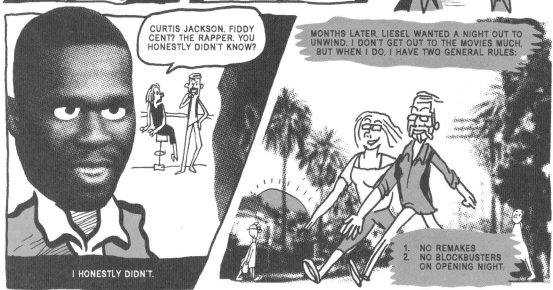

MONTHS LATER, LIESEL WANTED A NIGHT OUT TO UNWIND. I DON'T GET OUT TO THE MOVIES MUCH, BUT WHEN I DO, I HAVE TWO GENERAL RULES:

1. NO REMAKES
2. NO BLOCKBUSTERS ON OPENING NIGHT.

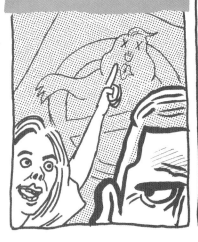

LIESEL WAS DEAD SET ON THE OPENING NIGHT SHOWING OF THE GHOSTBUSTERS REMAKE.

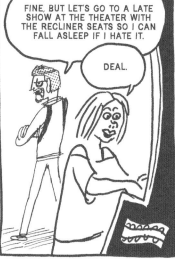

FINE, BUT LET'S GO TO A LATE SHOW AT THE THEATER WITH THE RECLINER SEATS SO I CAN FALL ASLEEP IF I HATE IT.

DEAL.

EACH TIME I AWOKE DURING THE FILM, KRISTIN WIIG, MELISSA MCCARTHY, AND KATE MCKINNON WERE DOING SOMETHING KOOKY THAT WASN'T QUITE ENOUGH TO KEEP ME FROM SLIDING BACK INTO UNCONSCIOUSNESS. I ASKED LIESEL WHAT "WE" THOUGHT OF IT AFTER AND SHE SAID "WE" THOUGHT IT WAS GOOFY FUN.

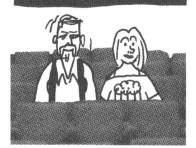

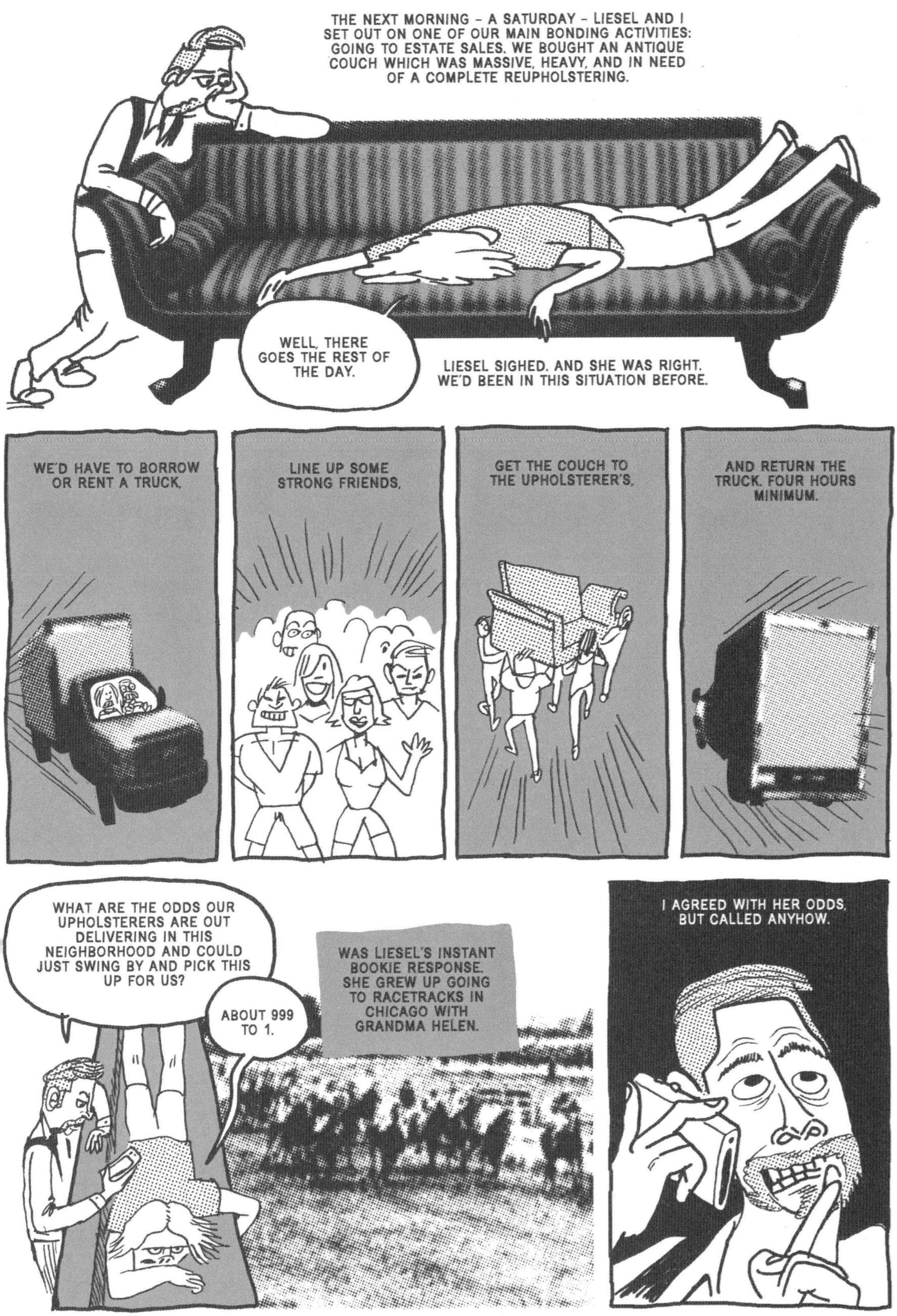
THE NEXT MORNING – A SATURDAY – LIESEL AND I SET OUT ON ONE OF OUR MAIN BONDING ACTIVITIES: GOING TO ESTATE SALES. WE BOUGHT AN ANTIQUE COUCH WHICH WAS MASSIVE, HEAVY, AND IN NEED OF A COMPLETE REUPHOLSTERING.
WELL, THERE GOES THE REST OF THE DAY.
LIESEL SIGHED. AND SHE WAS RIGHT. WE'D BEEN IN THIS SITUATION BEFORE.
WE'D HAVE TO BORROW OR RENT A TRUCK,
LINE UP SOME STRONG FRIENDS,
GET THE COUCH TO THE UPHOLSTERER'S,
AND RETURN THE TRUCK. FOUR HOURS MINIMUM.
WHAT ARE THE ODDS OUR UPHOLSTERERS ARE OUT DELIVERING IN THIS NEIGHBORHOOD AND COULD JUST SWING BY AND PICK THIS UP FOR US?
ABOUT 999 TO 1.
WAS LIESEL'S INSTANT BOOKIE RESPONSE. SHE GREW UP GOING TO RACETRACKS IN CHICAGO WITH GRANDMA HELEN.
I AGREED WITH HER ODDS, BUT CALLED ANYHOW.

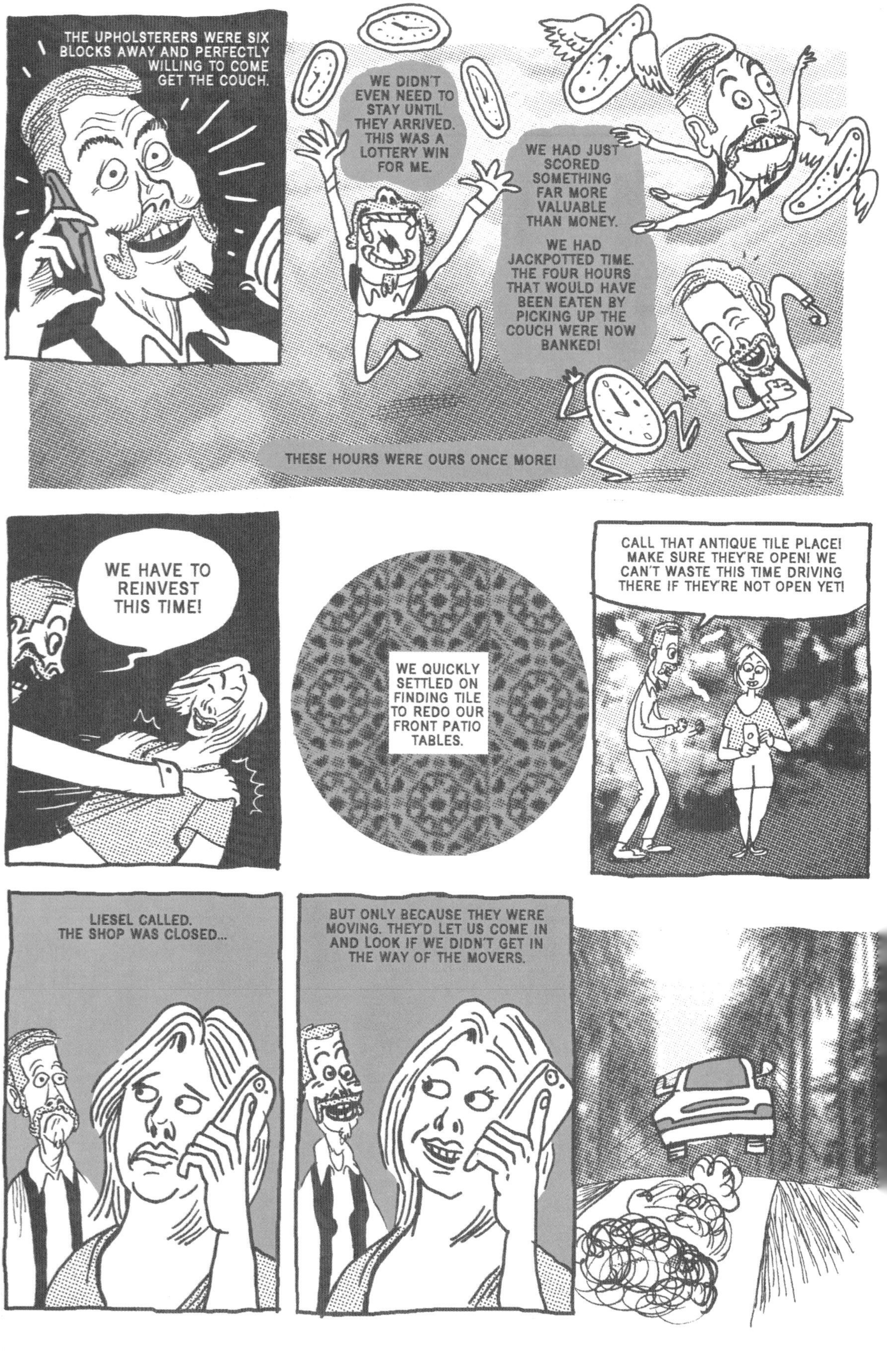
THE UPHOLSTERERS WERE SIX BLOCKS AWAY AND PERFECTLY WILLING TO COME GET THE COUCH.
WE DIDN'T EVEN NEED TO STAY UNTIL THEY ARRIVED. THIS WAS A LOTTERY WIN FOR ME.
WE HAD JUST SCORED SOMETHING FAR MORE VALUABLE THAN MONEY.
WE HAD JACKPOTTED TIME. THE FOUR HOURS THAT WOULD HAVE BEEN EATEN BY PICKING UP THE COUCH WERE NOW BANKED!
THESE HOURS WERE OURS ONCE MORE!
WE HAVE TO REINVEST THIS TIME!
WE QUICKLY SETTLED ON FINDING TILE TO REDO OUR FRONT PATIO TABLES.
CALL THAT ANTIQUE TILE PLACE! MAKE SURE THEY'RE OPEN! WE CAN'T WASTE THIS TIME DRIVING THERE IF THEY'RE NOT OPEN YET!
LIESEL CALLED. THE SHOP WAS CLOSED...
BUT ONLY BECAUSE THEY WERE MOVING. THEY'D LET US COME IN AND LOOK IF WE DIDN'T GET IN THE WAY OF THE MOVERS.

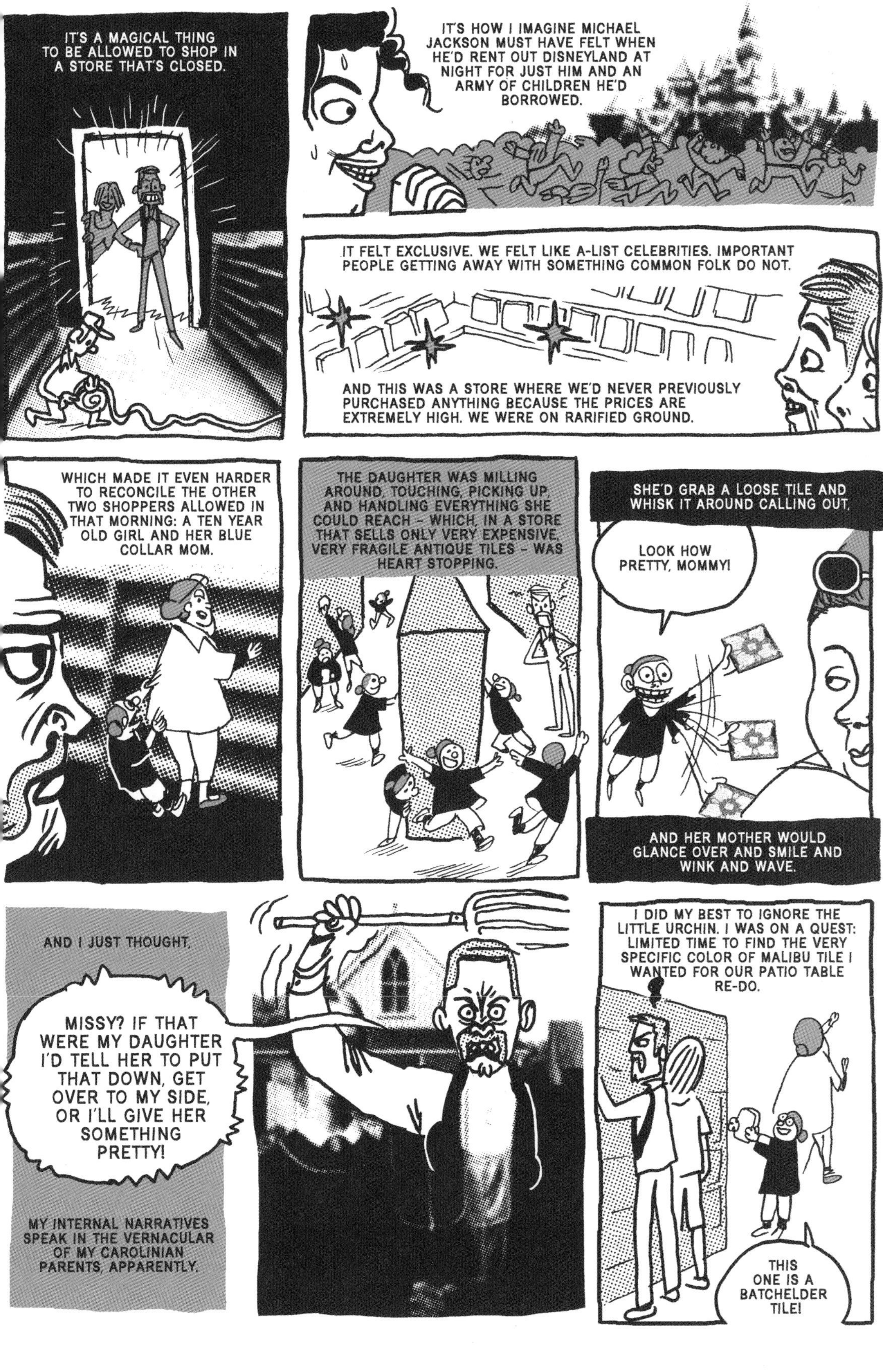
IT'S A MAGICAL THING TO BE ALLOWED TO SHOP IN A STORE THAT'S CLOSED.
IT'S HOW I IMAGINE MICHAEL JACKSON MUST HAVE FELT WHEN HE'D RENT OUT DISNEYLAND AT NIGHT FOR JUST HIM AND AN ARMY OF CHILDREN HE'D BORROWED.
IT FELT EXCLUSIVE. WE FELT LIKE A-LIST CELEBRITIES. IMPORTANT PEOPLE GETTING AWAY WITH SOMETHING COMMON FOLK DO NOT.
AND THIS WAS A STORE WHERE WE'D NEVER PREVIOUSLY PURCHASED ANYTHING BECAUSE THE PRICES ARE EXTREMELY HIGH. WE WERE ON RARIFIED GROUND.
WHICH MADE IT EVEN HARDER TO RECONCILE THE OTHER TWO SHOPPERS ALLOWED IN THAT MORNING: A TEN YEAR OLD GIRL AND HER BLUE COLLAR MOM.
THE DAUGHTER WAS MILLING AROUND, TOUCHING, PICKING UP, AND HANDLING EVERYTHING SHE COULD REACH – WHICH, IN A STORE THAT SELLS ONLY VERY EXPENSIVE, VERY FRAGILE ANTIQUE TILES – WAS HEART STOPPING.
SHE'D GRAB A LOOSE TILE AND WHISK IT AROUND CALLING OUT,
LOOK HOW PRETTY, MOMMY!
AND HER MOTHER WOULD GLANCE OVER AND SMILE AND WINK AND WAVE.
AND I JUST THOUGHT,
MISSY? IF THAT WERE MY DAUGHTER I'D TELL HER TO PUT THAT DOWN, GET OVER TO MY SIDE, OR I'LL GIVE HER SOMETHING PRETTY!
MY INTERNAL NARRATIVES SPEAK IN THE VERNACULAR OF MY CAROLINIAN PARENTS, APPARENTLY.
I DID MY BEST TO IGNORE THE LITTLE URCHIN. I WAS ON A QUEST: LIMITED TIME TO FIND THE VERY SPECIFIC COLOR OF MALIBU TILE I WANTED FOR OUR PATIO TABLE RE-DO.
THIS ONE IS A BATCHELDER TILE!

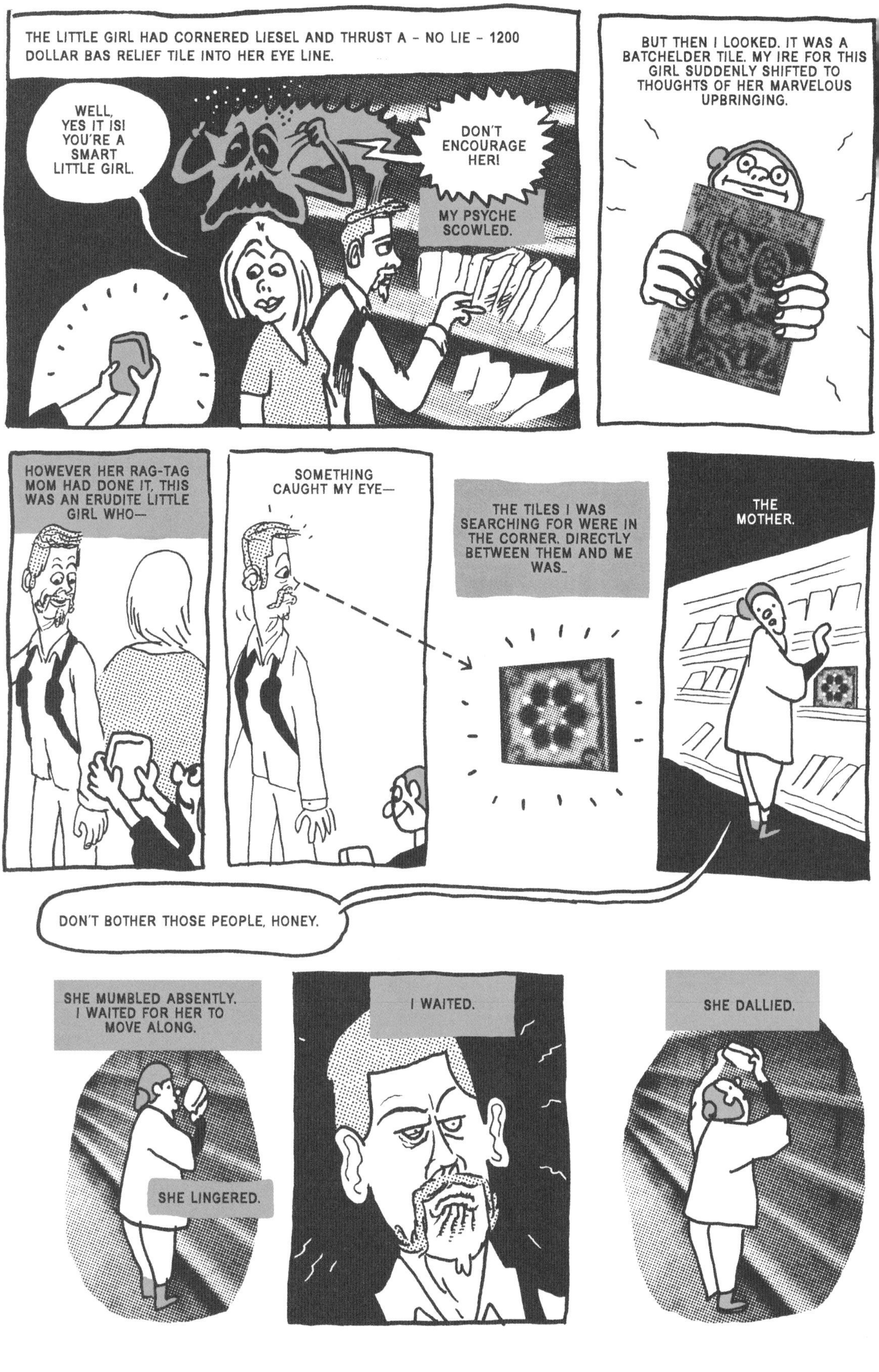
THE LITTLE GIRL HAD CORNERED LIESEL AND THRUST A - NO LIE - 1200 DOLLAR BAS RELIEF TILE INTO HER EYE LINE.
WELL, YES IT IS! YOU'RE A SMART LITTLE GIRL.
DON'T ENCOURAGE HER!
MY PSYCHE SCOWLED.
BUT THEN I LOOKED. IT WAS A BATCHELDER TILE. MY IRE FOR THIS GIRL SUDDENLY SHIFTED TO THOUGHTS OF HER MARVELOUS UPBRINGING.
HOWEVER HER RAG-TAG MOM HAD DONE IT, THIS WAS AN ERUDITE LITTLE GIRL WHO—
SOMETHING CAUGHT MY EYE—
THE TILES I WAS SEARCHING FOR WERE IN THE CORNER, DIRECTLY BETWEEN THEM AND ME WAS...
THE MOTHER.
DON'T BOTHER THOSE PEOPLE, HONEY.
SHE MUMBLED ABSENTLY. I WAITED FOR HER TO MOVE ALONG.
SHE LINGERED.
I WAITED.
SHE DALLIED.

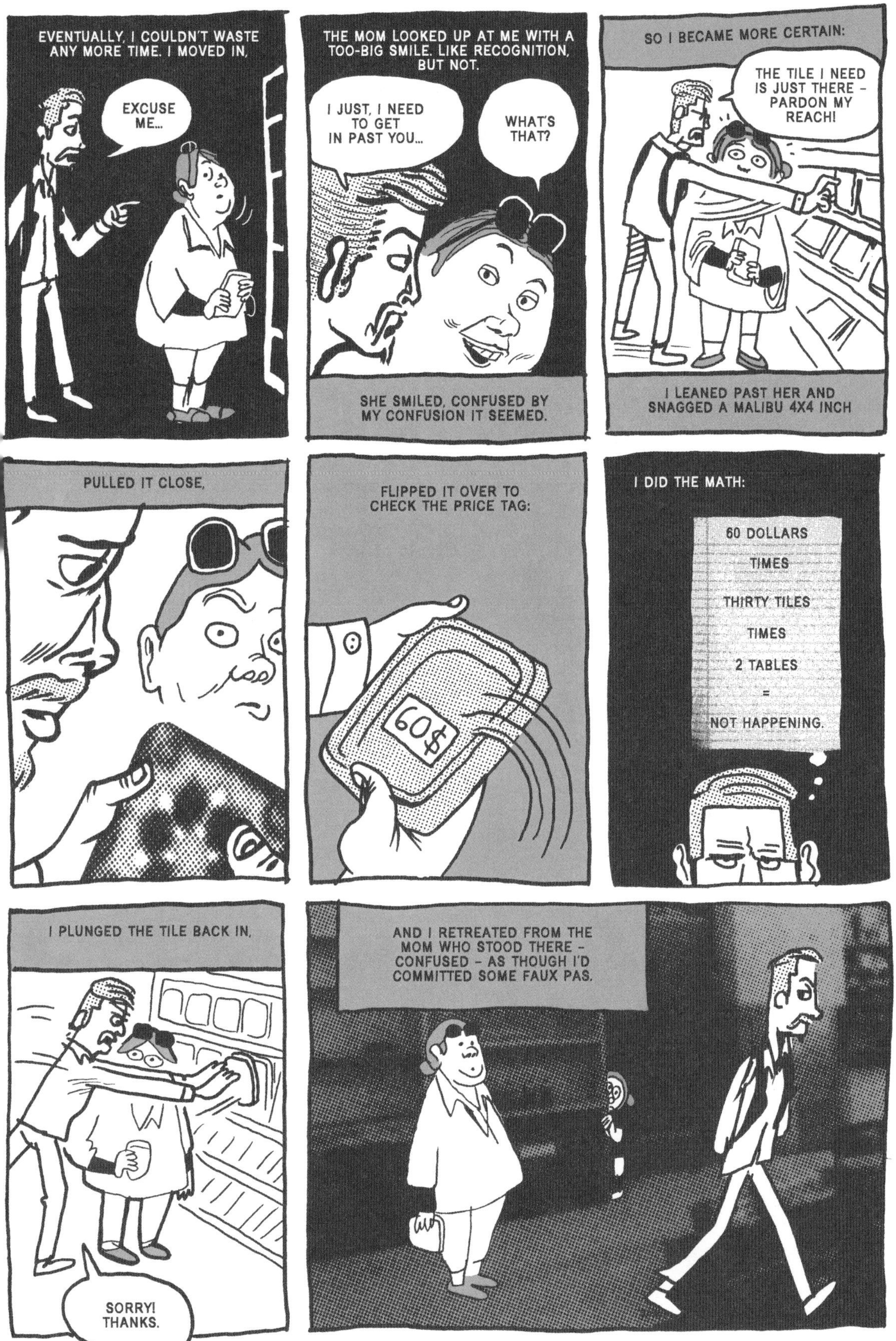
EVENTUALLY, I COULDN'T WASTE ANY MORE TIME. I MOVED IN,
EXCUSE ME...
THE MOM LOOKED UP AT ME WITH A TOO-BIG SMILE. LIKE RECOGNITION, BUT NOT.
I JUST, I NEED TO GET IN PAST YOU...
WHAT'S THAT?
SHE SMILED, CONFUSED BY MY CONFUSION IT SEEMED.
SO I BECAME MORE CERTAIN:
THE TILE I NEED IS JUST THERE – PARDON MY REACH!
I LEANED PAST HER AND SNAGGED A MALIBU 4X4 INCH
PULLED IT CLOSE,
FLIPPED IT OVER TO CHECK THE PRICE TAG:
60$
I DID THE MATH:
60 DOLLARS
TIMES
THIRTY TILES
TIMES
2 TABLES
=
NOT HAPPENING.
I PLUNGED THE TILE BACK IN,
SORRY! THANKS.
AND I RETREATED FROM THE MOM WHO STOOD THERE – CONFUSED – AS THOUGH I'D COMMITTED SOME FAUX PAS.

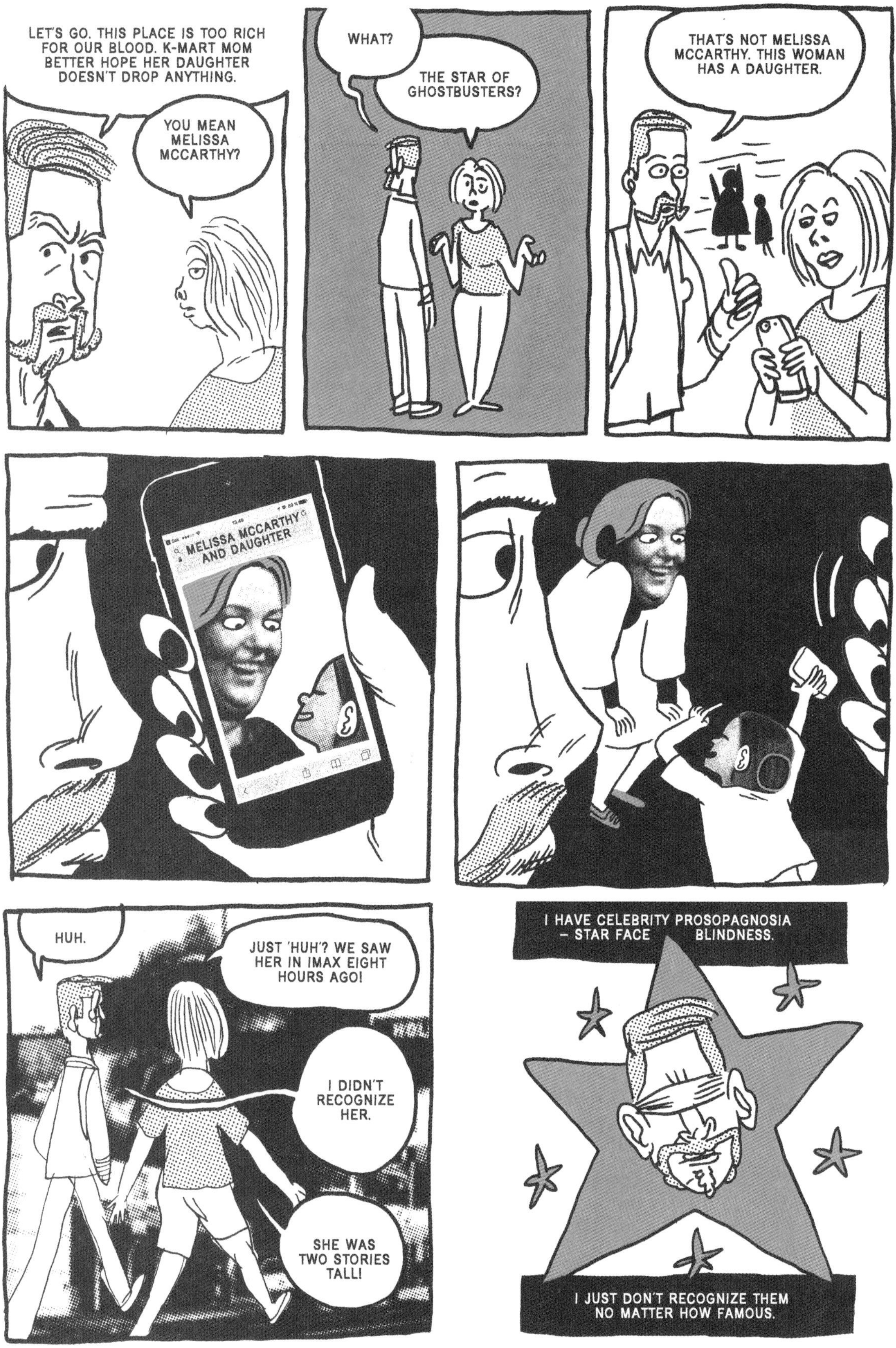
LET'S GO. THIS PLACE IS TOO RICH FOR OUR BLOOD. K-MART MOM BETTER HOPE HER DAUGHTER DOESN'T DROP ANYTHING.
YOU MEAN MELISSA MCCARTHY?
WHAT?
THE STAR OF GHOSTBUSTERS?
THAT'S NOT MELISSA MCCARTHY. THIS WOMAN HAS A DAUGHTER.
MELISSA MCCARTHY AND DAUGHTER
HUH.
JUST 'HUH'? WE SAW HER IN IMAX EIGHT HOURS AGO!
I DIDN'T RECOGNIZE HER.
SHE WAS TWO STORIES TALL!
I HAVE CELEBRITY PROSOPAGNOSIA – STAR FACE BLINDNESS.
I JUST DON'T RECOGNIZE THEM NO MATTER HOW FAMOUS.

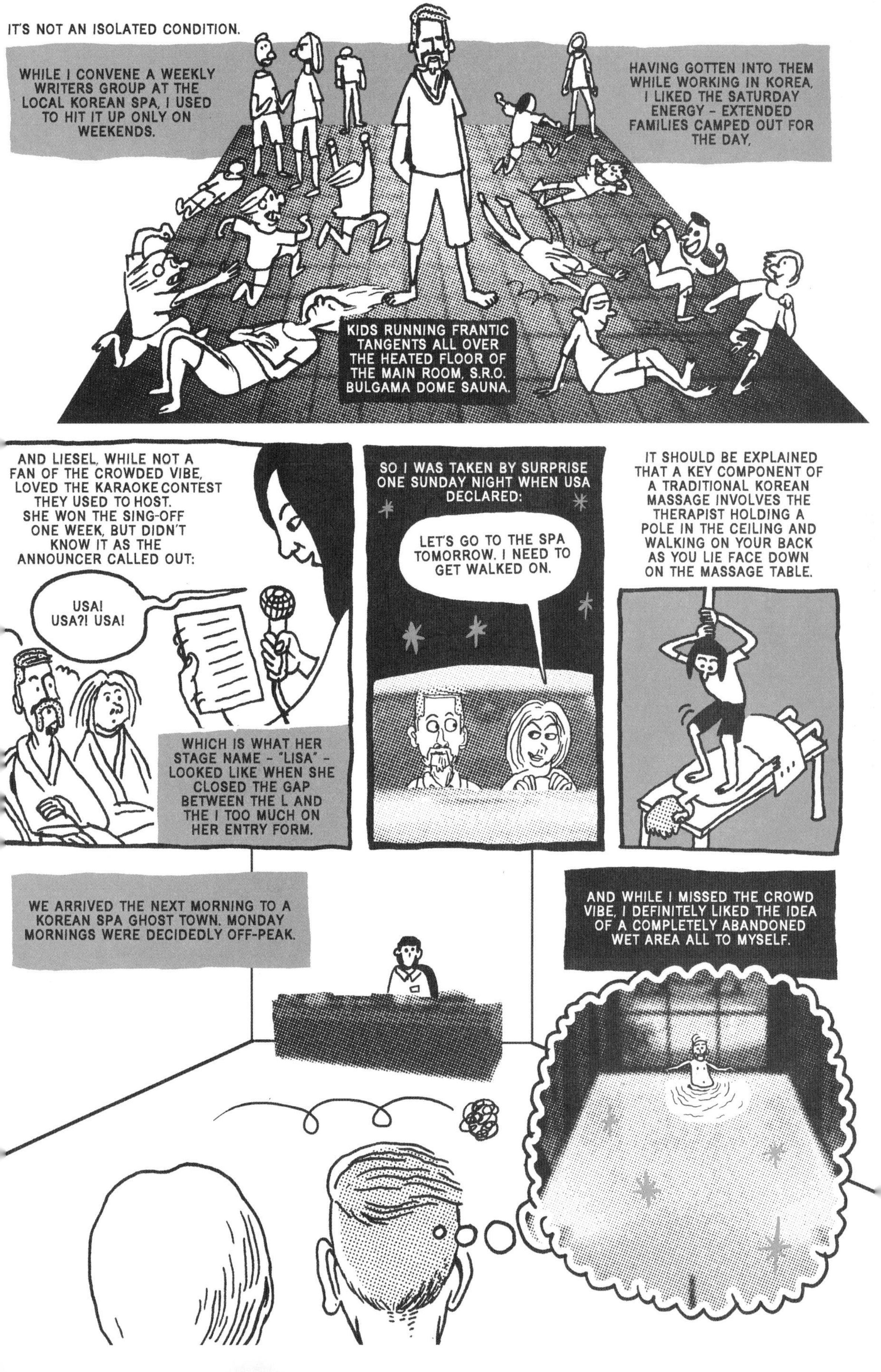
IT'S NOT AN ISOLATED CONDITION.
WHILE I CONVENE A WEEKLY WRITERS GROUP AT THE LOCAL KOREAN SPA, I USED TO HIT IT UP ONLY ON WEEKENDS.
HAVING GOTTEN INTO THEM WHILE WORKING IN KOREA, I LIKED THE SATURDAY ENERGY – EXTENDED FAMILIES CAMPED OUT FOR THE DAY,
KIDS RUNNING FRANTIC TANGENTS ALL OVER THE HEATED FLOOR OF THE MAIN ROOM, S.R.O. BULGAMA DOME SAUNA.
AND LIESEL, WHILE NOT A FAN OF THE CROWDED VIBE, LOVED THE KARAOKE CONTEST THEY USED TO HOST. SHE WON THE SING-OFF ONE WEEK, BUT DIDN'T KNOW IT AS THE ANNOUNCER CALLED OUT:
USA! USA?! USA!
WHICH IS WHAT HER STAGE NAME – "LISA" – LOOKED LIKE WHEN SHE CLOSED THE GAP BETWEEN THE L AND THE I TOO MUCH ON HER ENTRY FORM.
SO I WAS TAKEN BY SURPRISE ONE SUNDAY NIGHT WHEN USA DECLARED:
LET'S GO TO THE SPA TOMORROW. I NEED TO GET WALKED ON.
IT SHOULD BE EXPLAINED THAT A KEY COMPONENT OF A TRADITIONAL KOREAN MASSAGE INVOLVES THE THERAPIST HOLDING A POLE IN THE CEILING AND WALKING ON YOUR BACK AS YOU LIE FACE DOWN ON THE MASSAGE TABLE.
WE ARRIVED THE NEXT MORNING TO A KOREAN SPA GHOST TOWN. MONDAY MORNINGS WERE DECIDEDLY OFF-PEAK.
AND WHILE I MISSED THE CROWD VIBE, I DEFINITELY LIKED THE IDEA OF A COMPLETELY ABANDONED WET AREA ALL TO MYSELF.

I GOT NAKED,

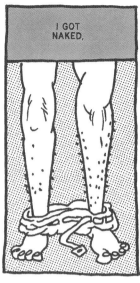

TOOK A SHOWER,

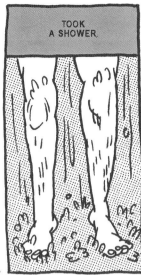

GRABBED A TOWEL,

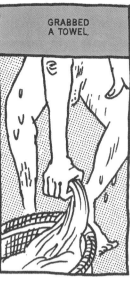

SANK INTO THE WARM TUB AND CLOSED MY EYES.

AAAAAAH!

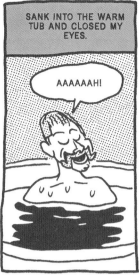

I IMMEDIATELY GOT THE FEELING THAT I WASN'T ALONE. I OPENED MY EYES AND SPOTTED... HIM.

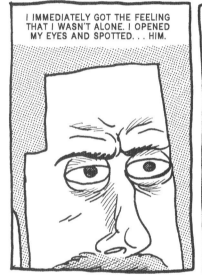

I LIKE TO THINK I TRY TO NOT PASS JUDGEMENTS, BUT I GOT A VIBE OFF OF HIM IMMEDIATELY AND NAMED HIM CREEPY GUY IN MY HEAD.

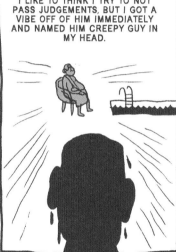

HE WAS SEATED IN THE WHITE PLASTIC CHAIRS TO THE SIDE OF THE COLD PLUNGE POOL ON THE FAR WALL. AND WHAT BOTHERED ME WAS THAT HE WAS WEARING A ROBE.

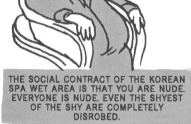

THE SOCIAL CONTRACT OF THE KOREAN SPA WET AREA IS THAT YOU ARE NUDE. EVERYONE IS NUDE. EVEN THE SHYEST OF THE SHY ARE COMPLETELY DISROBED.

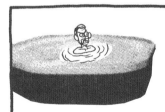

SO SEEING A LITERAL ROBE WAS UNNERVING. DOES HE NOT KNOW THE RULES? IT PUT ME ON EDGE WITH THIS GUY.

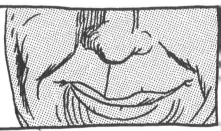

I MEAN, WHAT IS HE DOING HERE ON A MONDAY MORNING ANYWAY?

THE PLACE IS DESERTED.

DOESN'T HE HAVE A JOB? SHOULDN'T HE BE SOMEWHERE ELSE?

COMPLETELY LOST ON ME WAS THE FACT THAT THE SAME QUESTIONS COULD EASILY BE APPLIED TO ME.

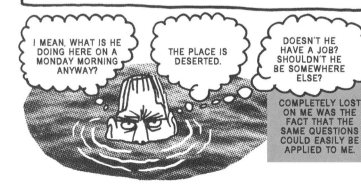

THERE WAS SOMETHING ELSE ABOUT HIM... I COULDN'T PEG WHAT IT WAS.

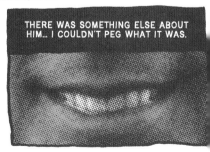

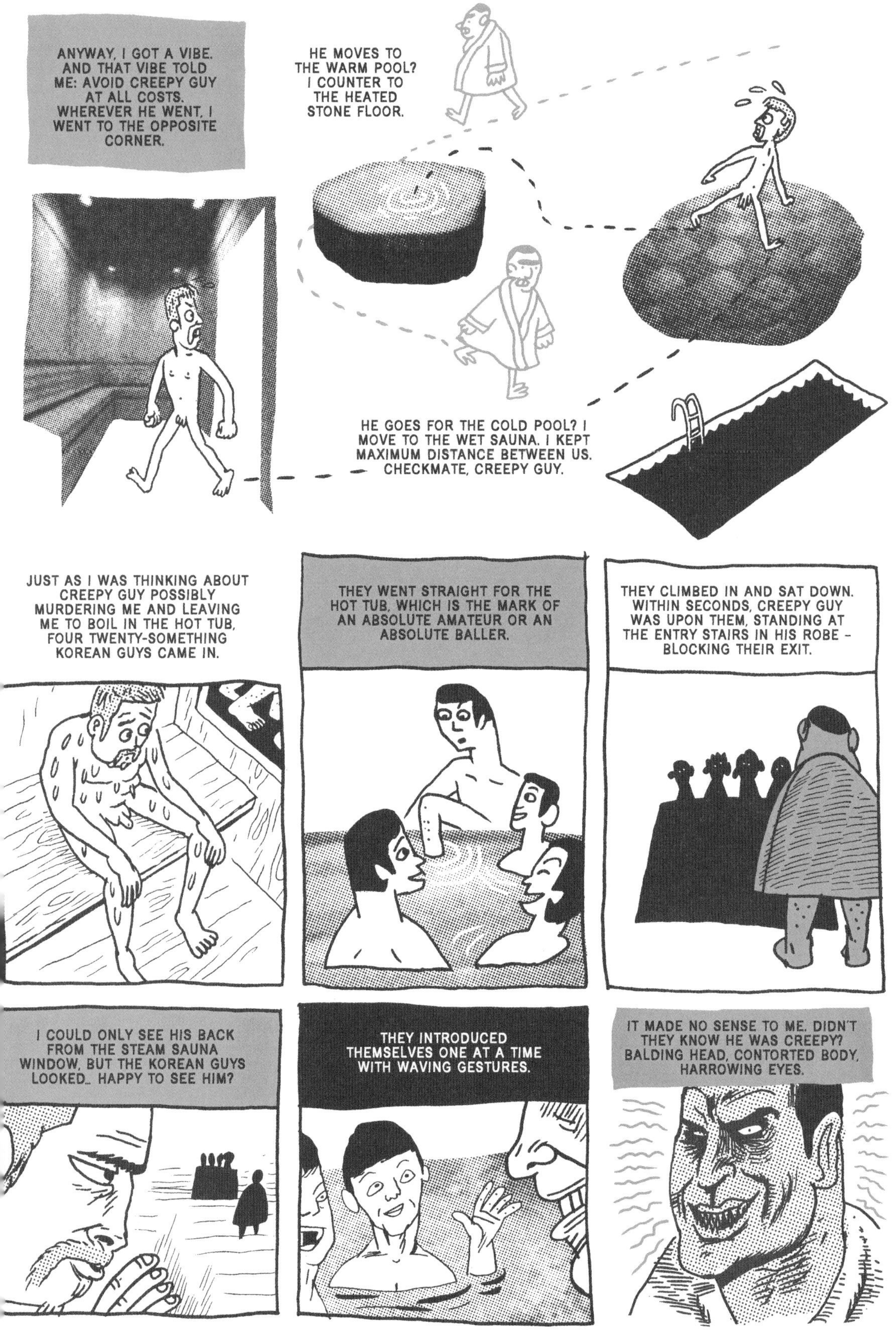
ANYWAY, I GOT A VIBE. AND THAT VIBE TOLD ME: AVOID CREEPY GUY AT ALL COSTS. WHEREVER HE WENT, I WENT TO THE OPPOSITE CORNER.
HE MOVES TO THE WARM POOL? I COUNTER TO THE HEATED STONE FLOOR.
HE GOES FOR THE COLD POOL? I MOVE TO THE WET SAUNA. I KEPT MAXIMUM DISTANCE BETWEEN US. CHECKMATE, CREEPY GUY.
JUST AS I WAS THINKING ABOUT CREEPY GUY POSSIBLY MURDERING ME AND LEAVING ME TO BOIL IN THE HOT TUB, FOUR TWENTY-SOMETHING KOREAN GUYS CAME IN.
THEY WENT STRAIGHT FOR THE HOT TUB, WHICH IS THE MARK OF AN ABSOLUTE AMATEUR OR AN ABSOLUTE BALLER.
THEY CLIMBED IN AND SAT DOWN. WITHIN SECONDS, CREEPY GUY WAS UPON THEM, STANDING AT THE ENTRY STAIRS IN HIS ROBE - BLOCKING THEIR EXIT.
I COULD ONLY SEE HIS BACK FROM THE STEAM SAUNA WINDOW, BUT THE KOREAN GUYS LOOKED... HAPPY TO SEE HIM?
THEY INTRODUCED THEMSELVES ONE AT A TIME WITH WAVING GESTURES.
IT MADE NO SENSE TO ME. DIDN'T THEY KNOW HE WAS CREEPY? BALDING HEAD, CONTORTED BODY, HARROWING EYES.

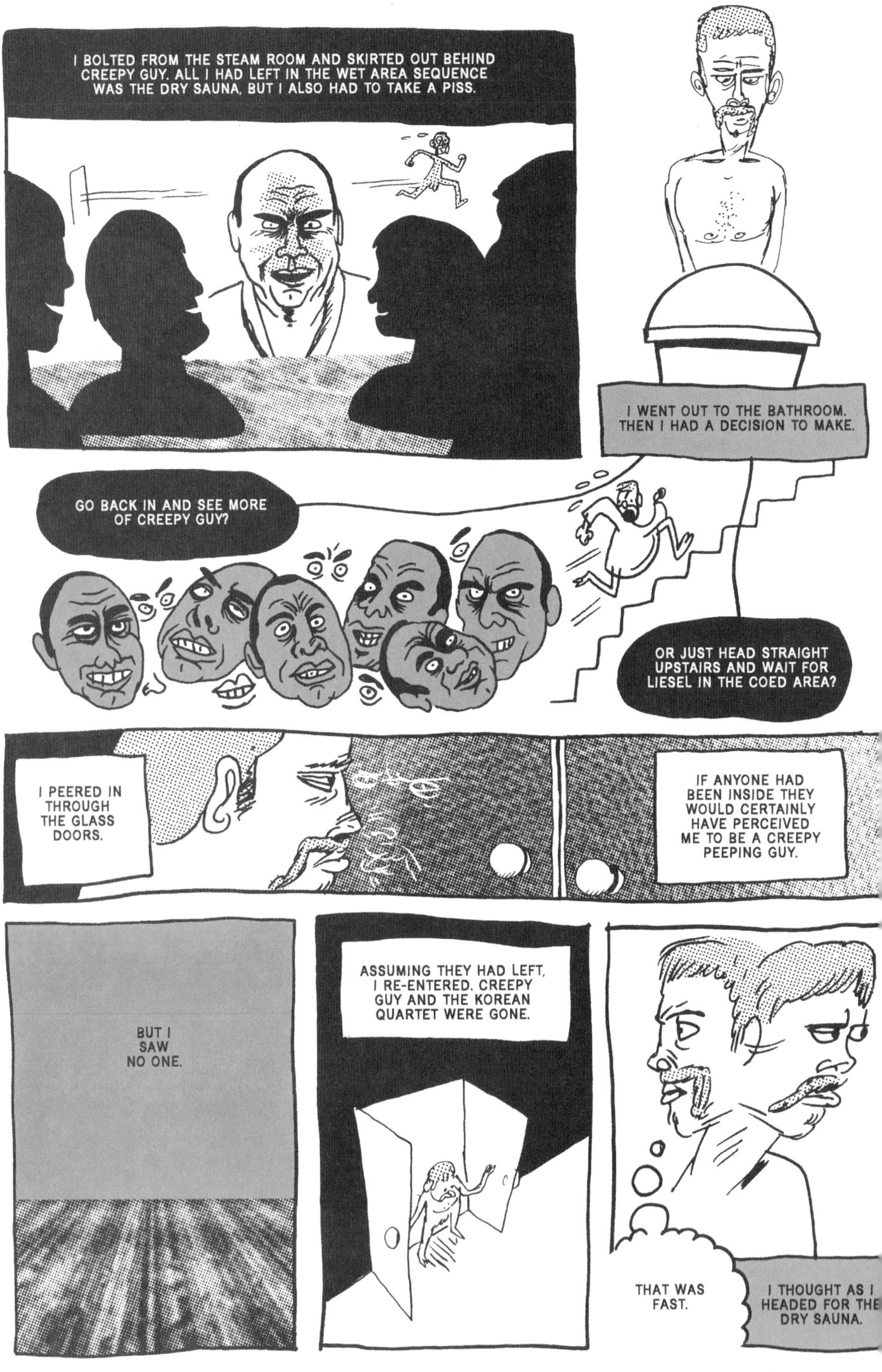

I BOLTED FROM THE STEAM ROOM AND SKIRTED OUT BEHIND CREEPY GUY. ALL I HAD LEFT IN THE WET AREA SEQUENCE WAS THE DRY SAUNA, BUT I ALSO HAD TO TAKE A PISS.
I WENT OUT TO THE BATHROOM. THEN I HAD A DECISION TO MAKE.
GO BACK IN AND SEE MORE OF CREEPY GUY?
OR JUST HEAD STRAIGHT UPSTAIRS AND WAIT FOR LIESEL IN THE COED AREA?
I PEERED IN THROUGH THE GLASS DOORS.
IF ANYONE HAD BEEN INSIDE THEY WOULD CERTAINLY HAVE PERCEIVED ME TO BE A CREEPY PEEPING GUY.
BUT I SAW NO ONE.
ASSUMING THEY HAD LEFT, I RE-ENTERED. CREEPY GUY AND THE KOREAN QUARTET WERE GONE.
THAT WAS FAST.
I THOUGHT AS I HEADED FOR THE DRY SAUNA.

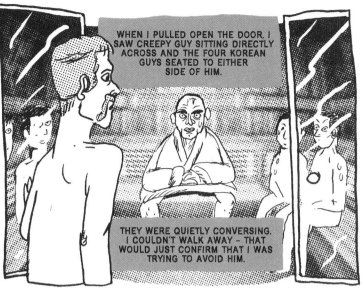

WHEN I PULLED OPEN THE DOOR, I SAW CREEPY GUY SITTING DIRECTLY ACROSS AND THE FOUR KOREAN GUYS SEATED TO EITHER SIDE OF HIM.

THEY WERE QUIETLY CONVERSING. I COULDN'T WALK AWAY – THAT WOULD JUST CONFIRM THAT I WAS TRYING TO AVOID HIM.

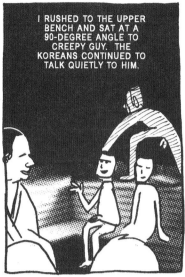

I RUSHED TO THE UPPER BENCH AND SAT AT A 90-DEGREE ANGLE TO CREEPY GUY. THE KOREANS CONTINUED TO TALK QUIETLY TO HIM.

HE ANSWERED QUIETLY WITH MALFORMED LIPS.

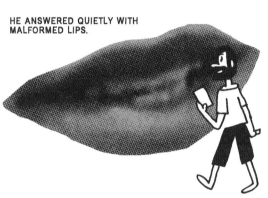

THEN, THE SPA'S SERVICE ATTENDANT CAME IN – BUT NOT TO DO A SWEEP FOR ABANDONED TOWELS. NO. HE WAS CARRYING PAPER AND PEN.

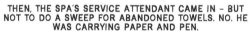

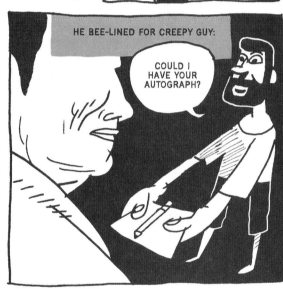

HE BEE-LINED FOR CREEPY GUY:

COULD I HAVE YOUR AUTOGRAPH?

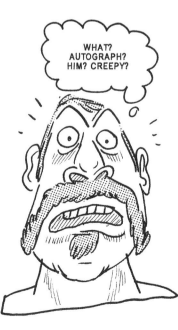

WHAT? AUTOGRAPH? HIM? CREEPY?

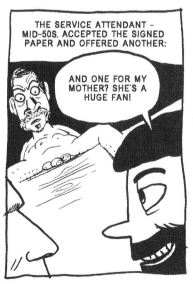

THE SERVICE ATTENDANT – MID-50S, ACCEPTED THE SIGNED PAPER AND OFFERED ANOTHER:

AND ONE FOR MY MOTHER? SHE'S A HUGE FAN!

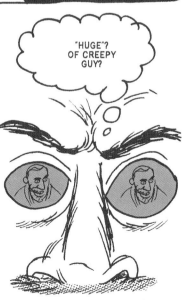

"HUGE"? OF CREEPY GUY?

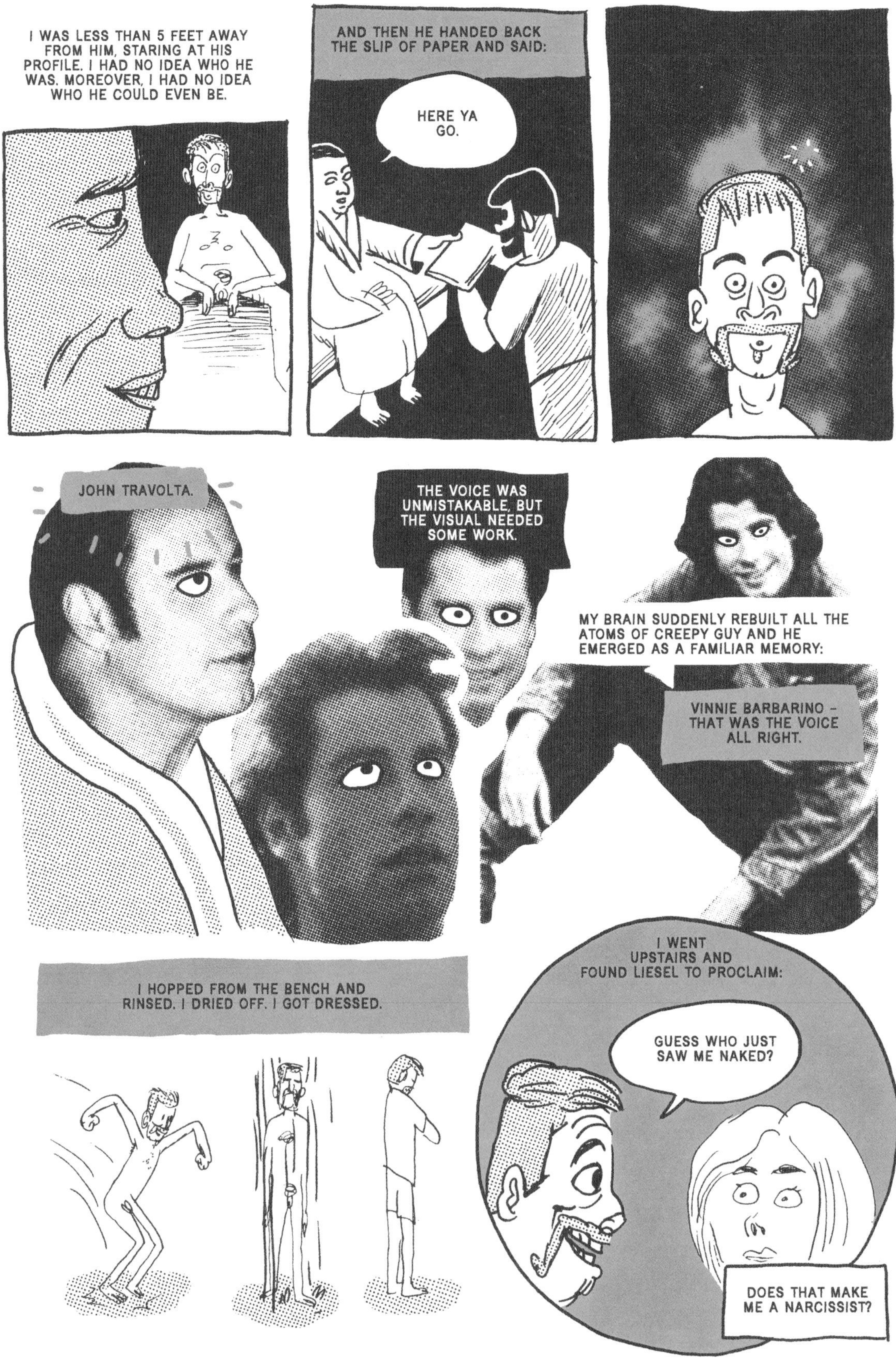

I WAS LESS THAN 5 FEET AWAY FROM HIM, STARING AT HIS PROFILE. I HAD NO IDEA WHO HE WAS. MOREOVER, I HAD NO IDEA WHO HE COULD EVEN BE.
AND THEN HE HANDED BACK THE SLIP OF PAPER AND SAID:
HERE YA GO.
JOHN TRAVOLTA.
THE VOICE WAS UNMISTAKABLE, BUT THE VISUAL NEEDED SOME WORK.
MY BRAIN SUDDENLY REBUILT ALL THE ATOMS OF CREEPY GUY AND HE EMERGED AS A FAMILIAR MEMORY:
VINNIE BARBARINO – THAT WAS THE VOICE ALL RIGHT.
I HOPPED FROM THE BENCH AND RINSED. I DRIED OFF. I GOT DRESSED.
I WENT UPSTAIRS AND FOUND LIESEL TO PROCLAIM:
GUESS WHO JUST SAW ME NAKED?
DOES THAT MAKE ME A NARCISSIST?

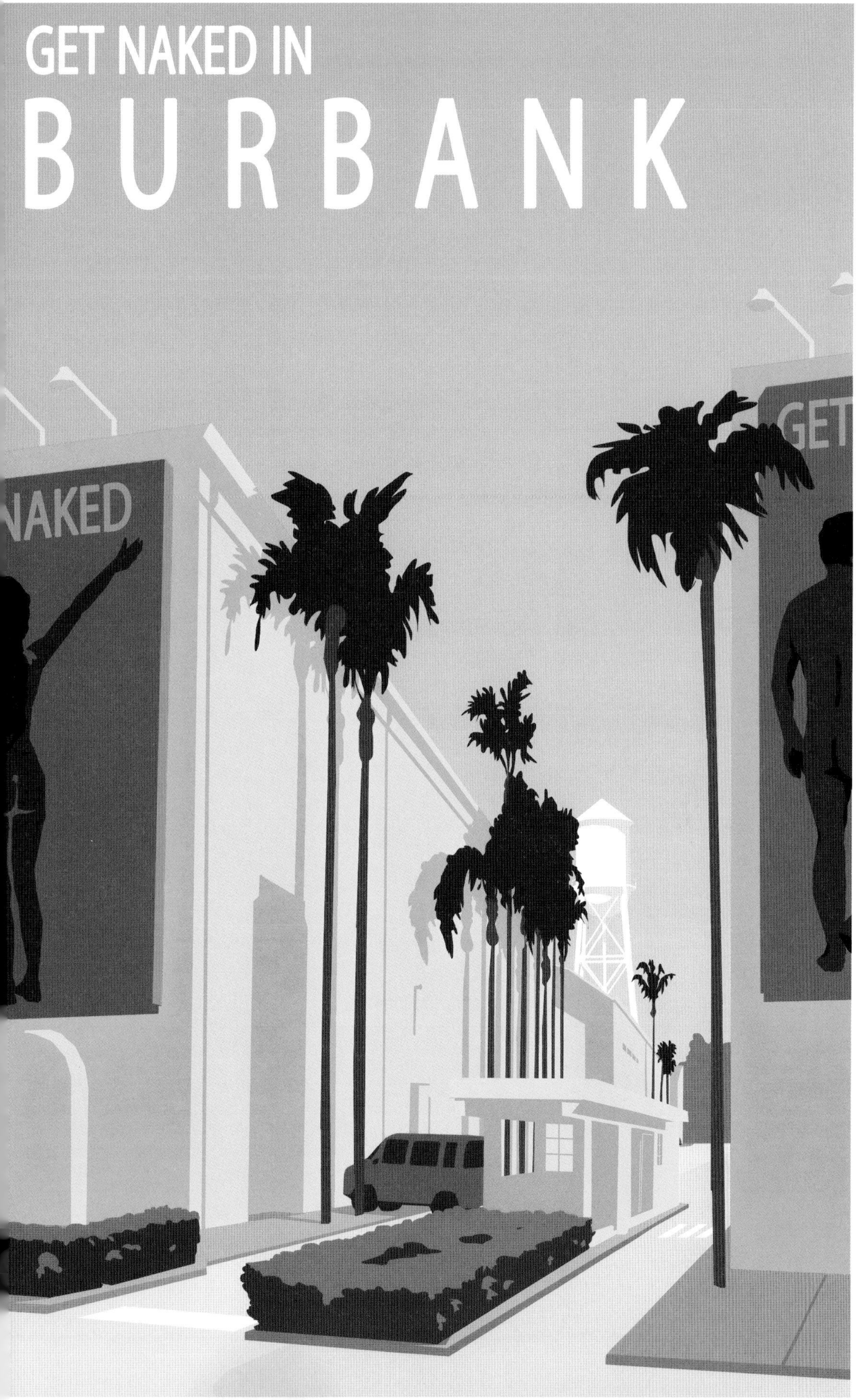
GET NAKED IN
BURBANK
NAKED
GET

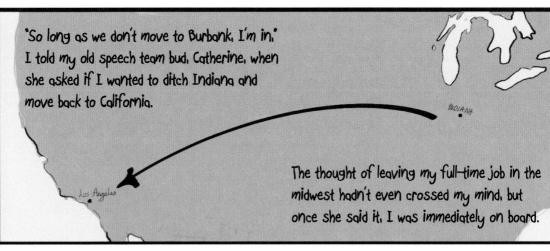

"So long as we don't move to Burbank, I'm in."
I told my old speech team bud, Catherine, when
she asked if I wanted to ditch Indiana and
move back to California.

The thought of leaving my full-time job in the
midwest hadn't even crossed my mind, but
once she said it, I was immediately on board.

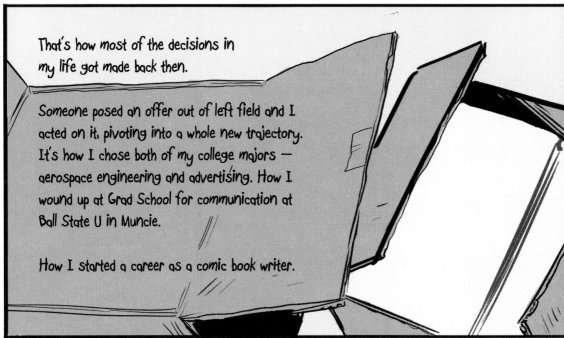

That's how most of the decisions in
my life got made back then.

Someone posed an offer out of left field and I
acted on it, pivoting into a whole new trajectory.
It's how I chose both of my college majors —
aerospace engineering and advertising. How I
wound up at Grad School for communication at
Ball State U in Muncie.

How I started a career as a comic book writer.

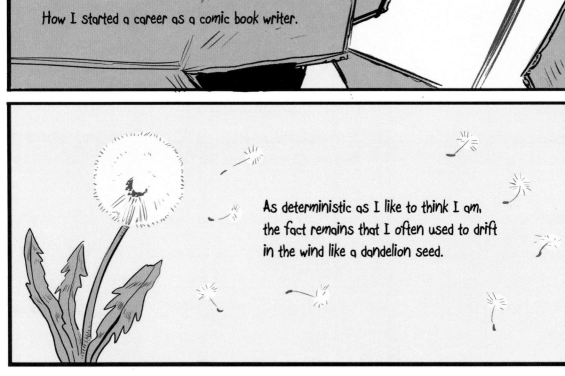

As deterministic as I like to think I am,
the fact remains that I often used to drift
in the wind like a dandelion seed.

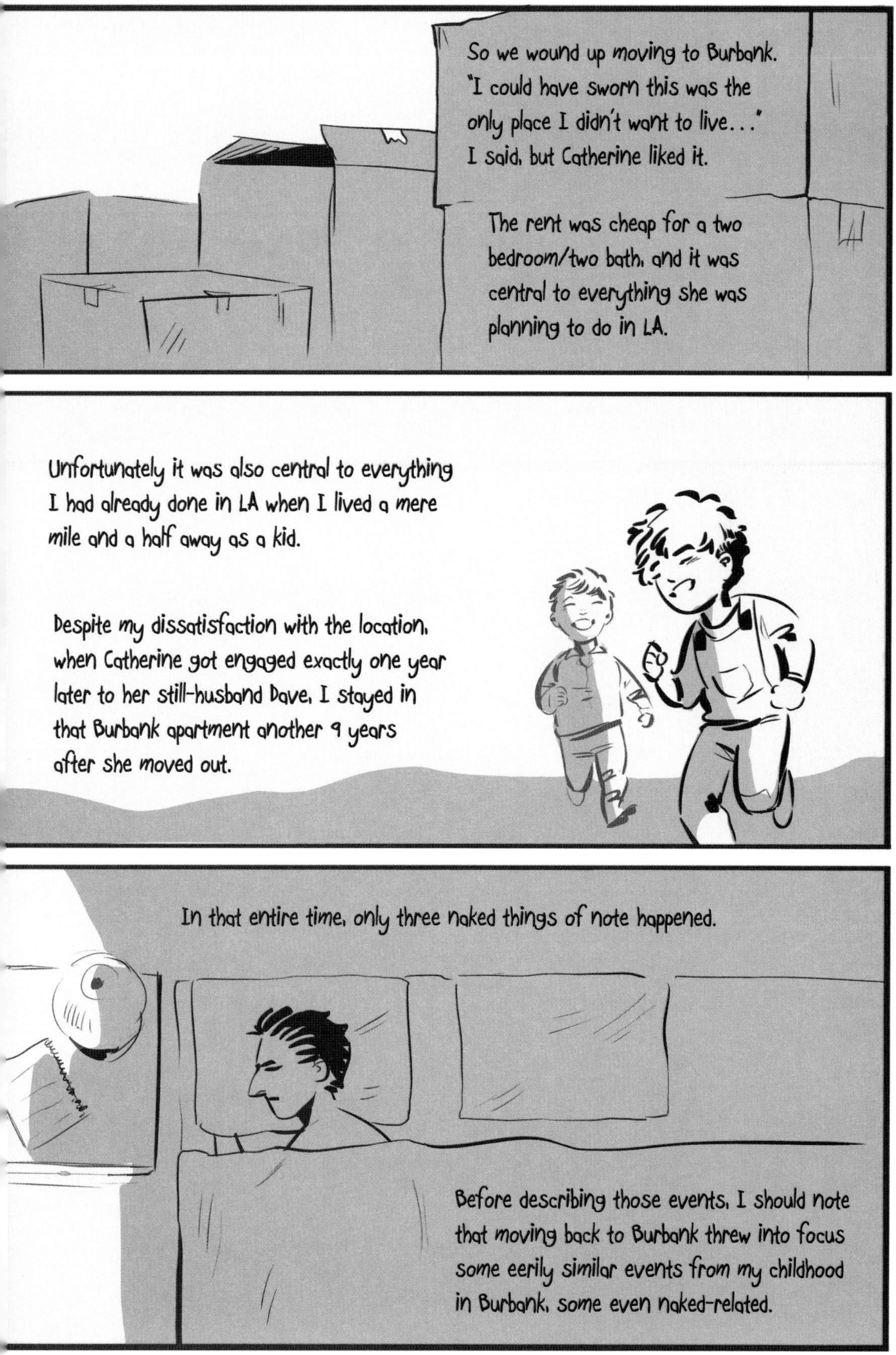
So we wound up moving to Burbank. "I could have sworn this was the only place I didn't want to live..." I said, but Catherine liked it.
The rent was cheap for a two bedroom/two bath, and it was central to everything she was planning to do in LA.
Unfortunately it was also central to everything I had already done in LA when I lived a mere mile and a half away as a kid.
Despite my dissatisfaction with the location, when Catherine got engaged exactly one year later to her still-husband Dave, I stayed in that Burbank apartment another 9 years after she moved out.
In that entire time, only three naked things of note happened.
Before describing those events, I should note that moving back to Burbank threw into focus some eerily similar events from my childhood in Burbank, some even naked-related.

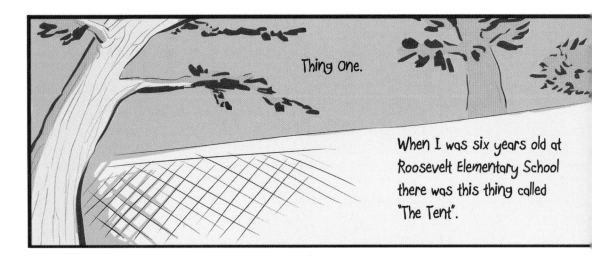

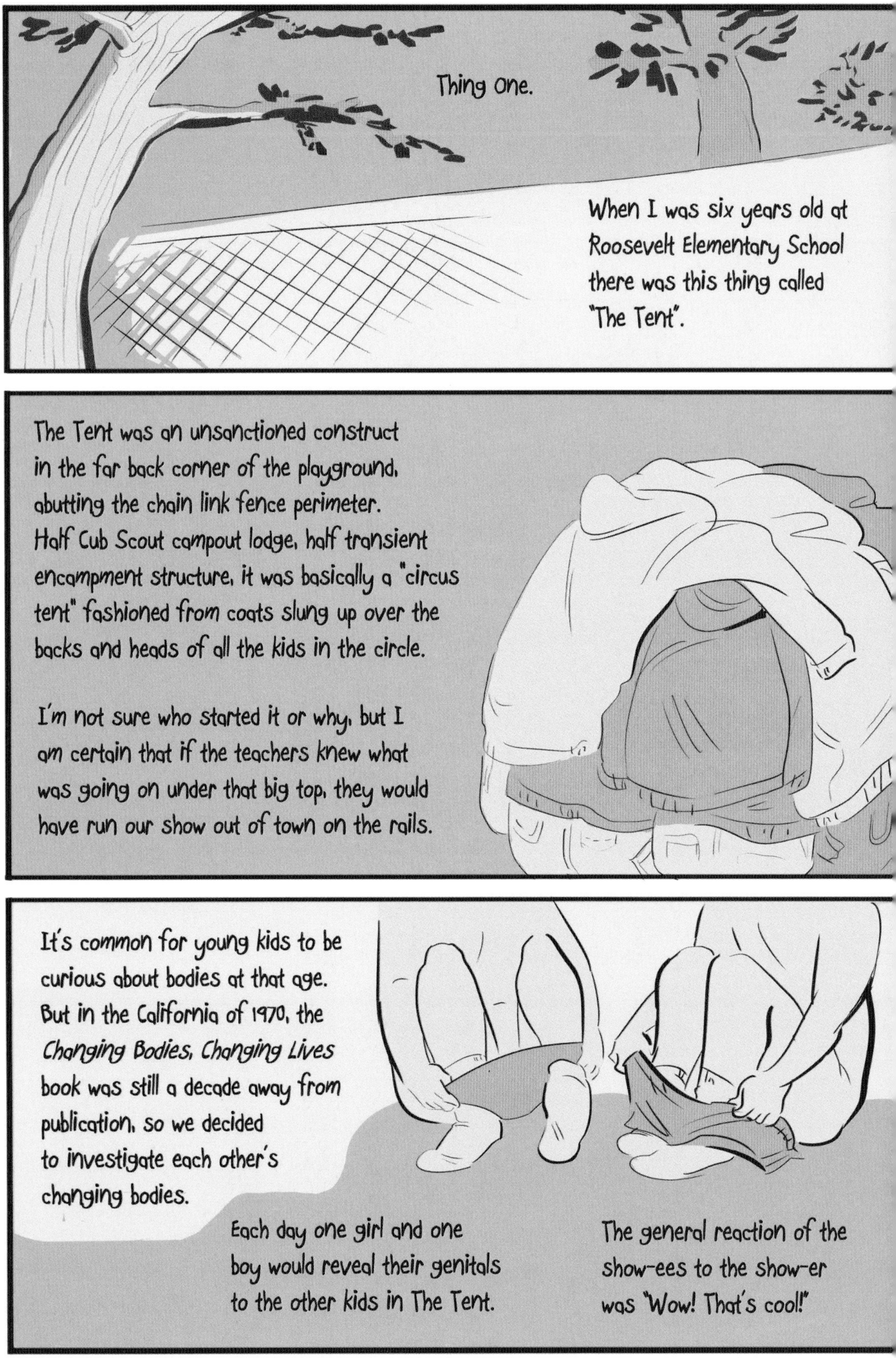

Thing One.

When I was six years old at Roosevelt Elementary School there was this thing called "The Tent".

The Tent was an unsanctioned construct in the far back corner of the playground, abutting the chain link fence perimeter. Half Cub Scout campout lodge, half transient encampment structure, it was basically a "circus tent" fashioned from coats slung up over the backs and heads of all the kids in the circle.

I'm not sure who started it or why, but I am certain that if the teachers knew what was going on under that big top, they would have run our show out of town on the rails.

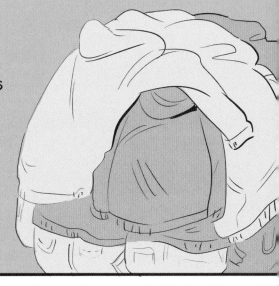

It's common for young kids to be curious about bodies at that age. But in the California of 1970, the *Changing Bodies, Changing Lives* book was still a decade away from publication, so we decided to investigate each other's changing bodies.

Each day one girl and one boy would reveal their genitals to the other kids in The Tent.

The general reaction of the show-ees to the show-er was "Wow! That's cool!"

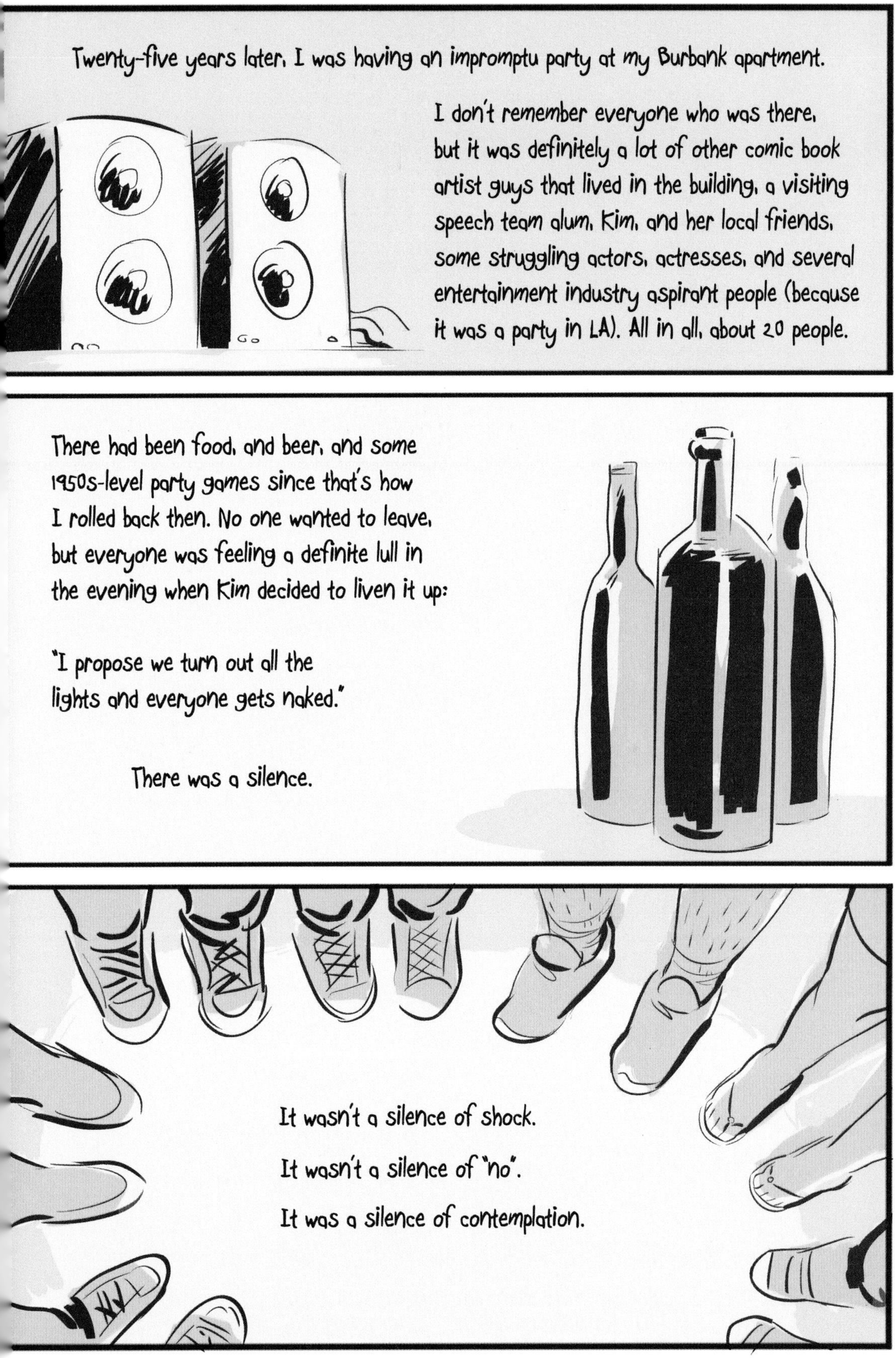
Twenty-five years later, I was having an impromptu party at my Burbank apartment.
I don't remember everyone who was there, but it was definitely a lot of other comic book artist guys that lived in the building, a visiting speech team alum, Kim, and her local friends, some struggling actors, actresses, and several entertainment industry aspirant people (because it was a party in LA). All in all, about 20 people.
There had been food, and beer, and some 1950s-level party games since that's how I rolled back then. No one wanted to leave, but everyone was feeling a definite lull in the evening when Kim decided to liven it up:
"I propose we turn out all the lights and everyone gets naked."
There was a silence.
It wasn't a silence of shock.
It wasn't a silence of "no".
It was a silence of contemplation.

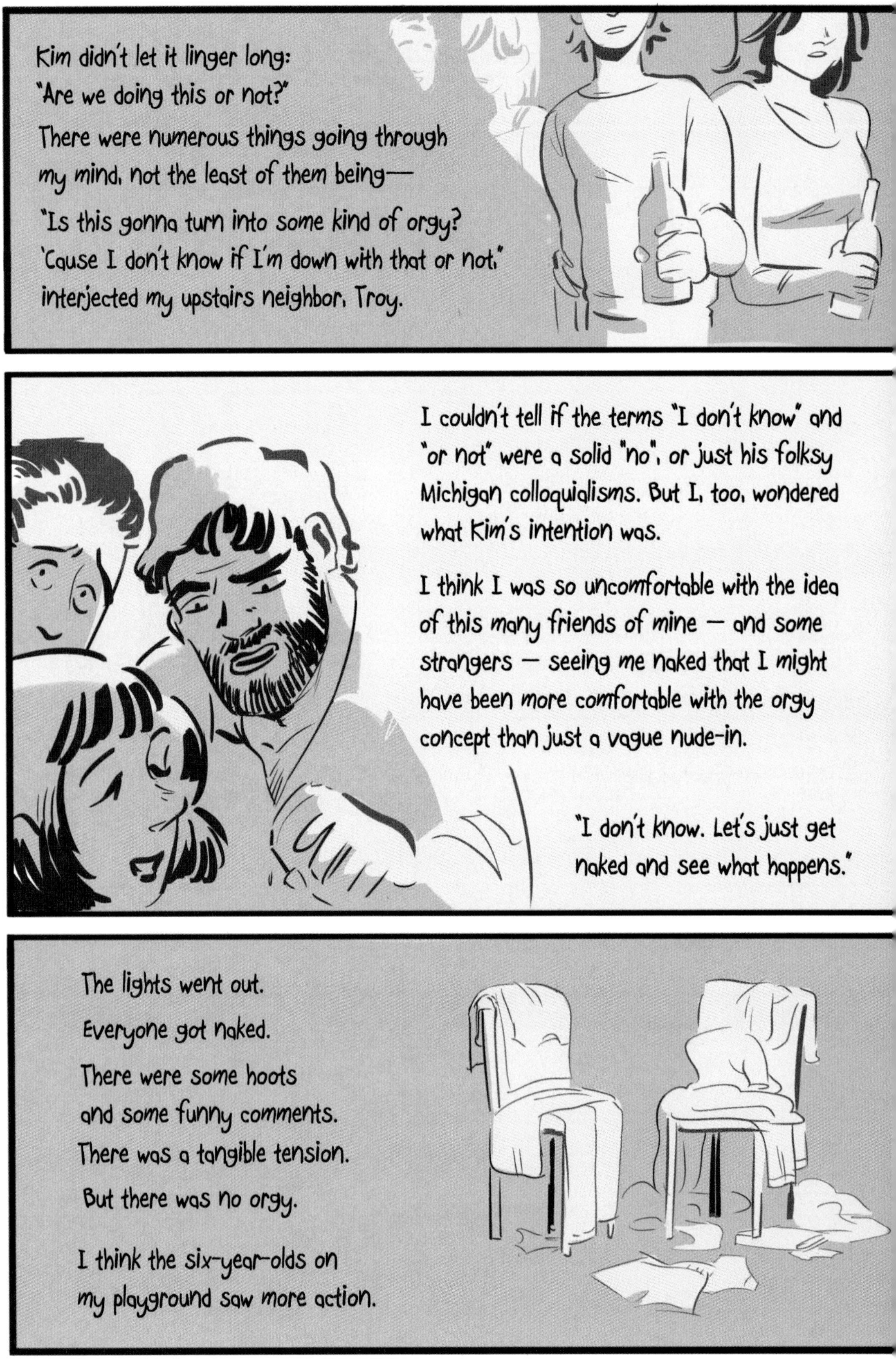
Kim didn't let it linger long:
"Are we doing this or not?"
There were numerous things going through my mind, not the least of them being—
"Is this gonna turn into some kind of orgy? 'Cause I don't know if I'm down with that or not,"
interjected my upstairs neighbor, Troy.
I couldn't tell if the terms "I don't know" and "or not" were a solid "no", or just his folksy Michigan colloquialisms. But I, too, wondered what Kim's intention was.
I think I was so uncomfortable with the idea of this many friends of mine — and some strangers — seeing me naked that I might have been more comfortable with the orgy concept than just a vague nude-in.
"I don't know. Let's just get naked and see what happens."
The lights went out.
Everyone got naked.
There were some hoots and some funny comments.
There was a tangible tension.
But there was no orgy.
I think the six-year-olds on my playground saw more action.

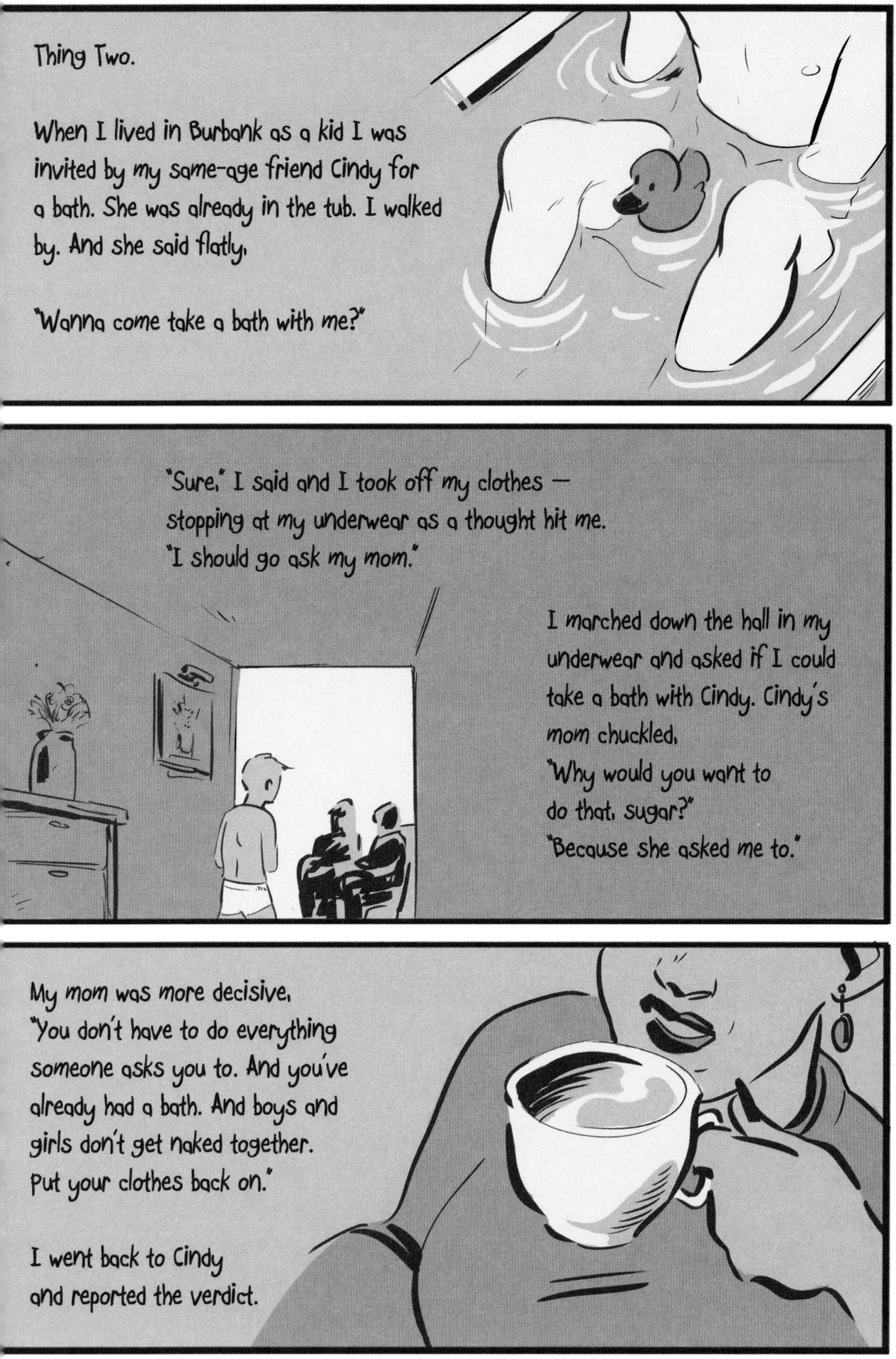

Thing Two.

When I lived in Burbank as a kid I was invited by my same-age friend Cindy for a bath. She was already in the tub. I walked by. And she said flatly,

"Wanna come take a bath with me?"

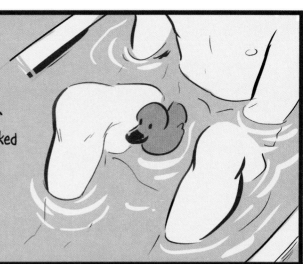

"Sure," I said and I took off my clothes — stopping at my underwear as a thought hit me. "I should go ask my mom."

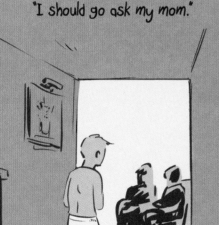

I marched down the hall in my underwear and asked if I could take a bath with Cindy. Cindy's mom chuckled, "Why would you want to do that, sugar?" "Because she asked me to."

My mom was more decisive, "You don't have to do everything someone asks you to. And you've already had a bath. And boys and girls don't get naked together. Put your clothes back on."

I went back to Cindy and reported the verdict.

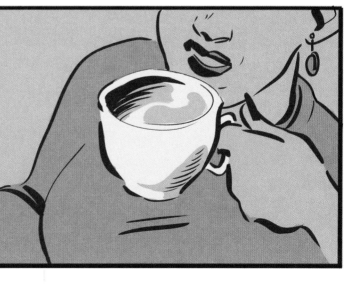

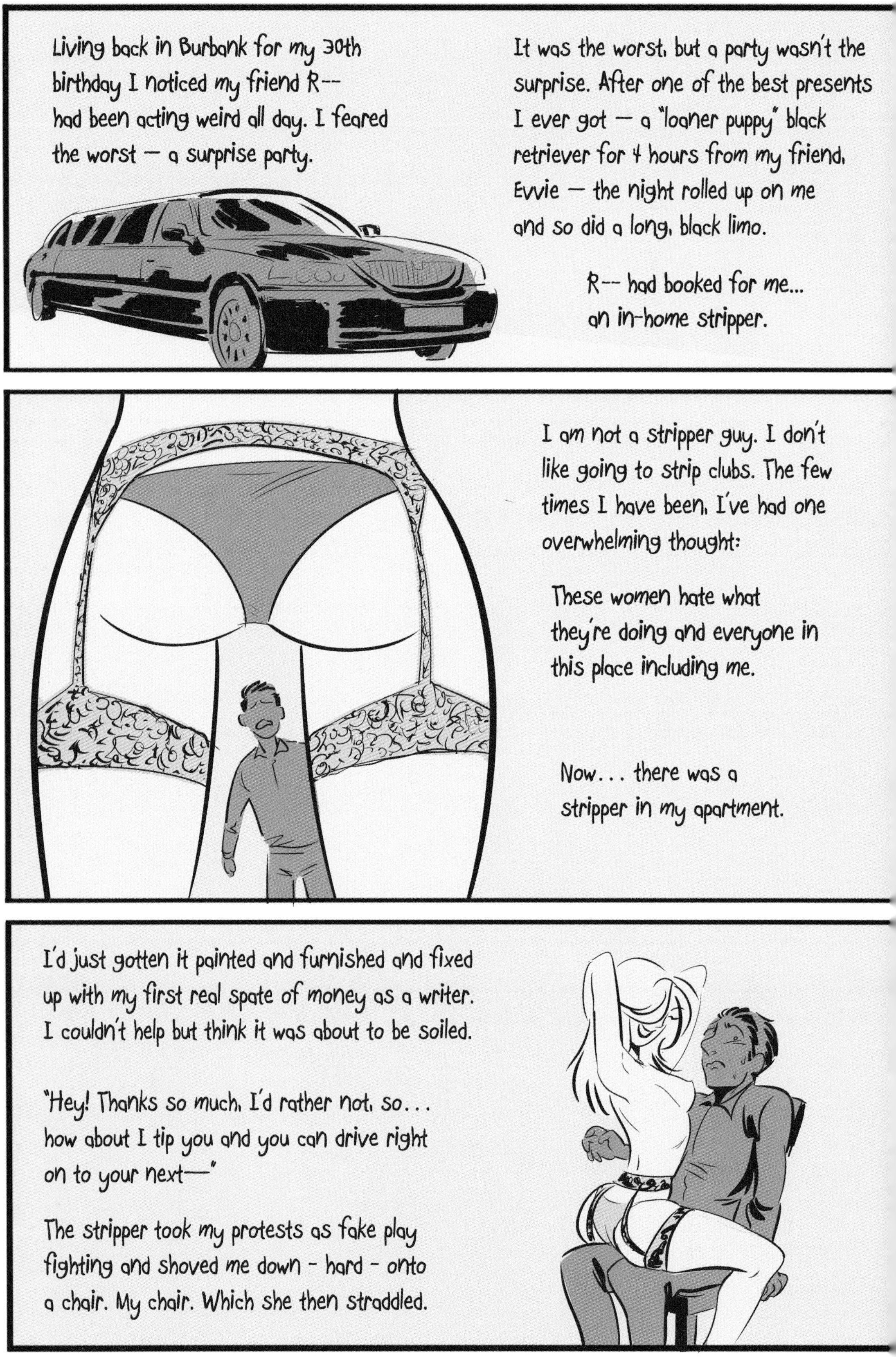

Living back in Burbank for my 30th birthday I noticed my friend R-- had been acting weird all day. I feared the worst — a surprise party.

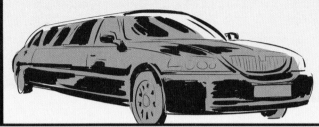

It was the worst, but a party wasn't the surprise. After one of the best presents I ever got — a "loaner puppy" black retriever for 4 hours from my friend, Evvie — the night rolled up on me and so did a long, black limo.

R-- had booked for me... an in-home stripper.

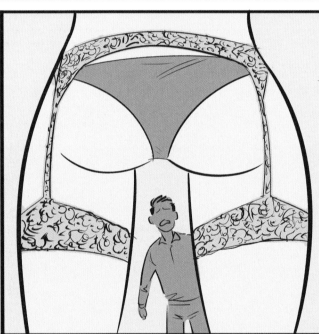

I am not a stripper guy. I don't like going to strip clubs. The few times I have been, I've had one overwhelming thought:

These women hate what they're doing and everyone in this place including me.

Now... there was a stripper in my apartment.

I'd just gotten it painted and furnished and fixed up with my first real spate of money as a writer. I couldn't help but think it was about to be soiled.

"Hey! Thanks so much, I'd rather not, so... how about I tip you and you can drive right on to your next—"

The stripper took my protests as fake play fighting and shoved me down - hard - onto a chair. My chair. Which she then straddled.

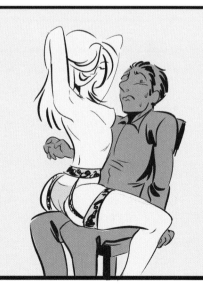

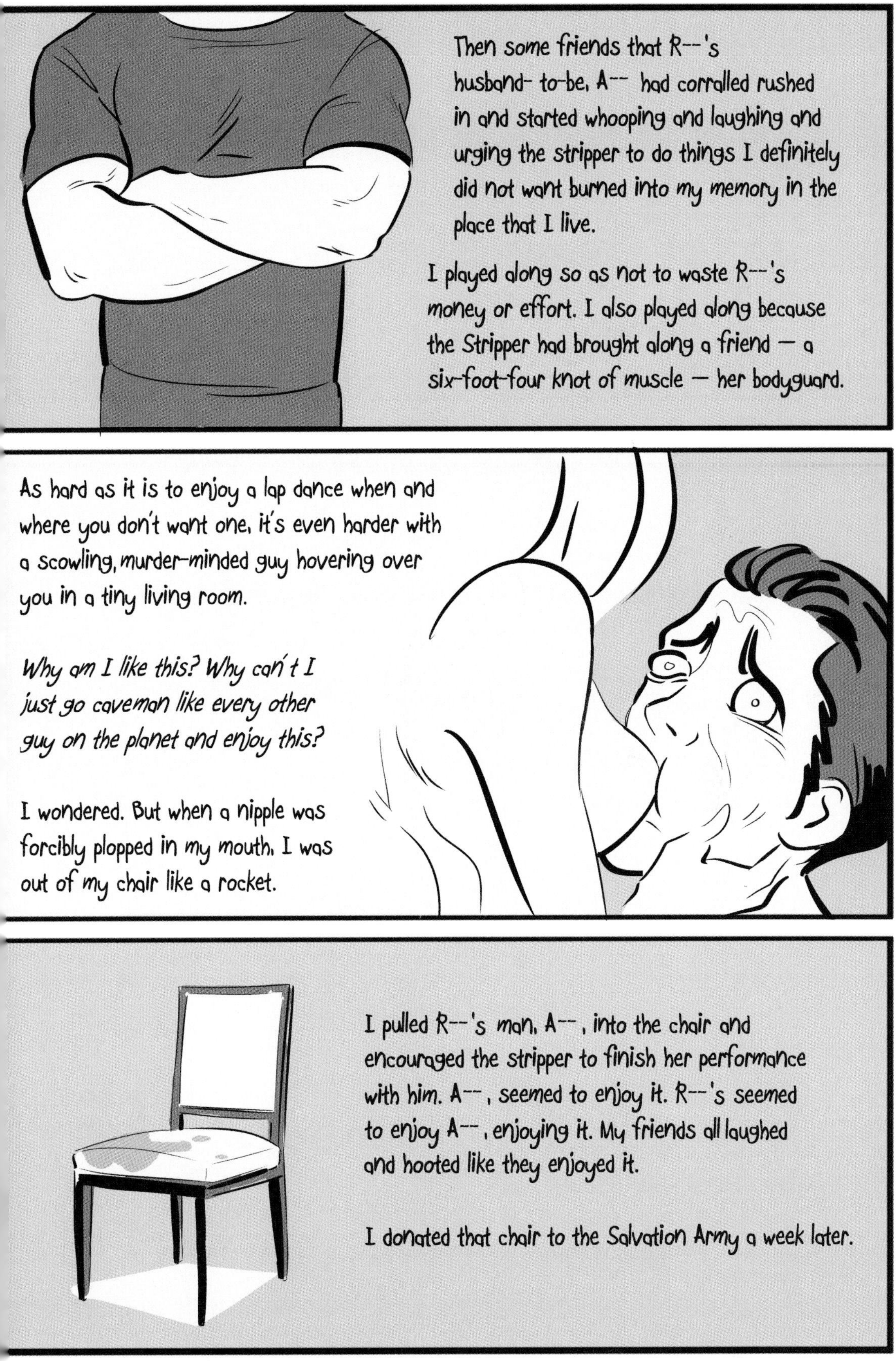
Then some friends that R--'s husband- to-be, A-- had corralled rushed in and started whooping and laughing and urging the stripper to do things I definitely did not want burned into my memory in the place that I live.
I played along so as not to waste R--'s money or effort. I also played along because the Stripper had brought along a friend — a six-foot-four knot of muscle — her bodyguard.
As hard as it is to enjoy a lap dance when and where you don't want one, it's even harder with a scowling, murder-minded guy hovering over you in a tiny living room.
Why am I like this? Why can't I just go caveman like every other guy on the planet and enjoy this?
I wondered. But when a nipple was forcibly plopped in my mouth, I was out of my chair like a rocket.
I pulled R--'s man, A--, into the chair and encouraged the stripper to finish her performance with him. A--, seemed to enjoy it. R--'s seemed to enjoy A--, enjoying it. My friends all laughed and hooted like they enjoyed it.
I donated that chair to the Salvation Army a week later.

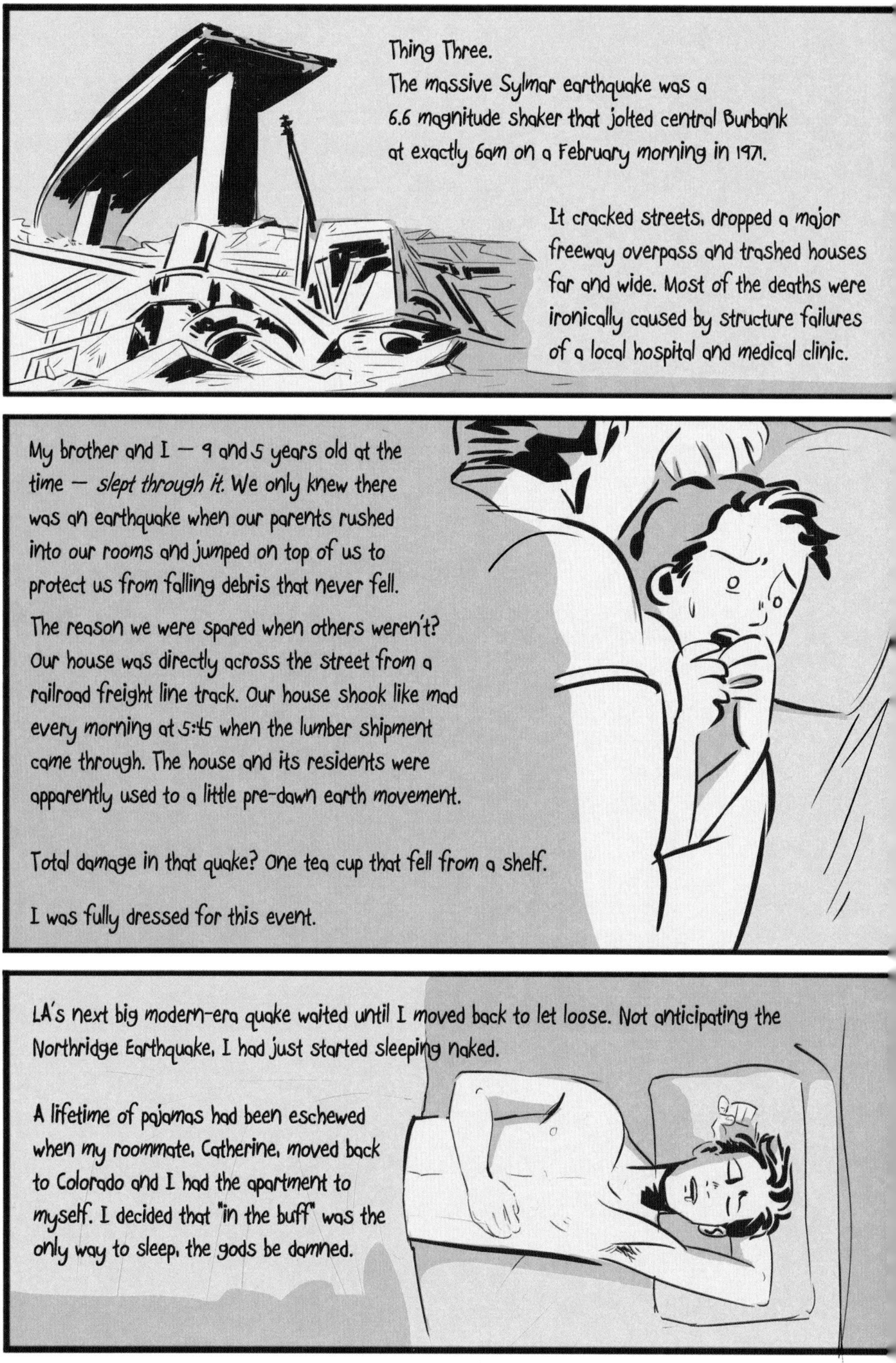
Thing Three.
The massive Sylmar earthquake was a 6.6 magnitude shaker that jolted central Burbank at exactly 6am on a February morning in 1971.
It cracked streets, dropped a major freeway overpass and trashed houses far and wide. Most of the deaths were ironically caused by structure failures of a local hospital and medical clinic.
My brother and I — 9 and 5 years old at the time — *slept through it.* We only knew there was an earthquake when our parents rushed into our rooms and jumped on top of us to protect us from falling debris that never fell.
The reason we were spared when others weren't? Our house was directly across the street from a railroad freight line track. Our house shook like mad every morning at 5:45 when the lumber shipment came through. The house and its residents were apparently used to a little pre-dawn earth movement.
Total damage in that quake? One tea cup that fell from a shelf.
I was fully dressed for this event.
LA's next big modern-era quake waited until I moved back to let loose. Not anticipating the Northridge Earthquake, I had just started sleeping naked.
A lifetime of pajamas had been eschewed when my roommate, Catherine, moved back to Colorado and I had the apartment to myself. I decided that "in the buff" was the only way to sleep, the gods be damned.

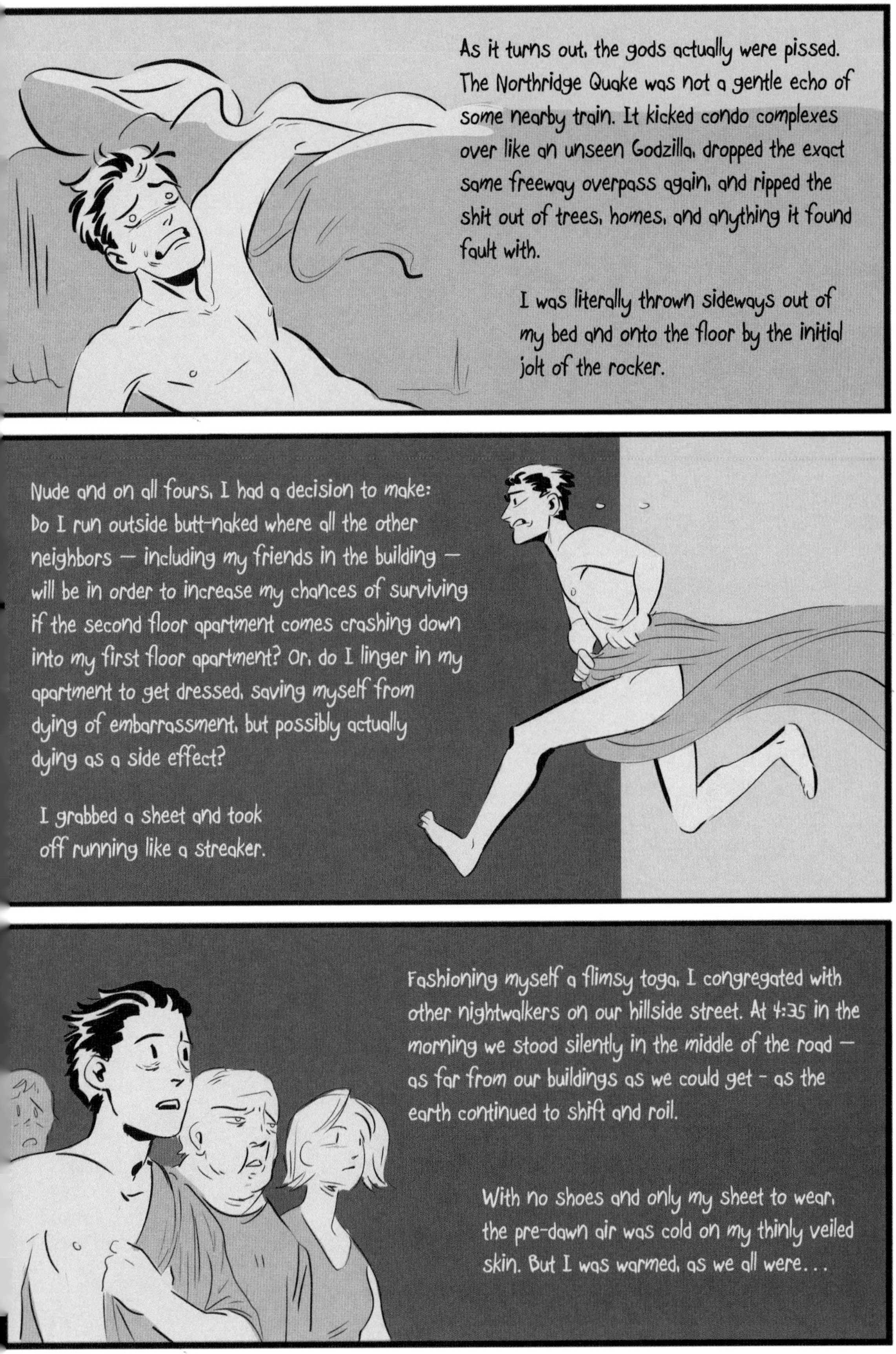
As it turns out, the gods actually were pissed. The Northridge Quake was not a gentle echo of some nearby train. It kicked condo complexes over like an unseen Godzilla, dropped the exact same freeway overpass again, and ripped the shit out of trees, homes, and anything it found fault with.
I was literally thrown sideways out of my bed and onto the floor by the initial jolt of the rocker.
Nude and on all fours, I had a decision to make: Do I run outside butt-naked where all the other neighbors — including my friends in the building — will be in order to increase my chances of surviving if the second floor apartment comes crashing down into my first floor apartment? Or, do I linger in my apartment to get dressed, saving myself from dying of embarrassment, but possibly actually dying as a side effect?
I grabbed a sheet and took off running like a streaker.
Fashioning myself a flimsy toga, I congregated with other nightwalkers on our hillside street. At 4:35 in the morning we stood silently in the middle of the road — as far from our buildings as we could get - as the earth continued to shift and roil.
With no shoes and only my sheet to wear, the pre-dawn air was cold on my thinly veiled skin. But I was warmed, as we all were…

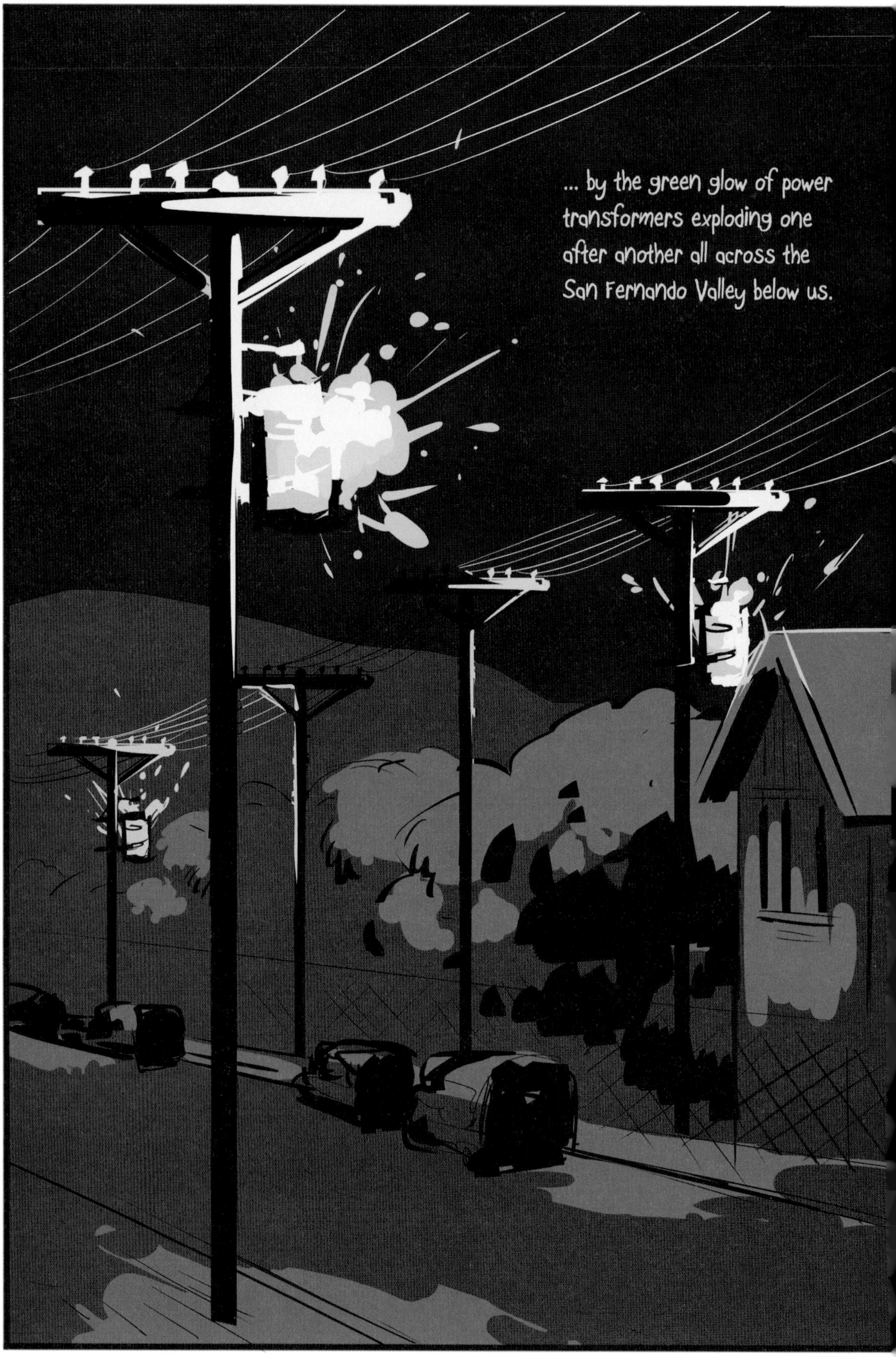
... by the green glow of power transformers exploding one after another all across the San Fernando Valley below us.

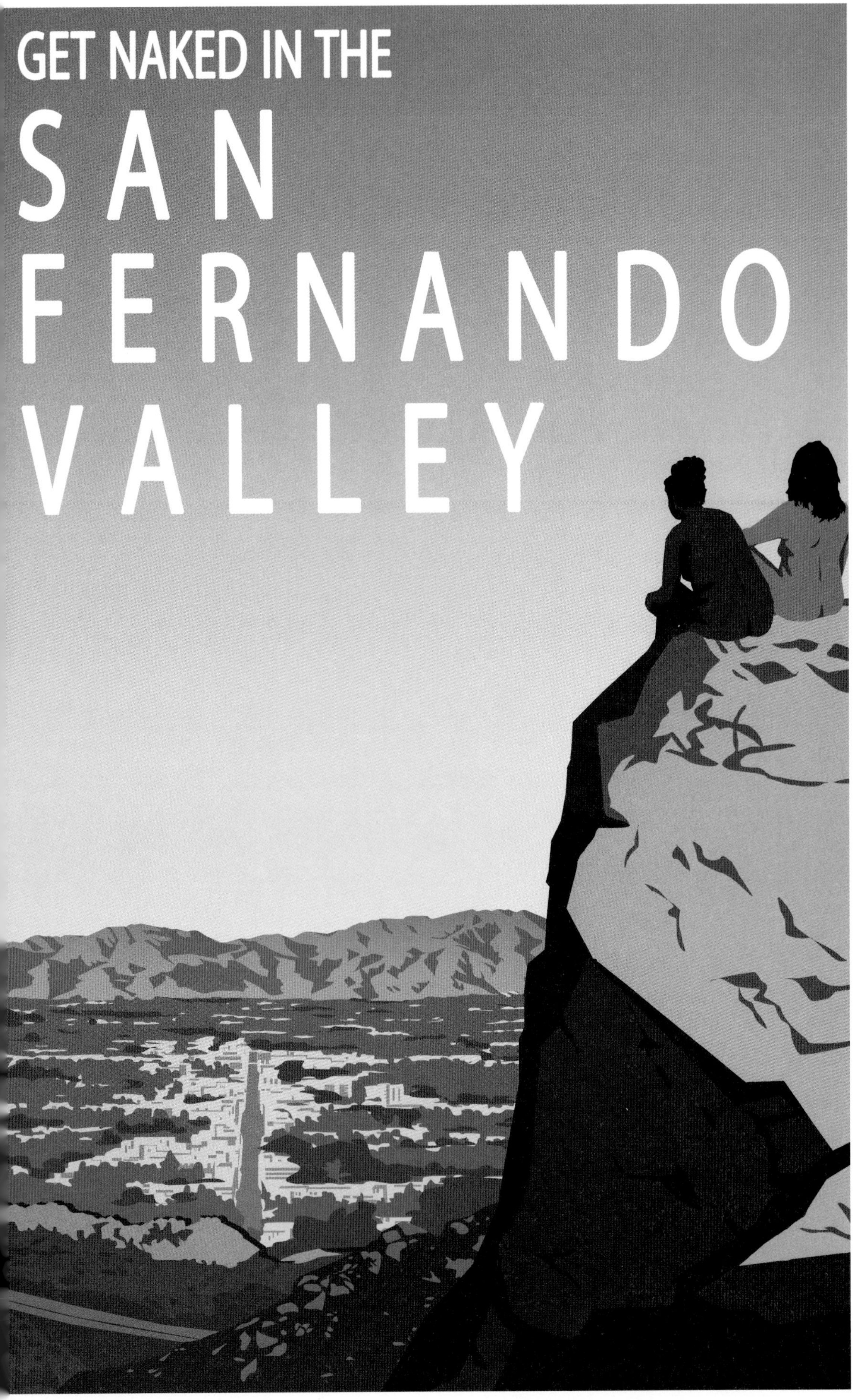
GET NAKED IN THE
SAN
FERNANDO
VALLEY

MY BEST FRIEND
WAS A KID NAMED
JOHN McHORNY.

NO LIE.

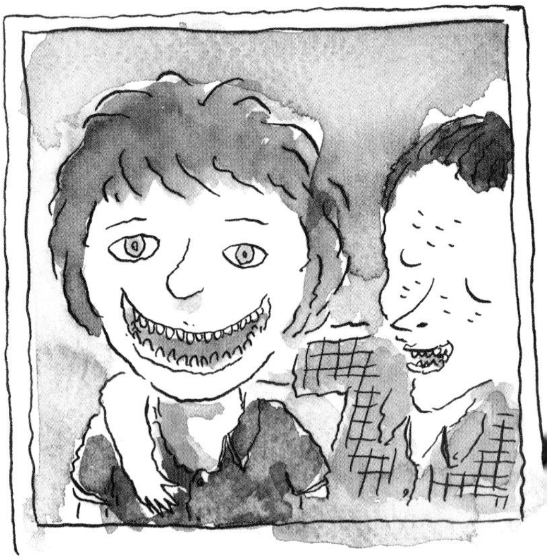

WE BECAME BEST
FRIENDS IN KINDERGARTEN. HE HAD
A HUGE SMILE, TWO BROTHERS, 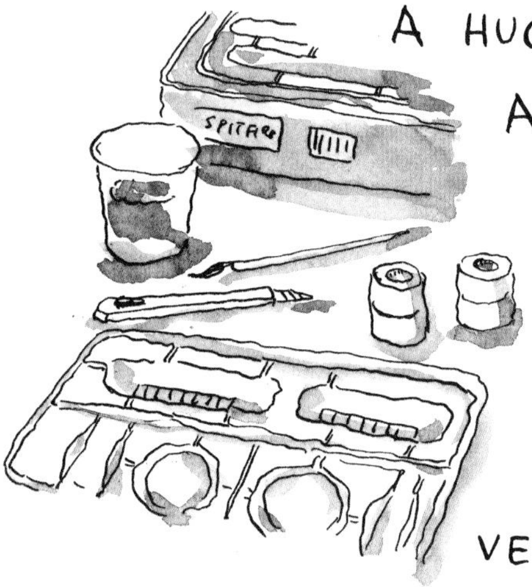
A SISTER, A MOM WHO'D WON
A DINING ROOM SET ON
THE TV GAME SHOW
LET'S MAKE A DEAL,
A DAD THAT I DIDN'T SEE
VERY OFTEN, AND THE BEST
COLLECTION OF PLAYABLE TOYS
IN THE ENTIRE SAN FERNANDO VALLEY.

WE WERE INSEPERABLE.

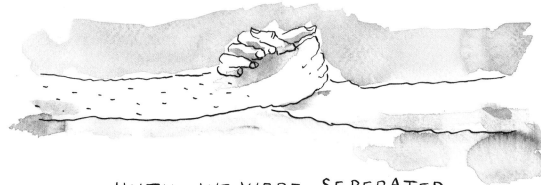

UNTIL WE WERE SEPERATED.

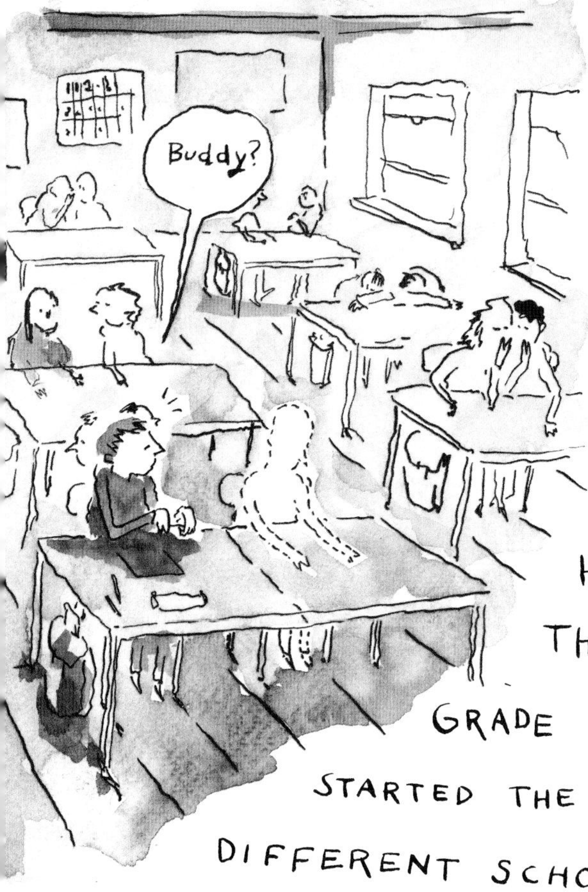
Buddy?

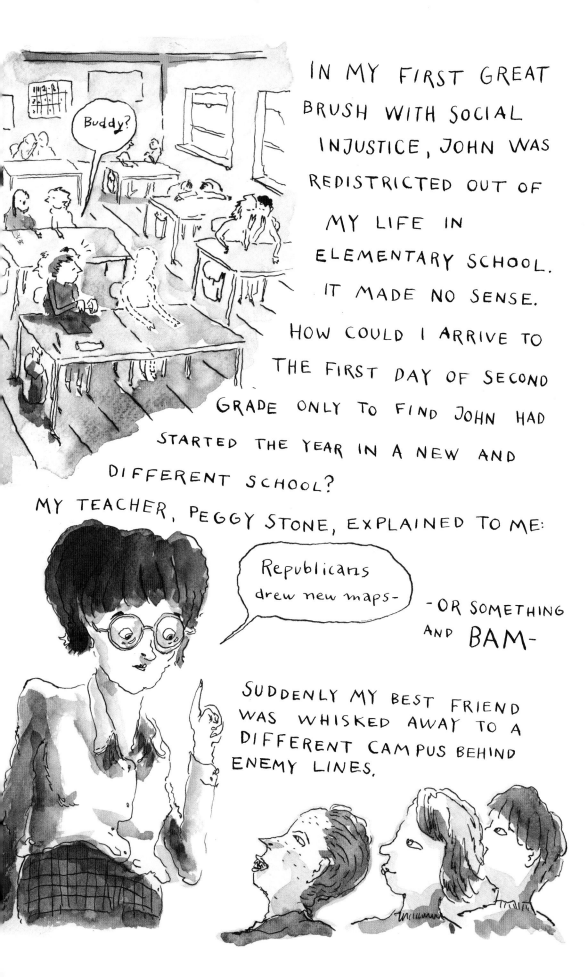

IN MY FIRST GREAT BRUSH WITH SOCIAL INJUSTICE, JOHN WAS REDISTRICTED OUT OF MY LIFE IN ELEMENTARY SCHOOL. IT MADE NO SENSE. HOW COULD I ARRIVE TO THE FIRST DAY OF SECOND GRADE ONLY TO FIND JOHN HAD STARTED THE YEAR IN A NEW AND DIFFERENT SCHOOL?

MY TEACHER, PEGGY STONE, EXPLAINED TO ME:

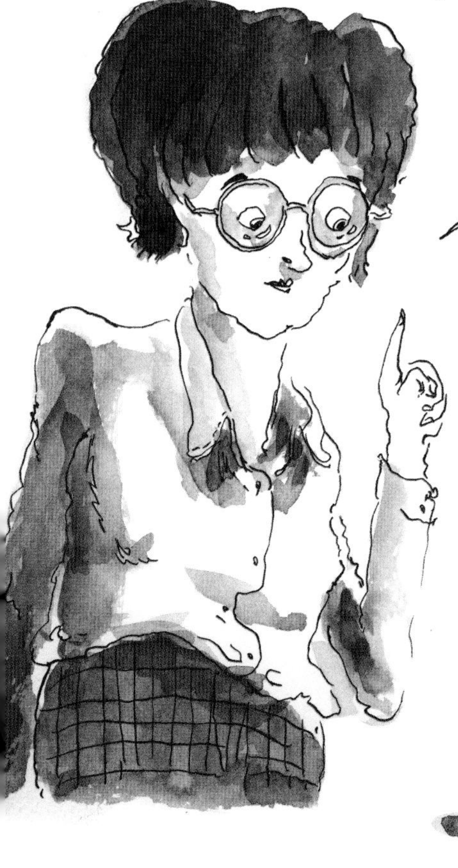
Republicans drew new maps-

-OR SOMETHING AND BAM-

SUDDENLY MY BEST FRIEND WAS WHISKED AWAY TO A DIFFERENT CAMPUS BEHIND ENEMY LINES.

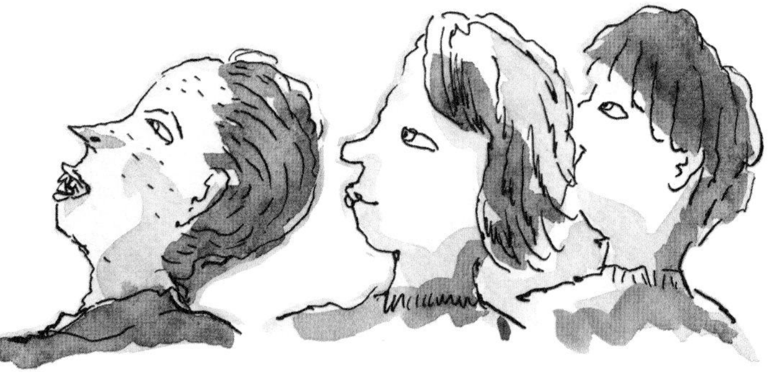

IN THE SAN FERNANDO VALLEY REDRAWING OF LINES, THE CITY OF BURBANK WAS BERLIN AND THE WALL THEY PUT UP WAS INSURMOUNTABLE FOR TWO SIX-YEAR-OLD BUDDIES.

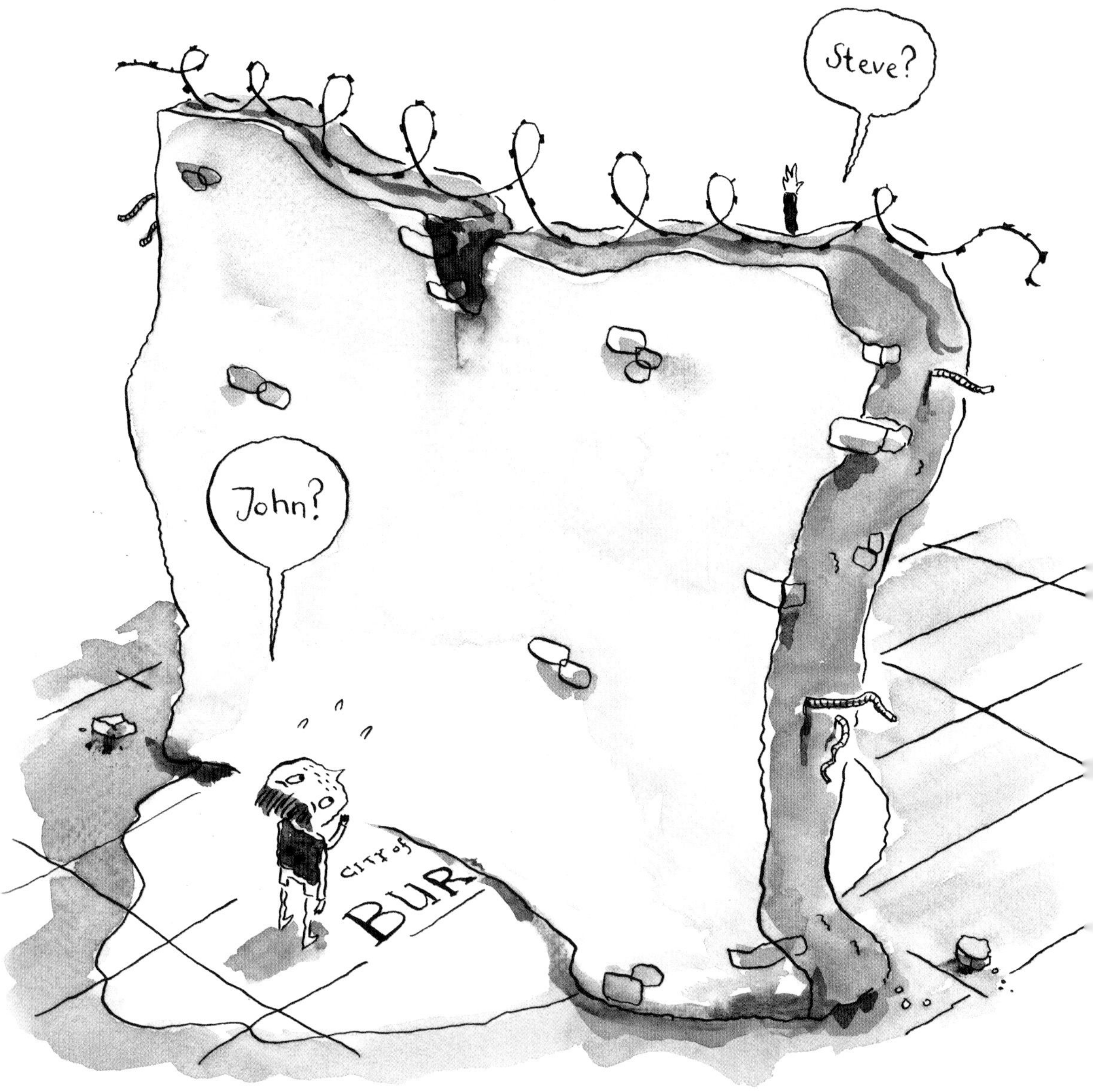
Steve?
John?
CITY OF
BUR

I BURST INTO TEARS, BUT MRS. STONE ASSURED ME I'D SEE MY BEST FRIEND AGAIN.

I DID. NOT EVERY DAY, BUT I STILL WENT OVER TO HIS HOUSE TO PLAY NOW AND THEN.

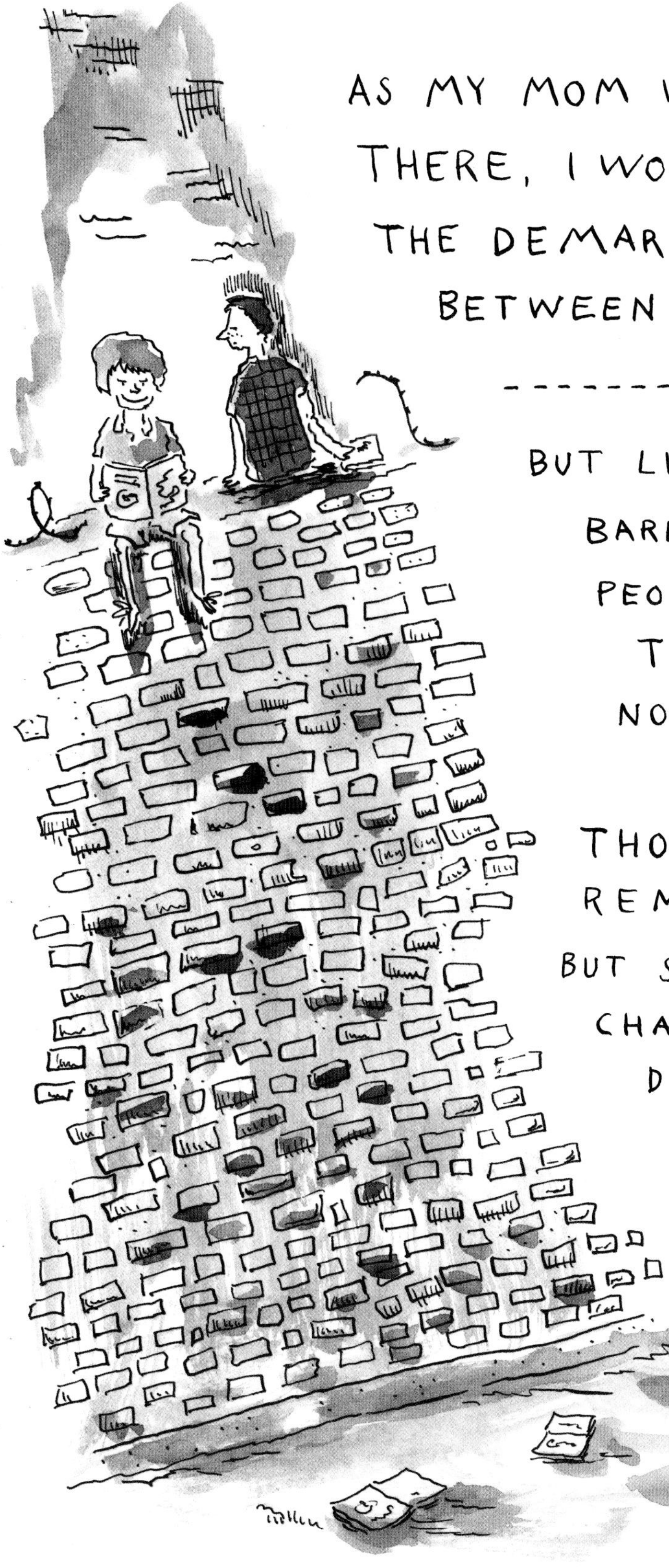

AS MY MOM WALKED ME THERE, I WOULD LOOK FOR THE DEMARCATION LINE BETWEEN OUR ZONES.

BUT LIKE MANY BARRIERS BETWEEN PEOPLE IT WAS THEORETICAL, NOT LITERAL.

THOSE PLAY DAYS REMAINED AWESOME, BUT SOMETHING CHANGES WHEN YOU DON'T SEE YOUR BEST FRIEND REGULARLY.

JOHN RARELY CAME TO PLAY AT MY HOUSE BUT THAT HAD MORE TO DO WITH DINNER.

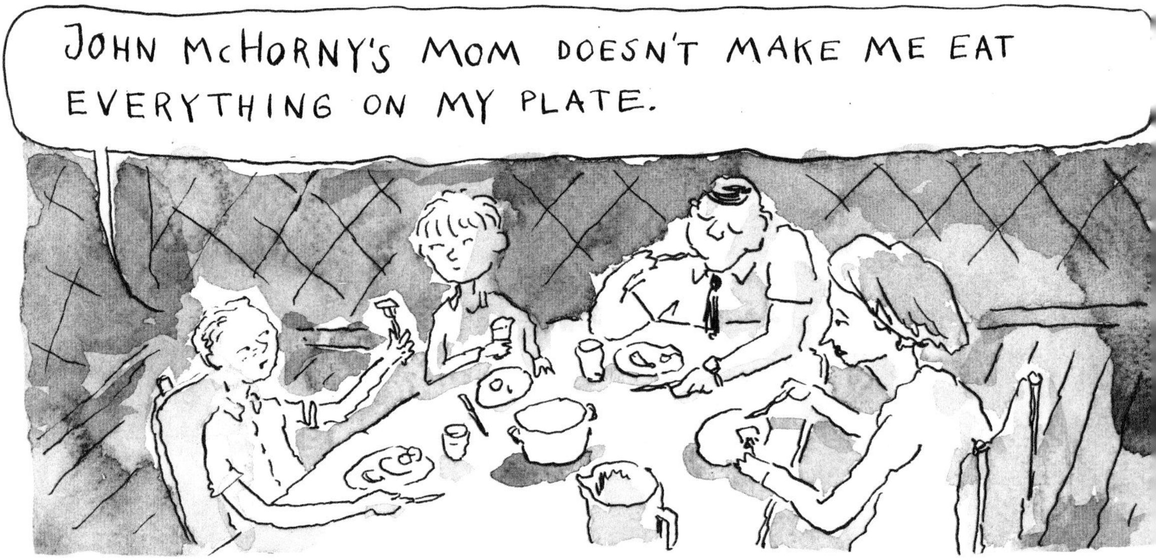
JOHN McHORNY'S MOM DOESN'T MAKE ME EAT EVERYTHING ON MY PLATE.

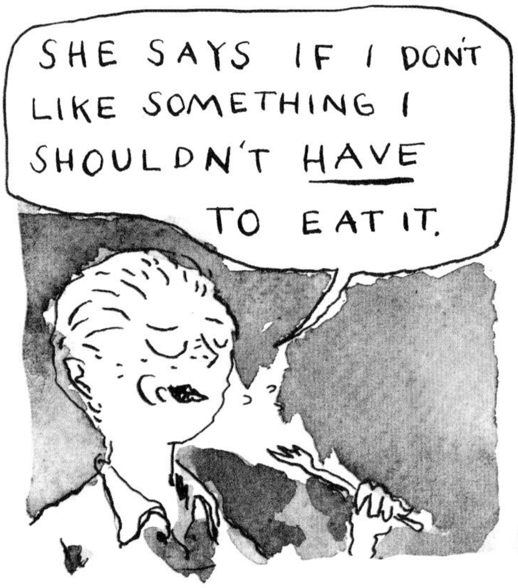
SHE SAYS IF I DON'T LIKE SOMETHING I SHOULDN'T HAVE TO EAT IT.

I WOULD PROCLAIM TO MY MOTHER AFTER A RETURN FROM A VISIT TO JOHN'S HOUSE.

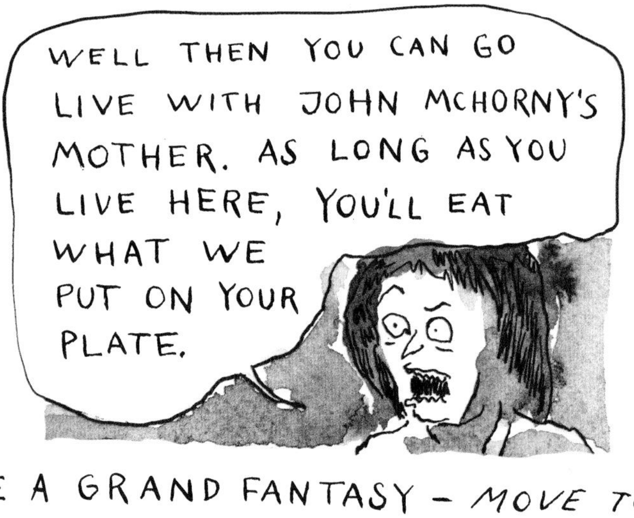
WELL THEN YOU CAN GO LIVE WITH JOHN MCHORNY'S MOTHER. AS LONG AS YOU LIVE HERE, YOU'LL EAT WHAT WE PUT ON YOUR PLATE.

IT SEEMED LIKE A GRAND FANTASY – *MOVE TO JOHN'S HOUSE... ONLY EAT WHAT I LIKE...* UTOPIA.

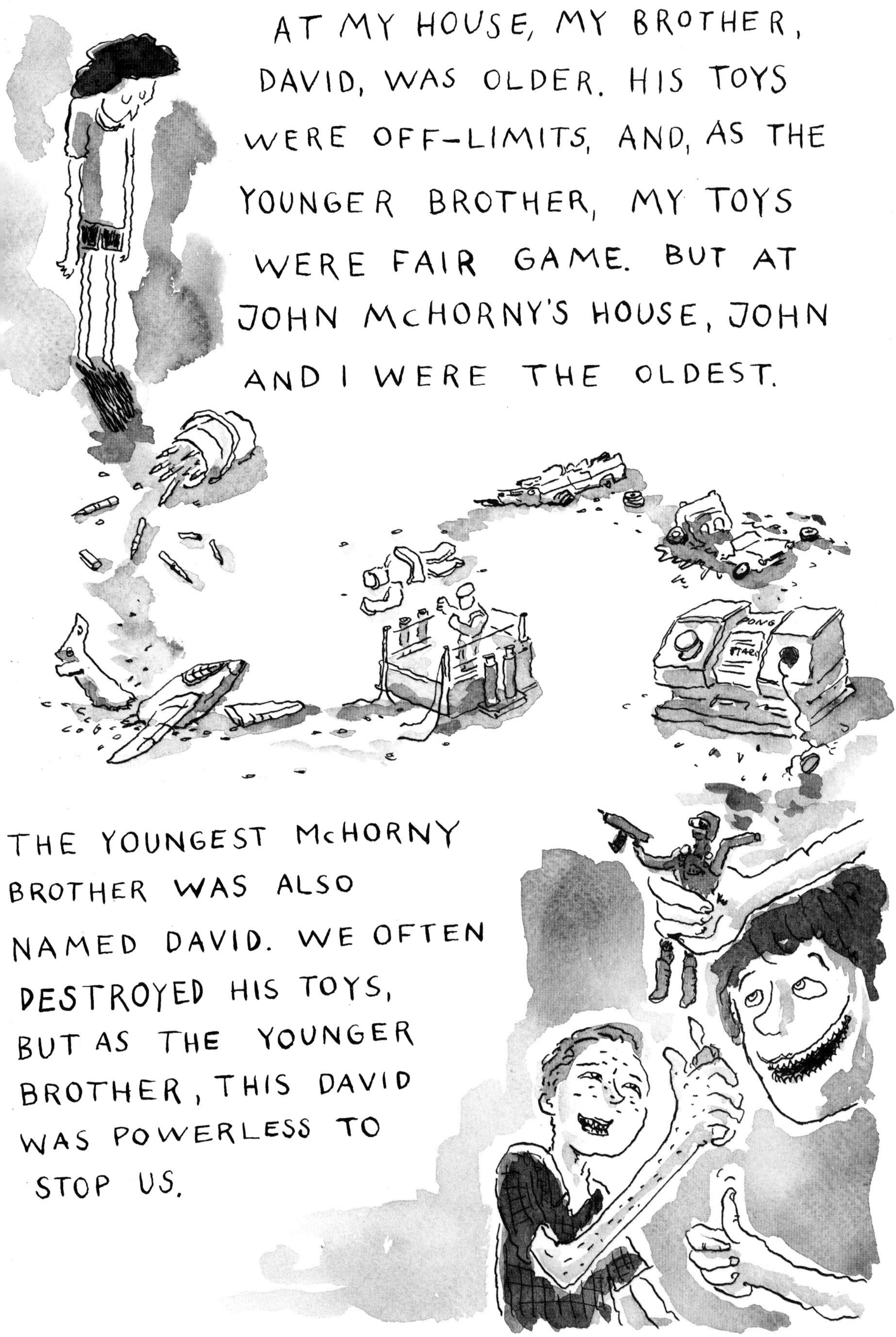
AT MY HOUSE, MY BROTHER, DAVID, WAS OLDER. HIS TOYS WERE OFF-LIMITS, AND, AS THE YOUNGER BROTHER, MY TOYS WERE FAIR GAME. BUT AT JOHN McHORNY'S HOUSE, JOHN AND I WERE THE OLDEST.
PONG
THE YOUNGEST McHORNY BROTHER WAS ALSO NAMED DAVID. WE OFTEN DESTROYED HIS TOYS, BUT AS THE YOUNGER BROTHER, THIS DAVID WAS POWERLESS TO STOP US.

NOT ONLY DID I NOT MOVE IN WITH JOHN McHORNY'S FAMILY, I MOVED AWAY FROM THEM COMPLETELY. MY DAD RETIRED FROM THE AIR FORCE AND WE MOVED TO COLORADO.

WE HAD TO - DUE TO COMPLICATIONS WITH ASTHMA THAT BOTH MY BROTHER AND I SUFFERED.

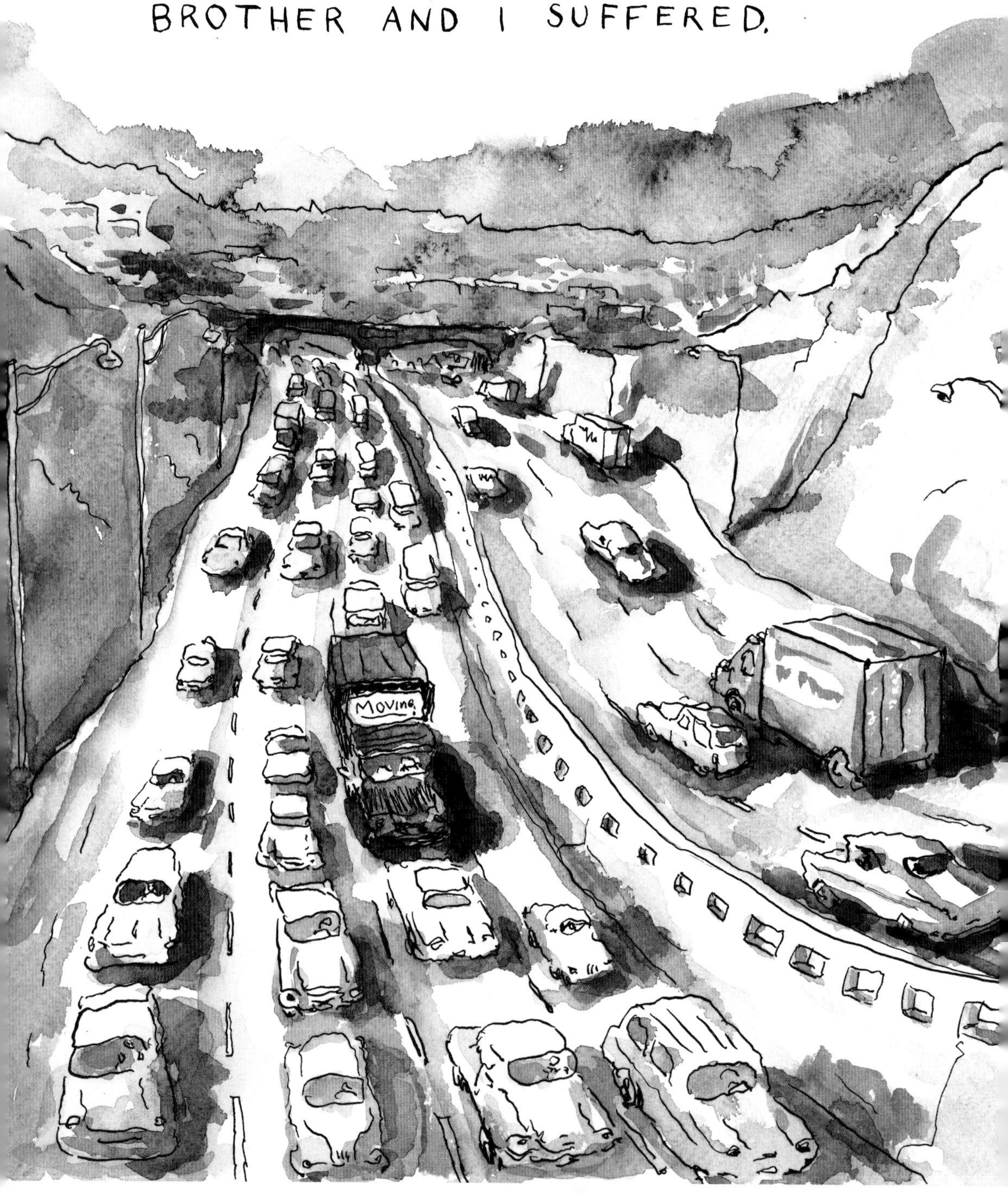
Moving

IT'S EASY TO FORGET NOW, BUT THE SMOG IN 1970s LOS ANGELES WAS ON PAR WITH WHAT WE SAW FOR THE BEIJING OLYMPICS IN CHINA.

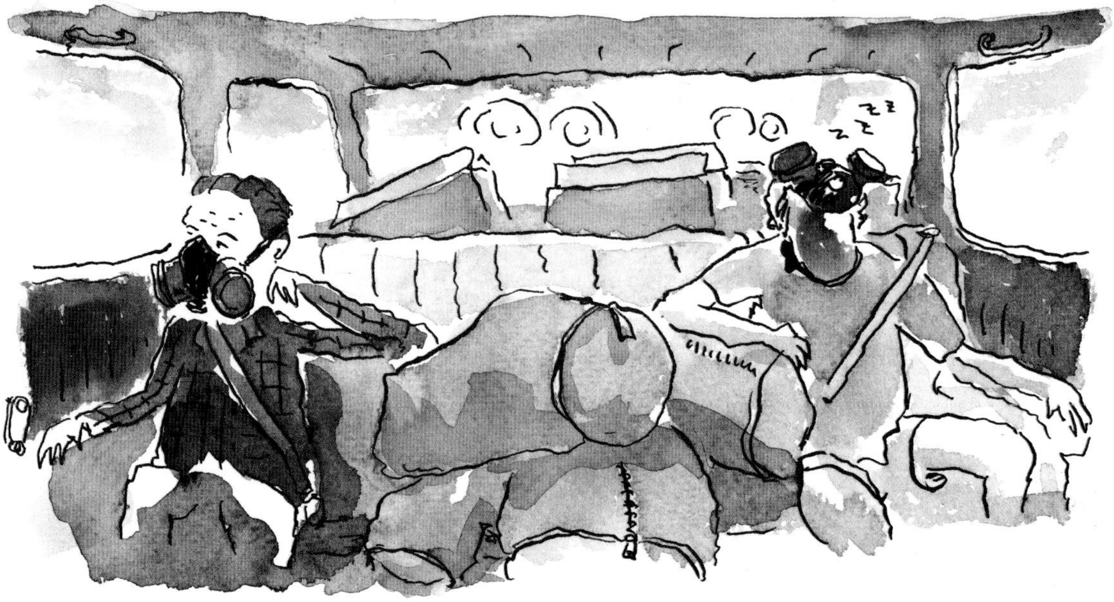

WHILE THE MIDWEST HAD "SNOW DAYS" WHERE KIDS GOT TO STAY HOME FROM SCHOOL DUE TO SNOW ACCUMULATIONS, WE CALIFORNIA KIDS HAD "SMOG DAYS" WHERE WE GOT TO STAY HOME FROM SCHOOL BECAUSE THE AIR WAS TOO FILTHY TO EXPOSE YOUNG LUNGS TO IT.

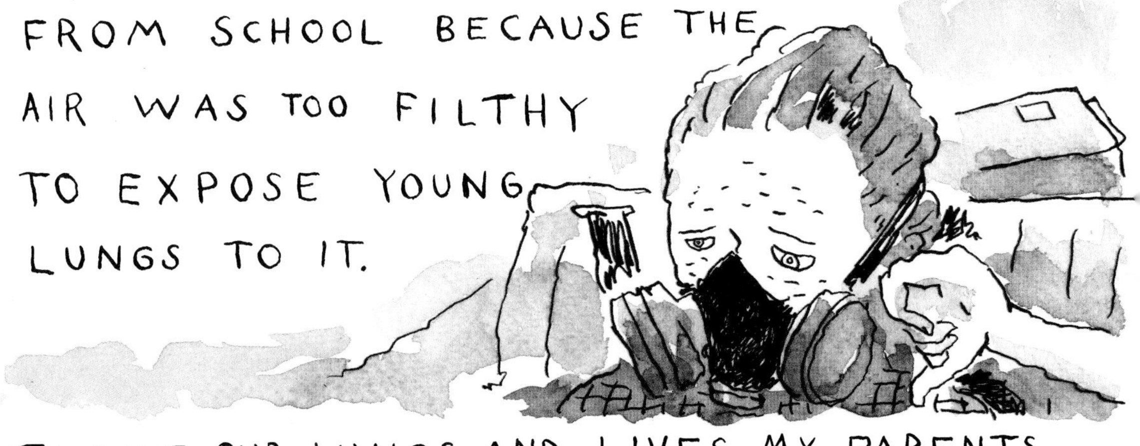

TO SAVE OUR LUNGS AND LIVES, MY PARENTS TRADED SMOG DAYS FOR SNOW DAYS AS WE RELOCATED TO COLORADO.

I SAW JOHN ONLY ONCE MORE. IT WAS ON A FAMILY TRIP BACK TO CALIFORNIA WHEN I WAS JUST STARTING HIGH SCHOOL.

I WAS SO EXCITED.

I'D BEEN A TERRIBLE PEN PAL. I'M FAIRLY SURE THE LAST LETTER WRITTEN WAS BY JOHN AND I'D DROPPED THE BALL AFTER THAT.

BUT THIS TRIP WAS A CHANCE TO REINSTATE OUR TIGHT BOND.

I WAS 15, WEIGHED ABOUT THE SAME AS I DID IN KINDERGARTEN, AND WAS ROCKING MY PRIDE-AND-JOY BAND JACKET.

I WAS <u>SO</u> INTERESTING THAT I WAS POSITIVE JOHN WOULD WANT TO BE MY BEST FRIEND AGAIN.

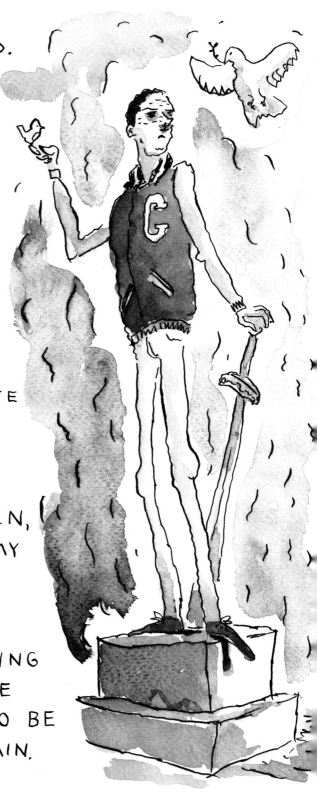

WE HAD TO GO TO THE
DEL TACO ON HOLLYWOOD WAY
TO SEE HIM BECAUSE THAT
WAS WERE HE WAS WORKING.

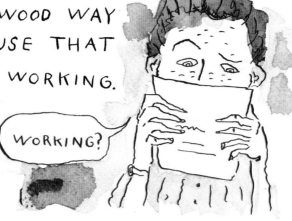

WORKING?

I WAS A COUPLE OF
YEARS AWAY FROM MY FIRST REAL
SUMMER JOB AND HE WAS ALREADY WORKING?

MY MOM WENT TO THE
COUNTER AND ASKED FOR
HIM, AND JOHN CAME
OUT FROM A
BACK ROOM.

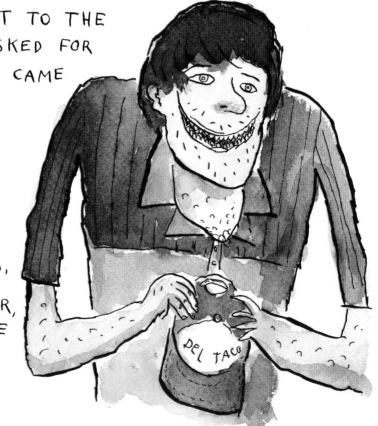

HE WAS WEARING
A FAIRLY HIDEOUS
POLYESTER UNIFORM,
THE UGLIEST
BASEBALL CAP EVER,
AND I COULDN'T HAVE
COVETED HIS
WARDROBE MORE.

HE HELD HIS HAT IN HIS HAND
AND SMILED BROADLY - THE EXACT SAME
SMILE HE HAD AS A SIX-YEAR OLD, EVEN
THOUGH HE NOW LOOKED LIKE A MAN.

HE WAS EXCITED TO SEE ME, AND WHILE I WAS EQUALLY EXCITED TO SEE HIM, I WAS ALSO INTIMIDATED.

HE SEEMED ABOUT FOUR YEARS OLDER THAN ME AND A DECADE MORE MATURE.

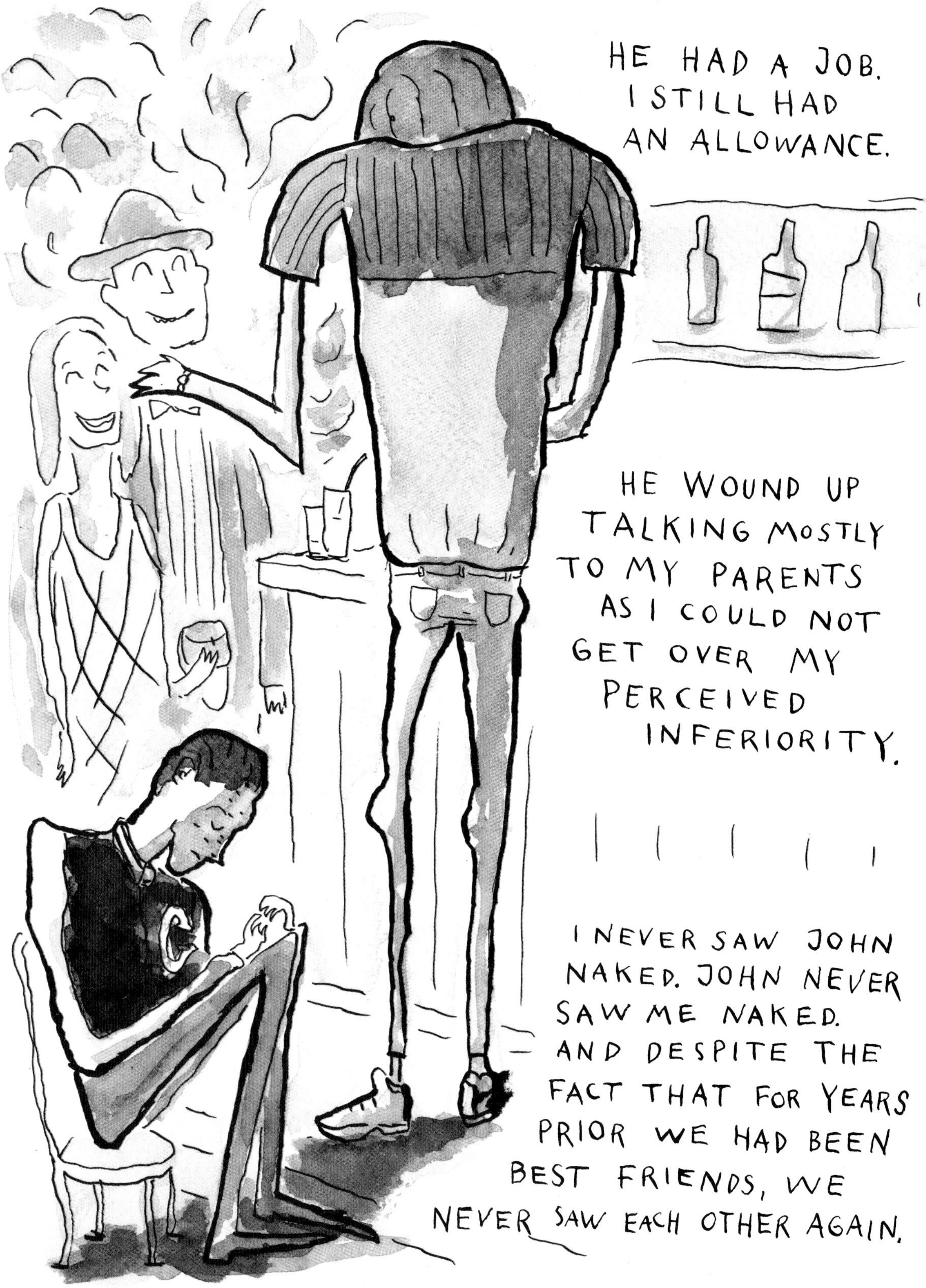
HE HAD A JOB. I STILL HAD AN ALLOWANCE.
HE WOUND UP TALKING MOSTLY TO MY PARENTS AS I COULD NOT GET OVER MY PERCEIVED INFERIORITY.
I NEVER SAW JOHN NAKED. JOHN NEVER SAW ME NAKED. AND DESPITE THE FACT THAT FOR YEARS PRIOR WE HAD BEEN BEST FRIENDS, WE NEVER SAW EACH OTHER AGAIN.

BUT I DID SEE MY SECOND GRADE TEACHER AGAIN - ALSO NOT NAKED - AND WE WERE BOTH PROBABLY THANKFUL FOR THAT.

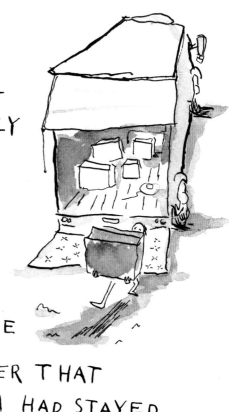

PEGGY STONE WOUND UP BEING MY NEIGHBOR WHEN I MOVED BACK TO BURBANK A DECADE AND A HALF AFTER THAT FAMILY TRIP. I HAD STAYED IN TOUCH WITH HER EVER SINCE LEAVING CALIFORNIA THE FIRST TIME -

MOSTLY BECAUSE MY MOM WAS MUCH BETTER AT WRITING LETTERS THAN I WAS AND ALWAYS SIGNED MY NAME AS WELL.

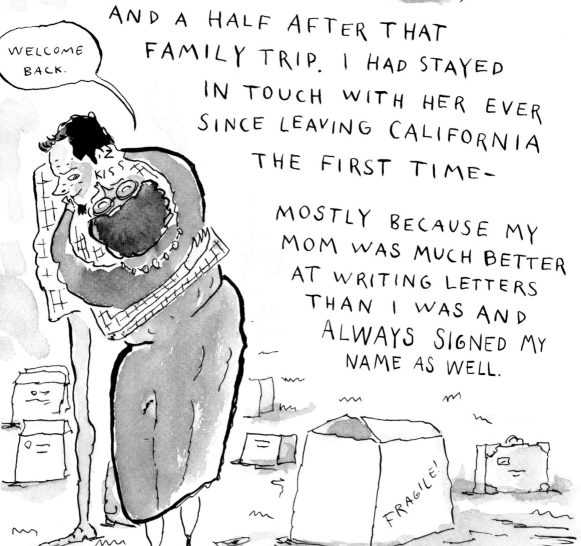

WELCOME BACK.

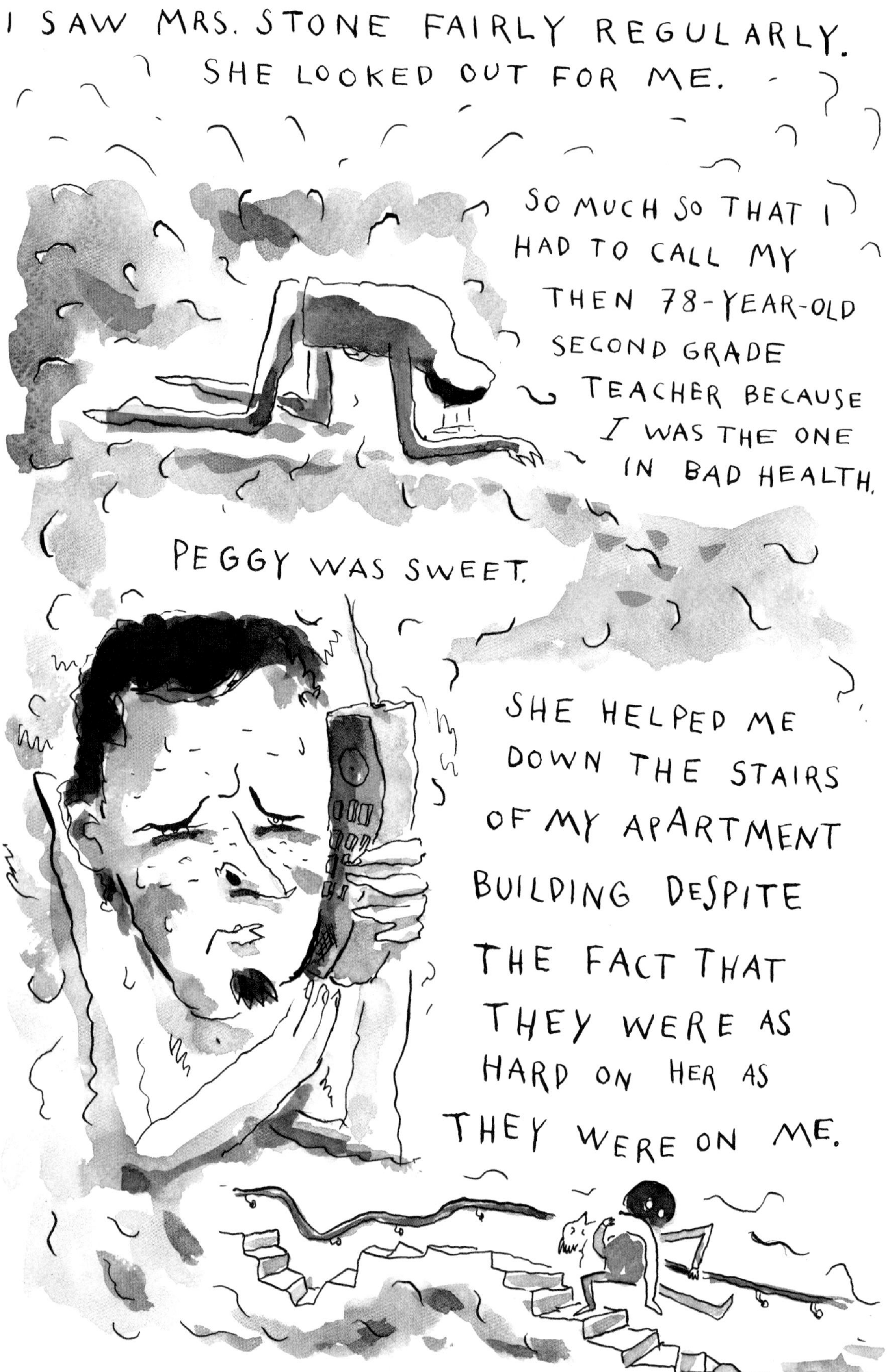
I SAW MRS. STONE FAIRLY REGULARLY.
SHE LOOKED OUT FOR ME.
SO MUCH SO THAT I HAD TO CALL MY THEN 78-YEAR-OLD SECOND GRADE TEACHER BECAUSE I WAS THE ONE IN BAD HEALTH.
PEGGY WAS SWEET.
SHE HELPED ME DOWN THE STAIRS OF MY APARTMENT BUILDING DESPITE THE FACT THAT THEY WERE AS HARD ON HER AS THEY WERE ON ME.

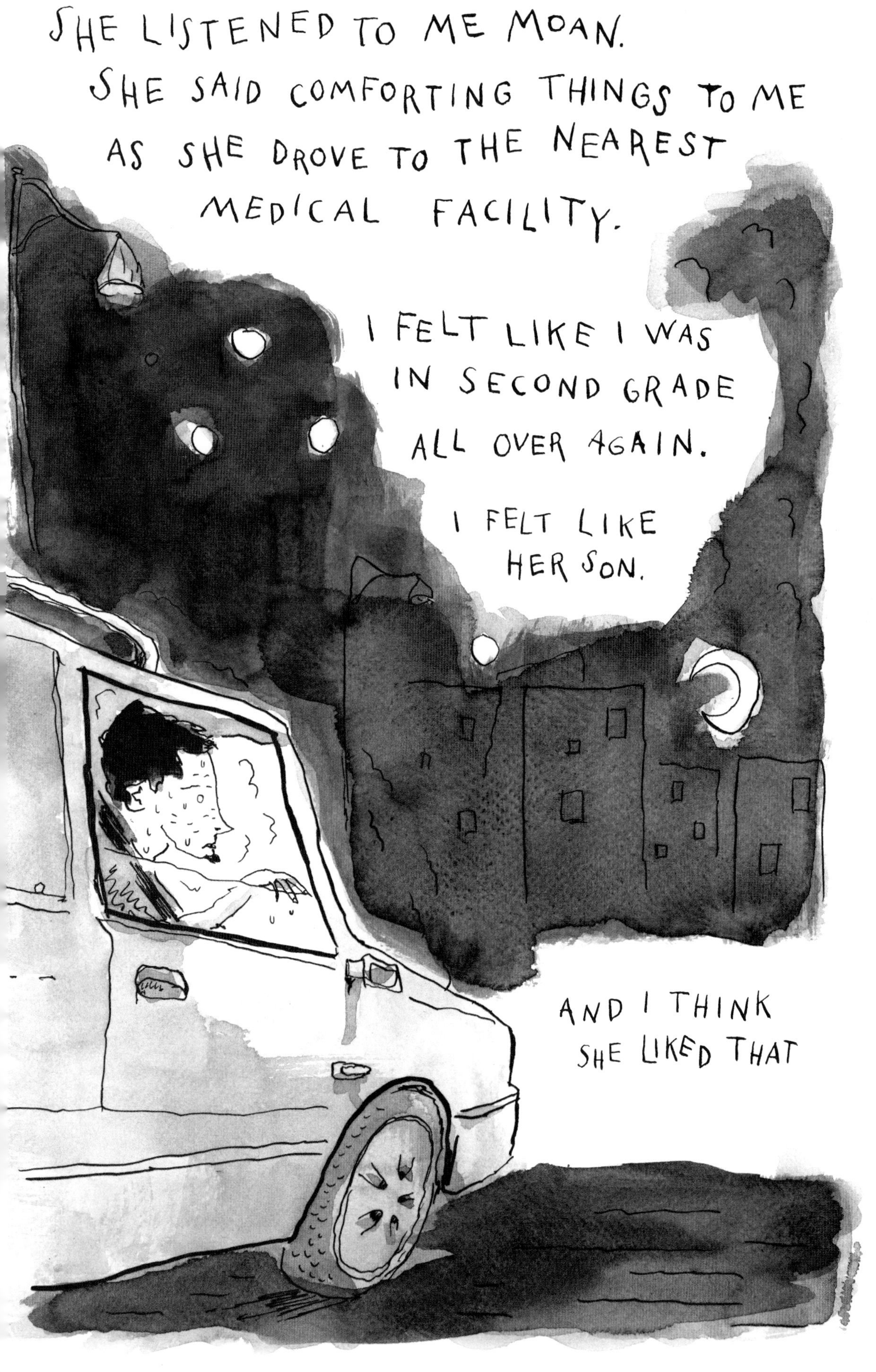
SHE LISTENED TO ME MOAN.
SHE SAID COMFORTING THINGS TO ME AS SHE DROVE TO THE NEAREST MEDICAL FACILITY.
I FELT LIKE I WAS IN SECOND GRADE ALL OVER AGAIN.
I FELT LIKE HER SON.
AND I THINK SHE LIKED THAT

MRS. STONE DELIVERED ME TO AN
URGENT CARE FACILITY ON
MAGNOLIA BOULEWARD
— BLOCKS FROM
WHERE I
LIVED AS
A KID.

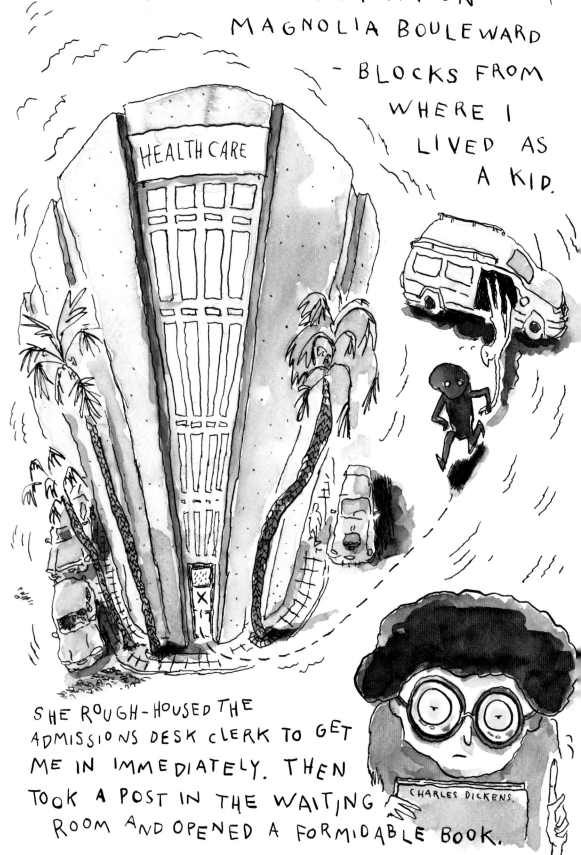

HEALTHCARE

SHE ROUGH-HOUSED THE
ADMISSIONS DESK CLERK TO GET
ME IN IMMEDIATELY. THEN
TOOK A POST IN THE WAITING
ROOM AND OPENED A FORMIDABLE BOOK.

CHARLES DICKENS.

MINUTES LATER I WAS ON MY SIDE, NAKED, IN A HOSPITAL BED. AND I WAS DRY. DESERT DRY. EVAPORATED.

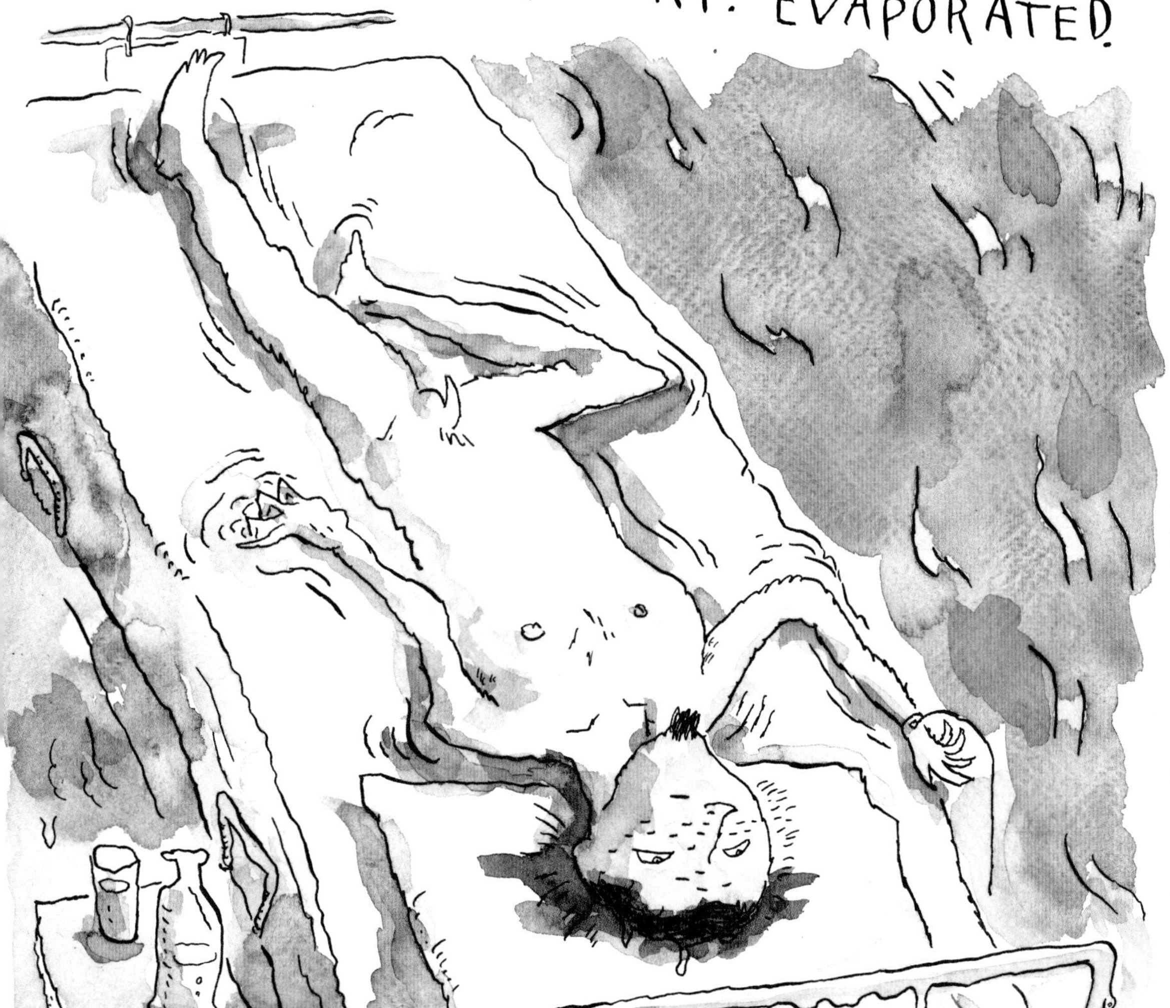

I DON'T KNOW HOW IT HAPPENED, BUT I WAS DANGEROUSLY DEHYDRATED. THAT WAS THE PROGNOSIS I HEARD RIGHT BEFORE I BLACKED OUT.

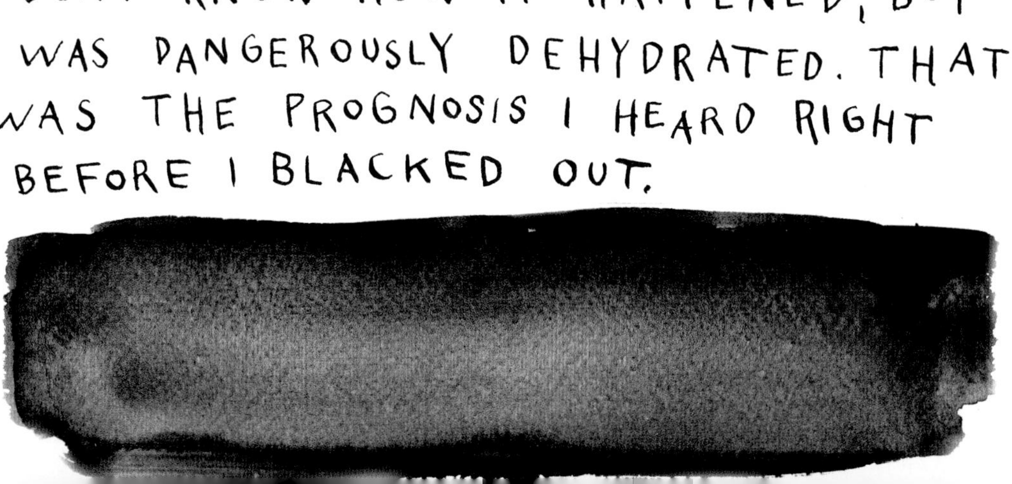

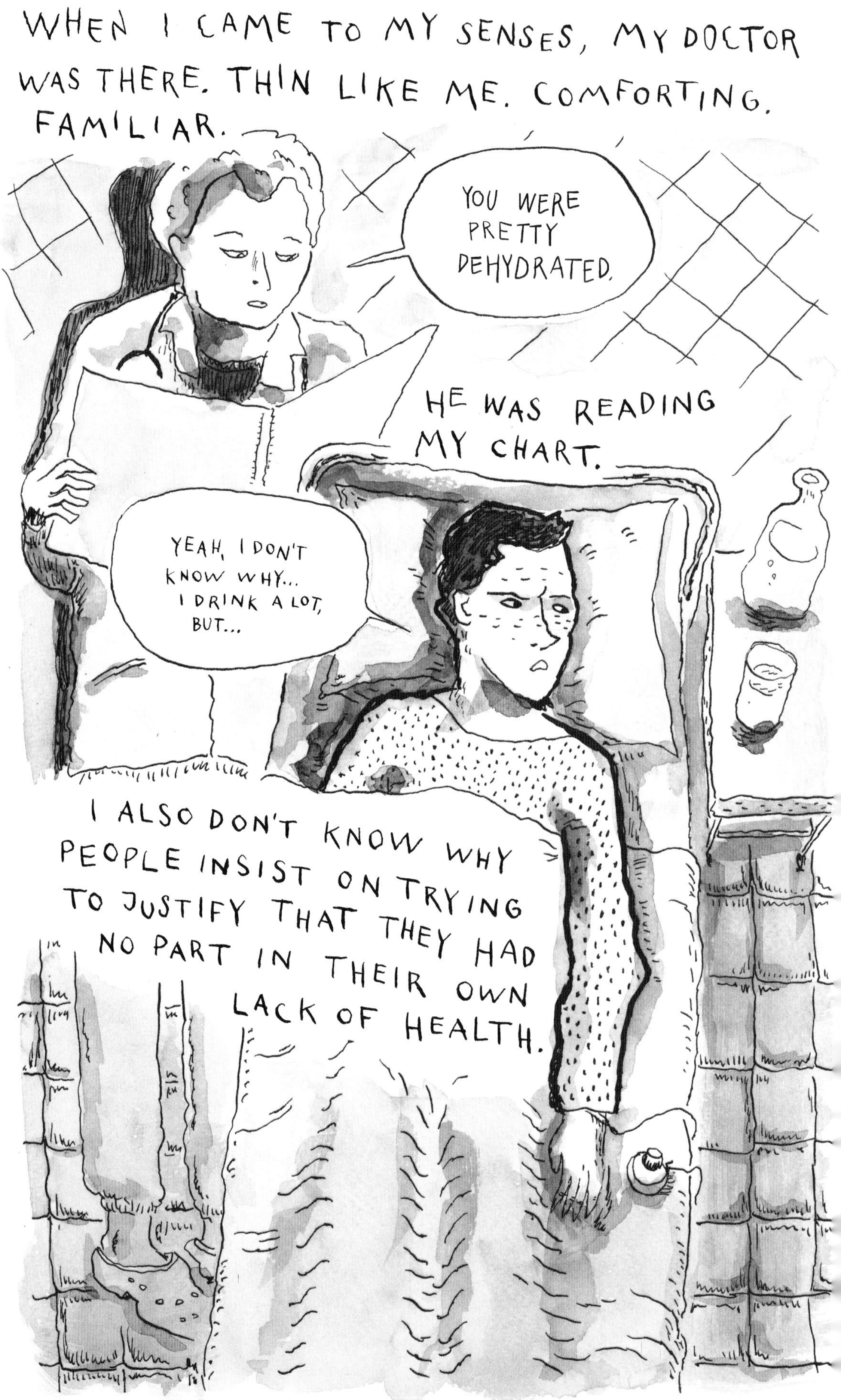
WHEN I CAME TO MY SENSES, MY DOCTOR WAS THERE. THIN LIKE ME. COMFORTING. FAMILIAR.
YOU WERE PRETTY DEHYDRATED.
HE WAS READING MY CHART.
YEAH, I DON'T KNOW WHY... I DRINK A LOT, BUT...
I ALSO DON'T KNOW WHY PEOPLE INSIST ON TRYING TO JUSTIFY THAT THEY HAD NO PART IN THEIR OWN LACK OF HEALTH.

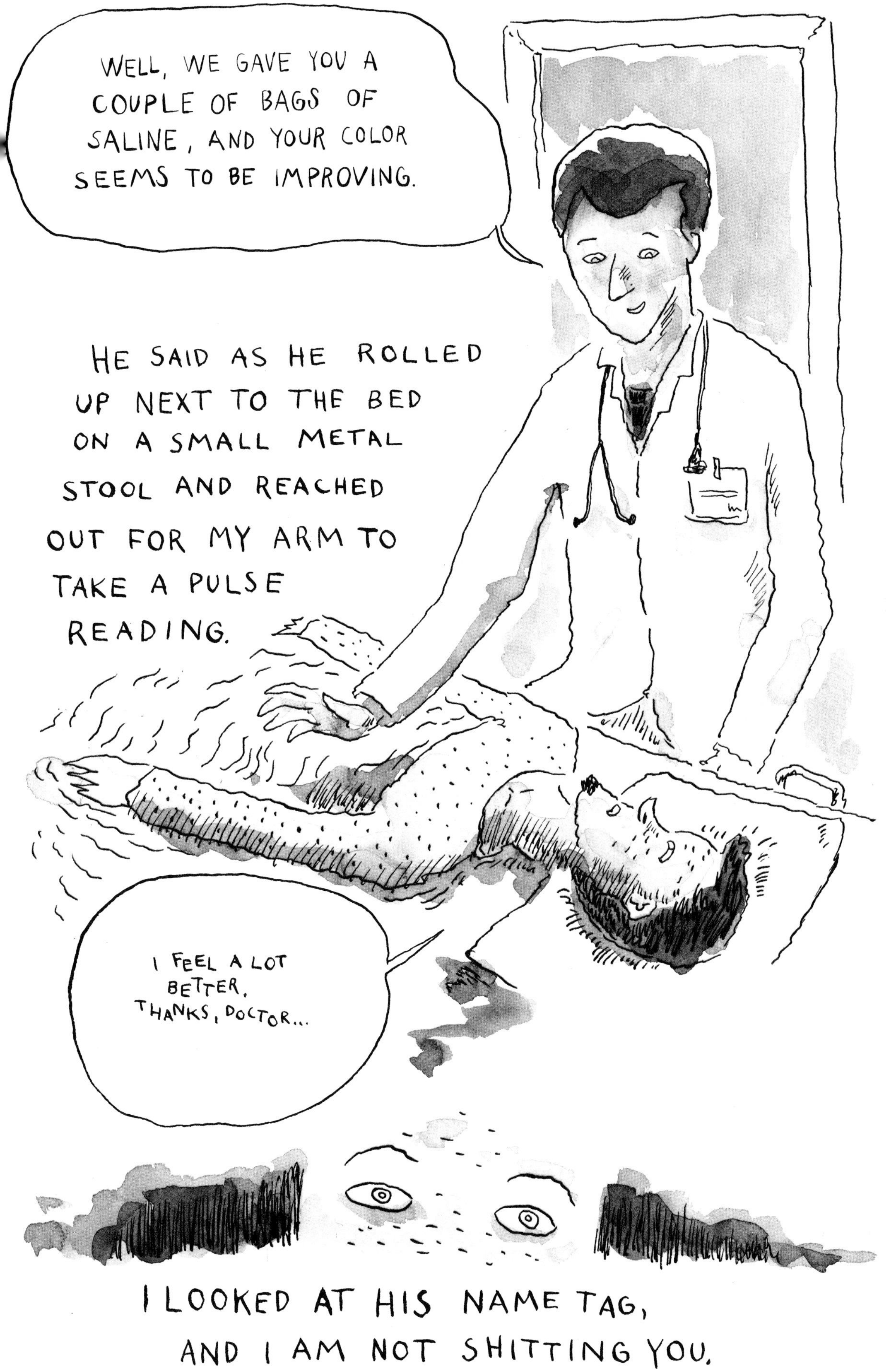

WELL, WE GAVE YOU A COUPLE OF BAGS OF SALINE, AND YOUR COLOR SEEMS TO BE IMPROVING.
HE SAID AS HE ROLLED UP NEXT TO THE BED ON A SMALL METAL STOOL AND REACHED OUT FOR MY ARM TO TAKE A PULSE READING.
I FEEL A LOT BETTER. THANKS, DOCTOR...
I LOOKED AT HIS NAME TAG, AND I AM NOT SHITTING YOU.

I'M IN A HOSPITAL IN THE SAN FERNANDO VALLEY—
NOT FAR FROM WHERE I GREW UP — AND MY
VISION IS A LITTLE WOOZY...

I'VE JUST COME TO MY SENSES FROM
A DEHYDRATION BLACK OUT... AND I SQUINT
TO FOCUS THROUGH MY WEAKNESS TO
READ A NAME:

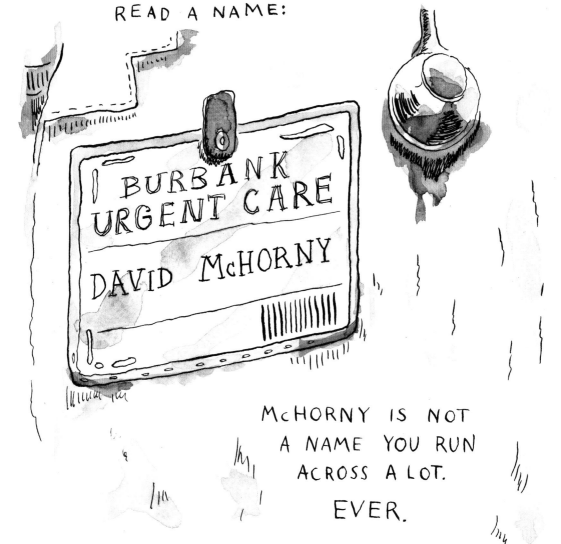

BURBANK
URGENT CARE

DAVID McHORNY

McHORNY IS NOT
A NAME YOU RUN
ACROSS A LOT.
EVER.

AND *DAVID McHORNY* IS VERY SPECIFIC.
AND I AM IN BURBANK
AND IT'S 30 YEARS LATER
AND I'M OUT OF IT

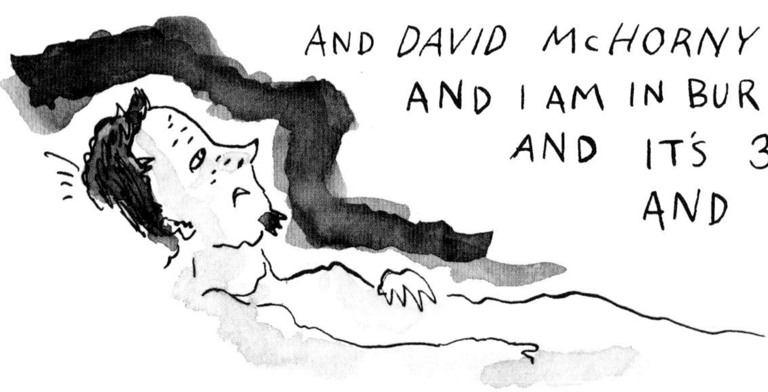

AND I SAY:

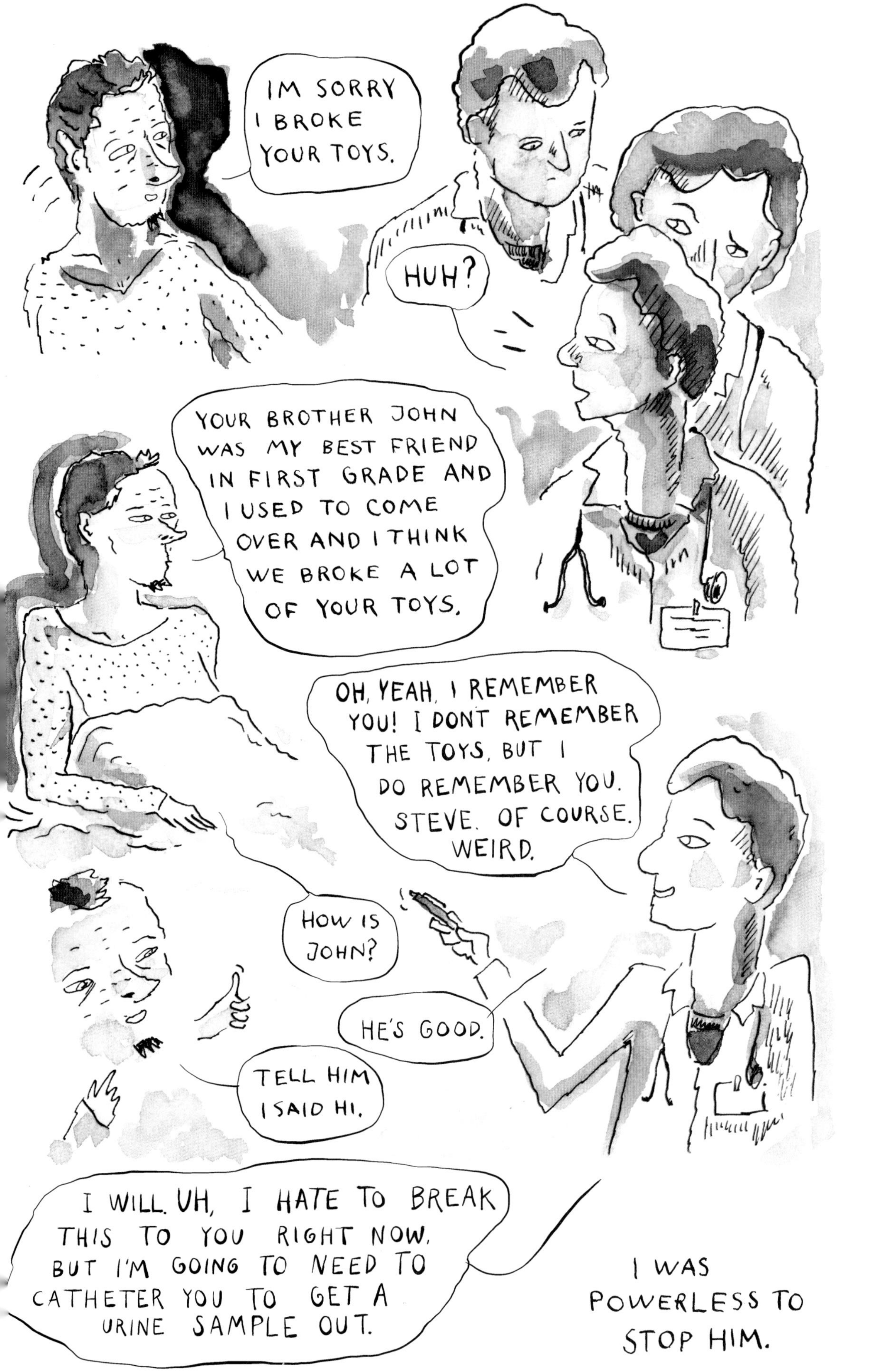
IM SORRY I BROKE YOUR TOYS.
HUH?
YOUR BROTHER JOHN WAS MY BEST FRIEND IN FIRST GRADE AND I USED TO COME OVER AND I THINK WE BROKE A LOT OF YOUR TOYS.
OH, YEAH, I REMEMBER YOU! I DONT REMEMBER THE TOYS, BUT I DO REMEMBER YOU. STEVE. OF COURSE. WEIRD.
HOW IS JOHN?
HE'S GOOD.
TELL HIM I SAID HI.
I WILL. UH, I HATE TO BREAK THIS TO YOU RIGHT NOW, BUT I'M GOING TO NEED TO CATHETER YOU TO GET A URINE SAMPLE OUT.
I WAS POWERLESS TO STOP HIM.

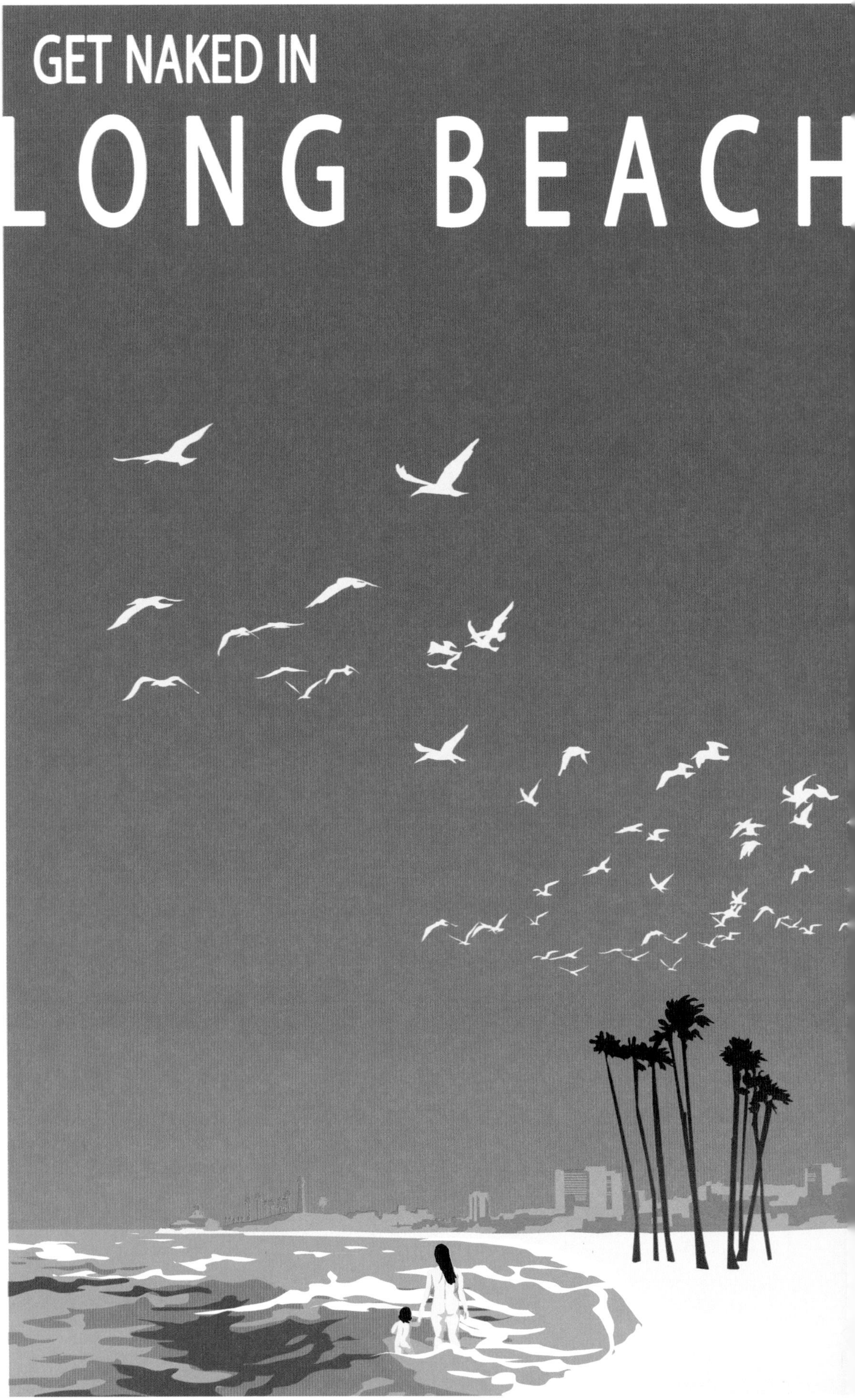
GET NAKED IN
LONG BEACH

I smelled like shit.

I'd showered. I'd put on clean clothes tumbled dry with Bounce fabric softener sheets. I'd brushed my teeth with Crest toothpaste and gargled with minty-septic Listerine mouthwash. I was wearing Axe deodorant and a light spritz of Hugo Boss cologne.

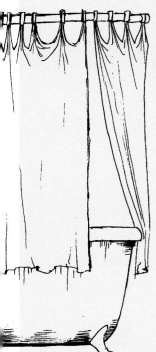
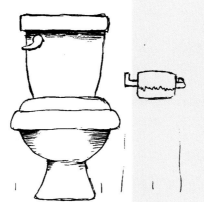
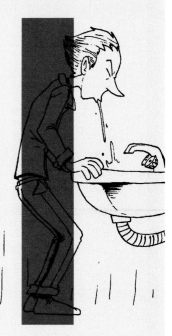

And yet, against that insurmountable ocean of unnatural, flavor-fueled fragrance, the predominant odor emanating from me was...   *shit.*

I only noticed this when I was steps away from the driver sent to take me to the Long Beach Airport for a five-plus hour flight to New York. There was no time to go back inside, and investigate. To probe the cause of the sudden fecal flora would be to miss my flight which was not an option.

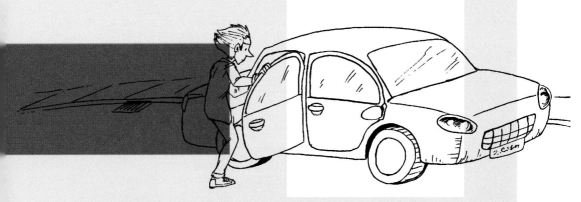

I had to climb in to the car knowing I smelled like a freshly fertilized lawn.

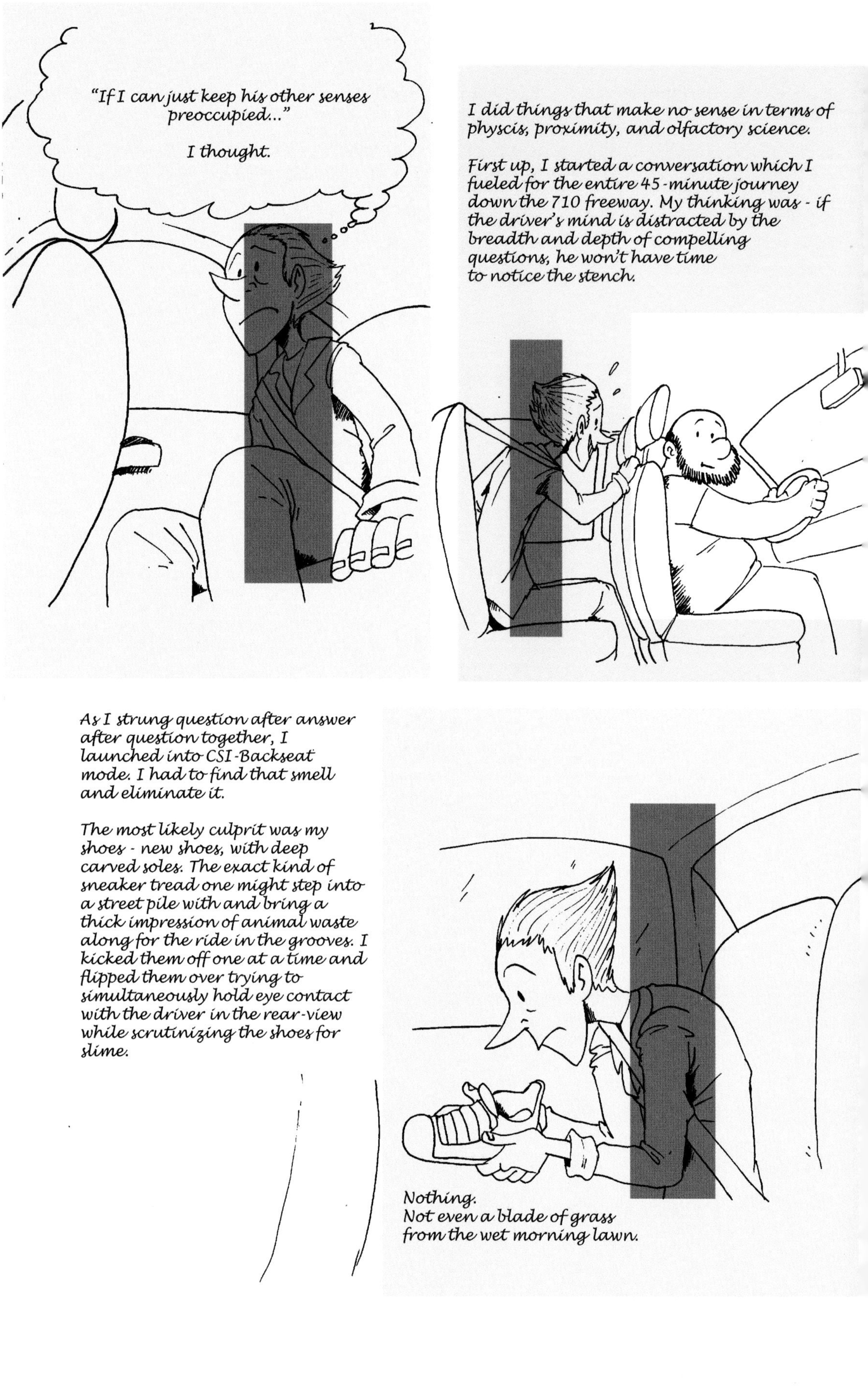

"If I can just keep his other senses preoccupied..."
I thought.
I did things that make no sense in terms of physcis, proximity, and olfactory science.
First up, I started a conversation which I fueled for the entire 45-minute journey down the 710 freeway. My thinking was - if the driver's mind is distracted by the breadth and depth of compelling questions, he won't have time to notice the stench.
As I strung question after answer after question together, I launched into CSI-Backseat mode. I had to find that smell and eliminate it.
The most likely culprit was my shoes - new shoes, with deep carved soles. The exact kind of sneaker tread one might step into a street pile with and bring a thick impression of animal waste along for the ride in the grooves. I kicked them off one at a time and flipped them over trying to simultaneously hold eye contact with the driver in the rear-view while scrutinizing the shoes for slime.
Nothing.
Not even a blade of grass from the wet morning lawn.

At the airport, I tipped the driver heavily - hazard pay - for not saying he smelt what I surely dealt. I bee-lined around the curb check-in cabbies and avoided all the human attendants.

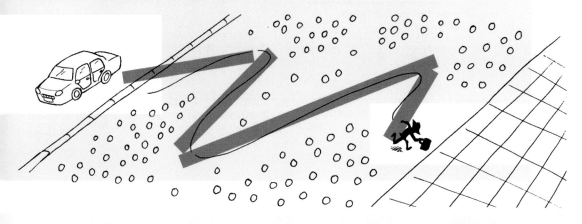

I stopped at the farthest Jet Blue self-check in kiosk. I tried to look confused as if to telegraph: "Don't get in line behind me! I have no idea what I'm doing! Keep your distance, 'cause I could be here for hours!"

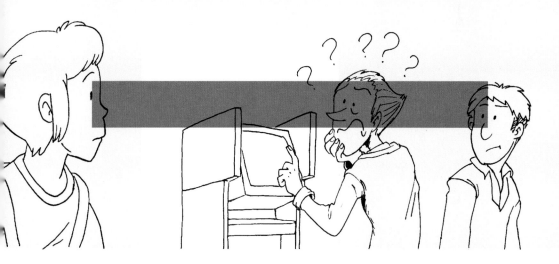

I inserted my credit card. "Did you step in something?" responded the screen.

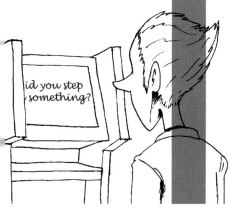

I broke into a cold sweat.

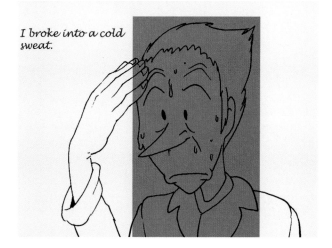

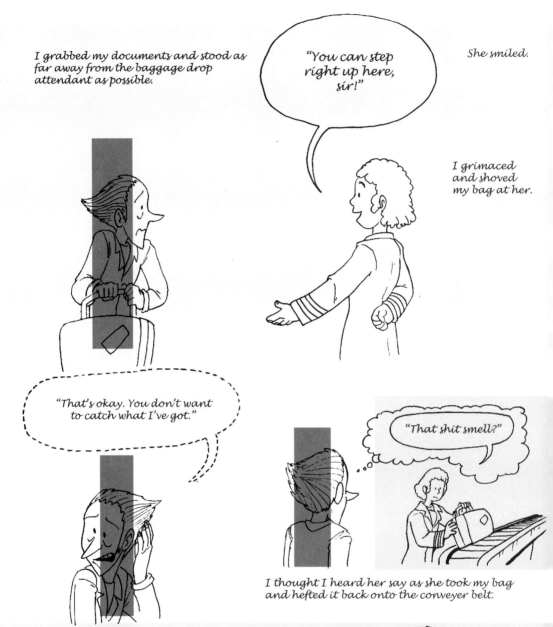

I grabbed my documents and stood as far away from the baggage drop attendant as possible.

"You can step right up here, sir!"

She smiled.

I grimaced and shoved my bag at her.

"That's okay. You don't want to catch what I've got."

"That shit smell?"

I thought I heard her say as she took my bag and hefted it back onto the conveyer belt.

I took off running.

If I weren't so panicked about the increasing likelihood that I had - unbeknownst to myself - crapped my pants, I would have paused and taken in the burnished beauty that is the Long Beach Airport. It's a later-period American Art Deco building. The kind of charming little fliery that populates movies of the 40s where New Yorkers make their way from the hustle of the east to the open air of the west.

And then they step in some shit and everything goes to hell.

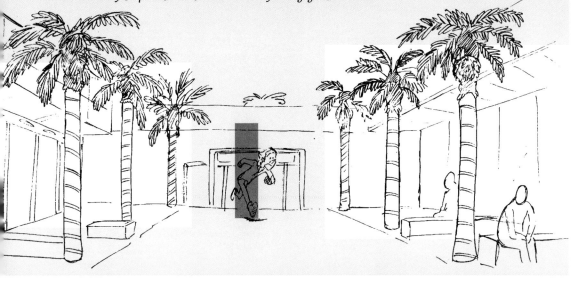

I made my way to the most out of the way men's room I could find - upstairs, south end by the restaurant. I took the most cloistered stall available - sided by a wall and a handicap crapper. Finally, sweet, sweet isolation.

If I couldn't locate and eradicate the offending smear of fecal fungus I'd somehow contracted between my shower and the forty foot walk to my shuttle I would be a pariah, an outcast - a literal shitbag on a plane. Making small talk with the passenger next to me.

"You live in Chicago?"
"I do, just outside of Oakbrook. And how about you? Did you sleep in a pit of human excrement?"

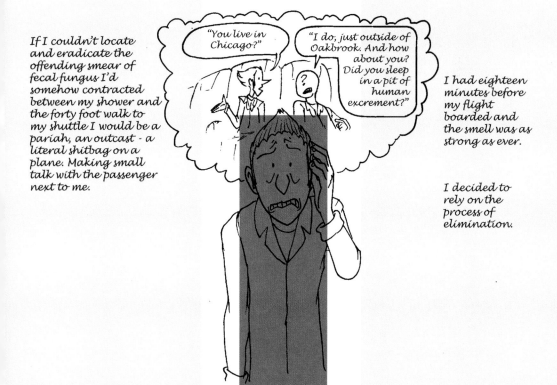

I had eighteen minutes before my flight boarded and the smell was as strong as ever.

I decided to rely on the process of elimination.

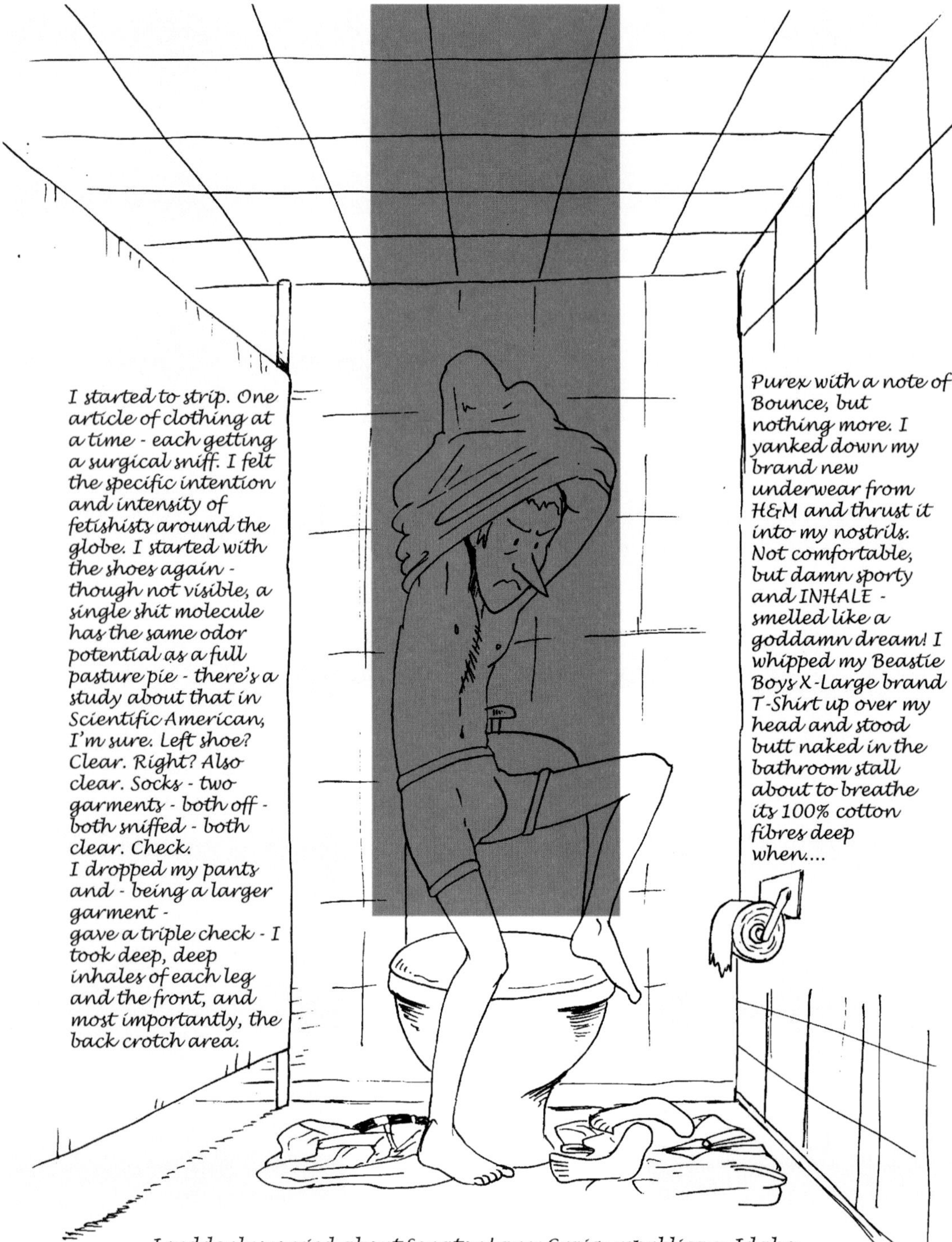
I started to strip. One article of clothing at a time - each getting a surgical sniff. I felt the specific intention and intensity of fetishists around the globe. I started with the shoes again - though not visible, a single shit molecule has the same odor potential as a full pasture pie - there's a study about that in Scientific American, I'm sure. Left shoe? Clear. Right? Also clear. Socks - two garments - both off - both sniffed - both clear. Check.
I dropped my pants and - being a larger garment - gave a triple check - I took deep, deep inhales of each leg and the front, and most importantly, the back crotch area.
Purex with a note of Bounce, but nothing more. I yanked down my brand new underwear from H&M and thrust it into my nostrils. Not comfortable, but damn sporty and INHALE - smelled like a goddamn dream! I whipped my Beastie Boys X-Large brand T-Shirt up over my head and stood butt naked in the bathroom stall about to breathe its 100% cotton fibres deep when....

I suddenly worried about Senator Larry Craig, republican, Idaho.

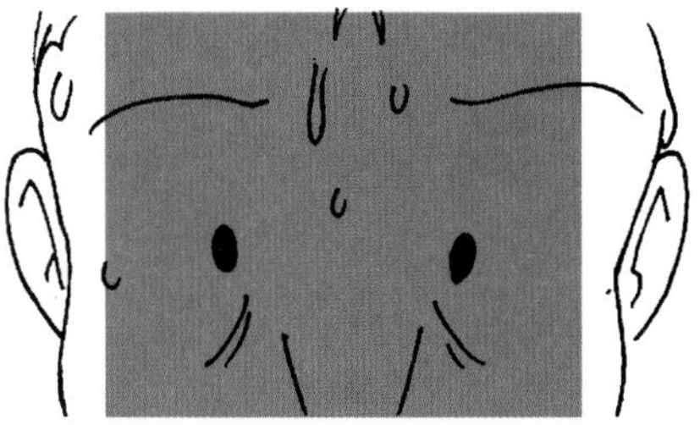

Not so much worried about him, as worried about what had happened to him in a public toilet.

The senator - by the media's account - was in a men's room at the Minneapolis/St. Paul International Airport and he - his foot - jittered like - you know - as if he were practicing quickstep.

Was it nerves? A mild palsy? The onset of Parkinson's so bravely championed by Michael J Fox? We would understand and accept any of those.

But the senator's hand was dangling. Sitting on a toilet, your hands are kind of - "where do we go?" When you're a kid, a male kid, you need at least one hand to keep your then short buddy from pissing straight out and dowsing the door of the stall. As teenagers, many of us try this just to see if it will make it that far.

It does.

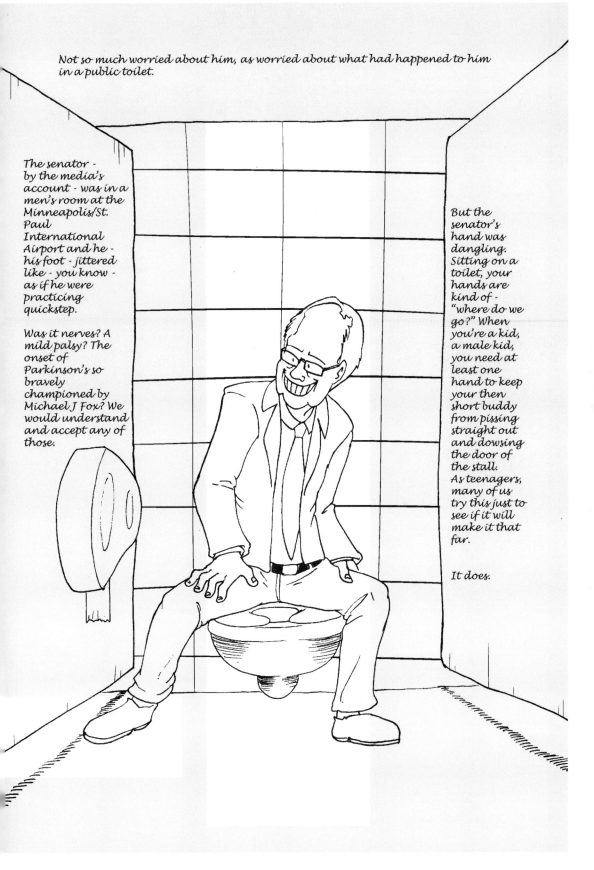

The Senator was tapping and then his hand stretched down. Not only dangling, but by accounts of subsequent police reports, moving up under the adjacent stall. It was a thing of Congress at that time to just invade the space of others and apparently, latrines were included in the war initiative.

The senator, not knowing an officer of the law trained to pick up on solicitations of homosexual sex in aiport men's rooms, had intercepted the tapping and interpreted it as bathroom Morse code for:

"Hey, how'd you like to mile-high club? You know, minus the mile?"

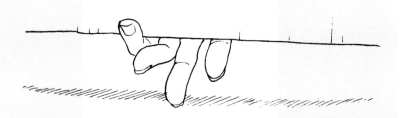

If tapping and arm dragging could result in the termination of a Congressional career, what would be the penalty for full-on nudity?

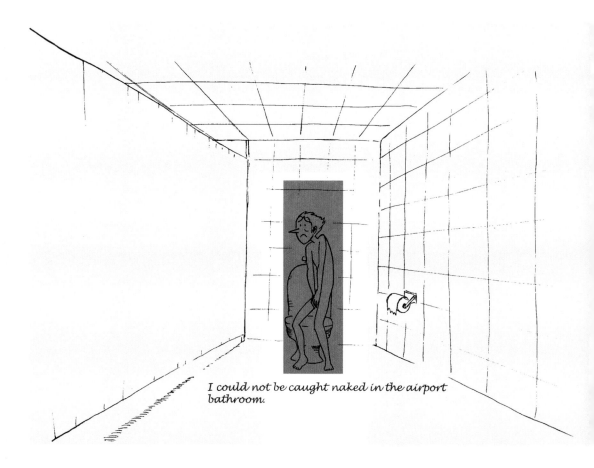

I could not be caught naked in the airport bathroom.

I smelled the shirt.

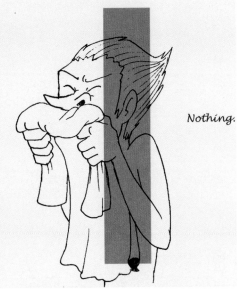

Nothing.

I sniffed my skin to the degree possible - pits, arms, legs, the U-turn...

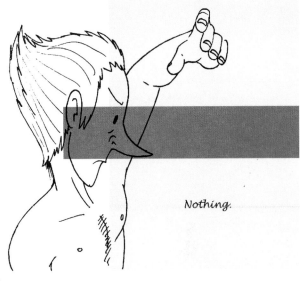

Nothing.

I pulled my clothes back on and grimly accepted that wherever the smell was hiding, it was in deep cover that Navy Seals couldn't extract.

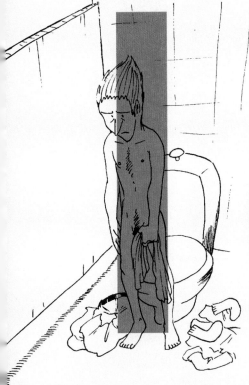

As a child I was haunted by the Dr. Seuss story The Pale Green Pants. A young kid is stalked by a pair of disembodied pants in a pea-soup shade. They're always creeping up on him and he's terrified by their unholy presence. He resolves this phobia by befriending the satanic garments as only a Suess protagonist could. I always thought the story must be methaphorical. I now realize it was - for an untraceable shit molecule with the full explosive force of its source material.

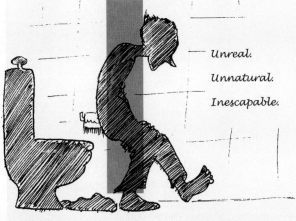

Unreal.

Unnatural.

Inescapable.

I boarded the plane.

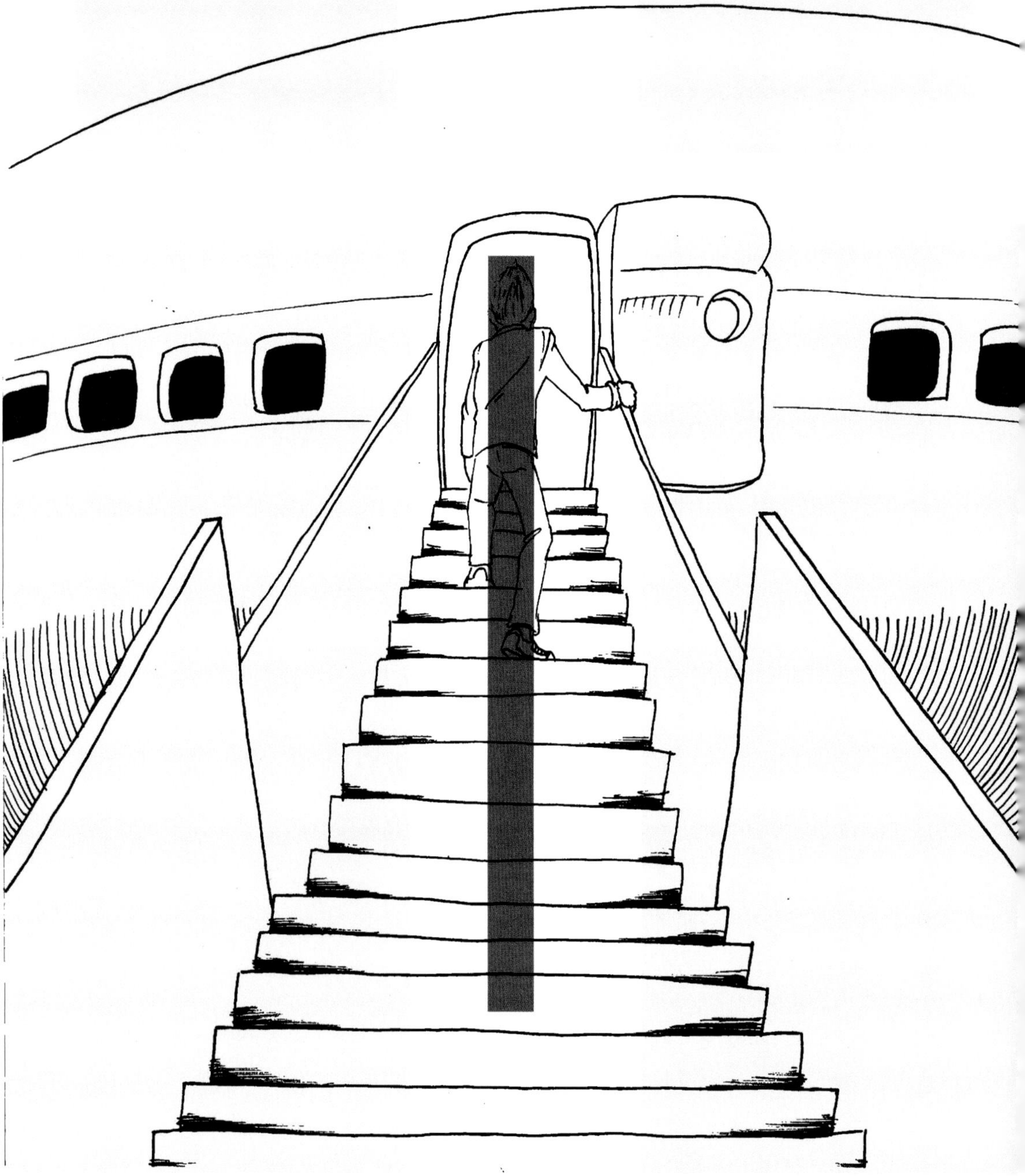

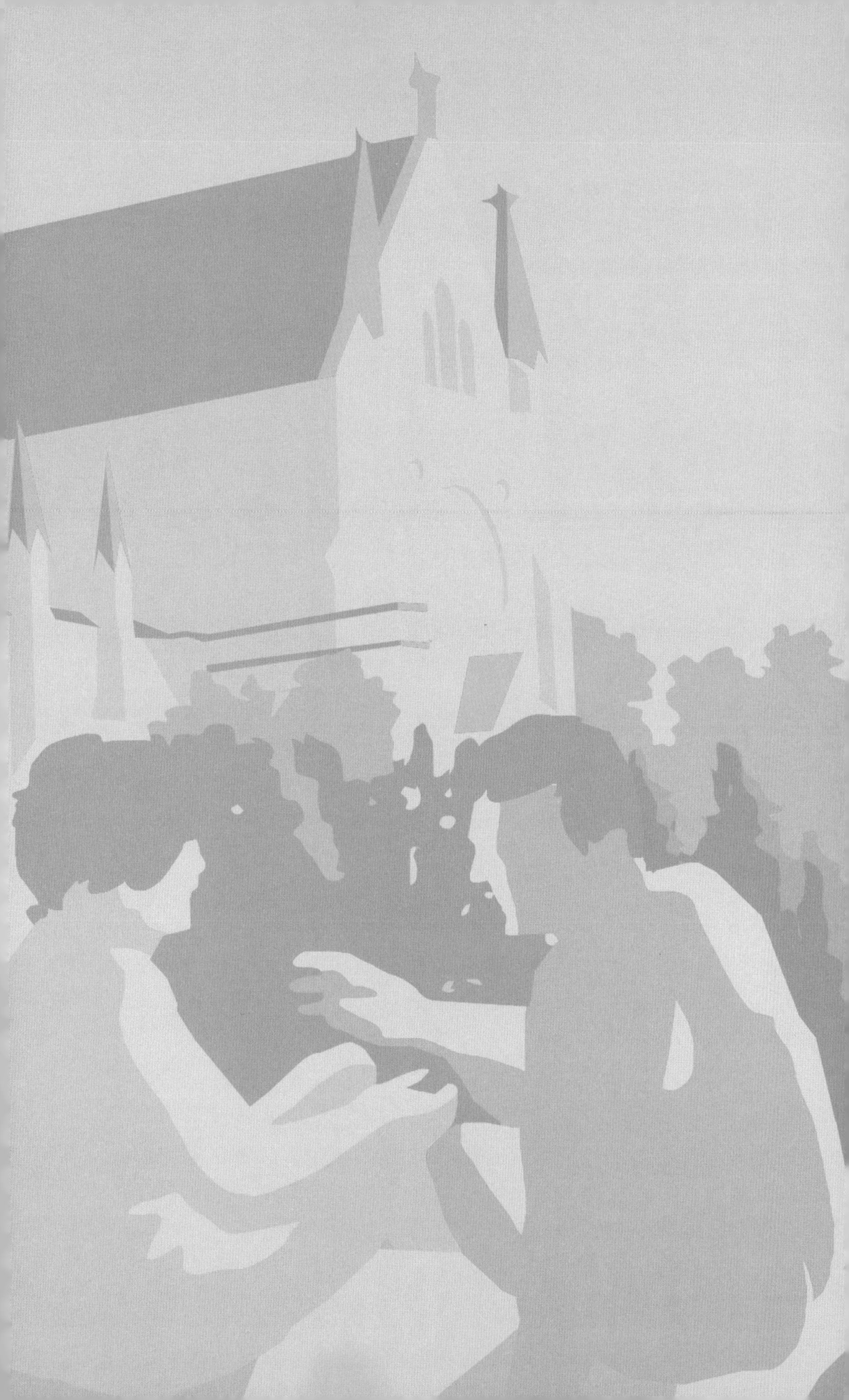

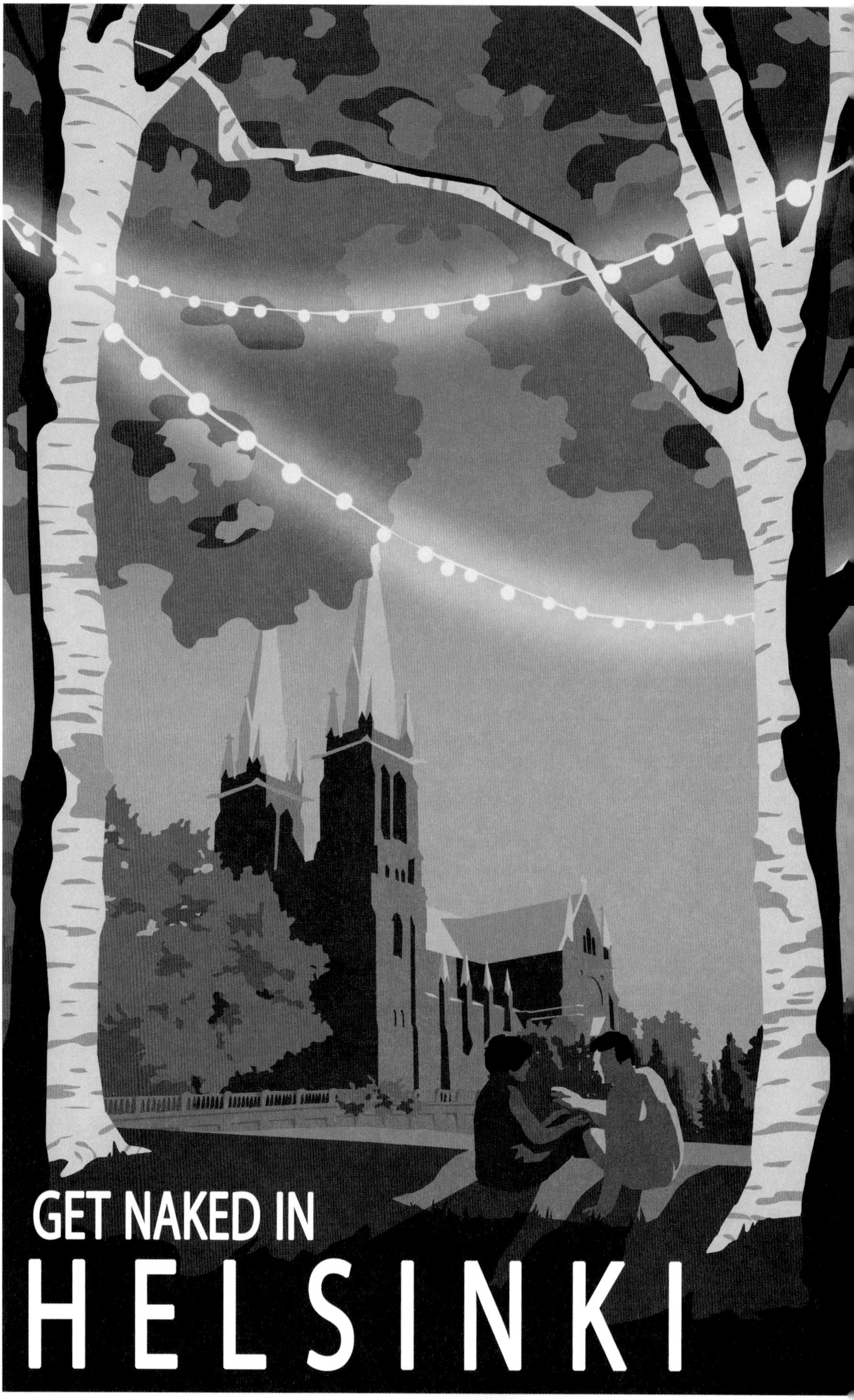
GET NAKED IN
HELSINKI

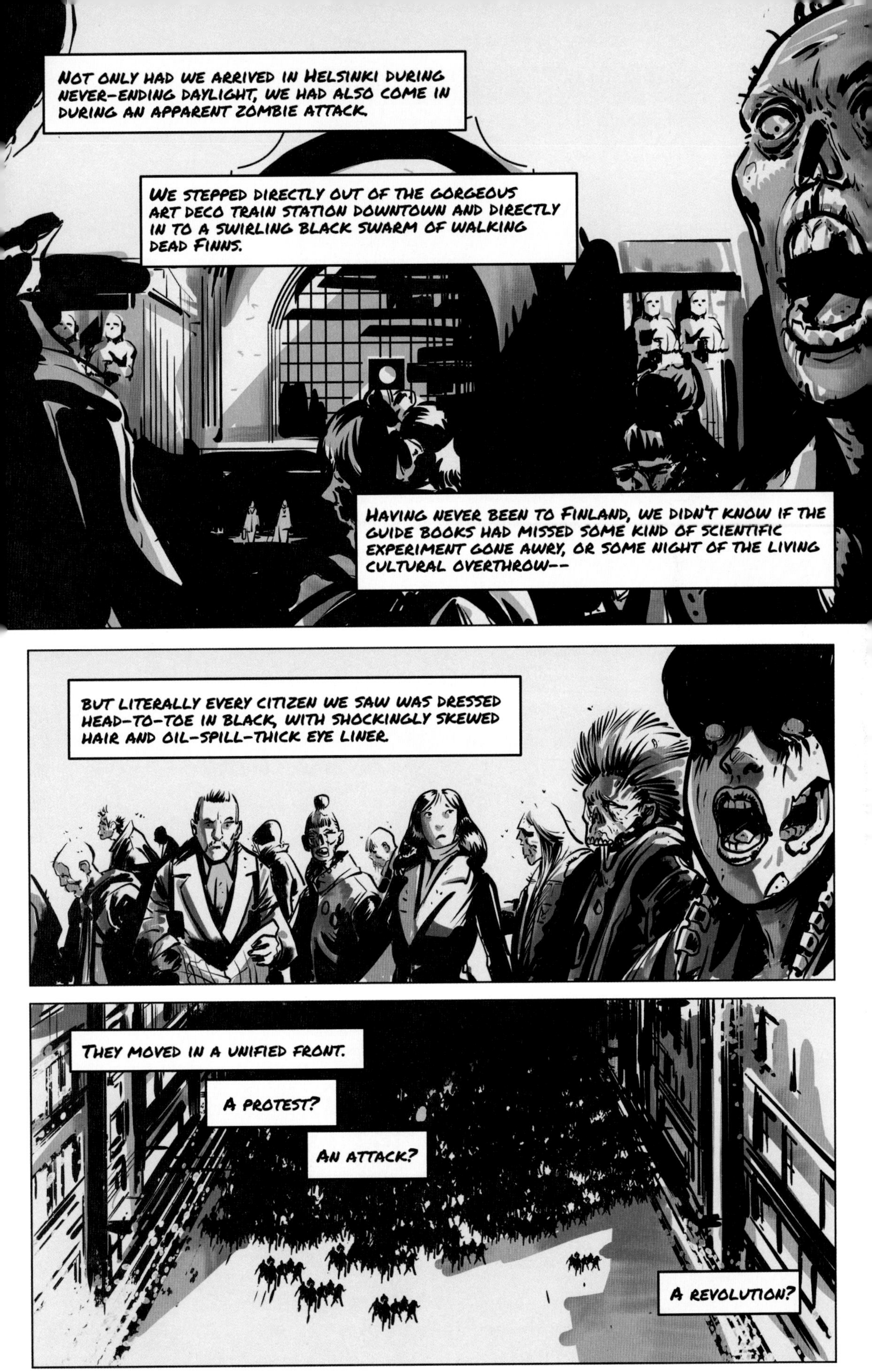
NOT ONLY HAD WE ARRIVED IN HELSINKI DURING NEVER-ENDING DAYLIGHT, WE HAD ALSO COME IN DURING AN APPARENT ZOMBIE ATTACK.
WE STEPPED DIRECTLY OUT OF THE GORGEOUS ART DECO TRAIN STATION DOWNTOWN AND DIRECTLY IN TO A SWIRLING BLACK SWARM OF WALKING DEAD FINNS.
HAVING NEVER BEEN TO FINLAND, WE DIDN'T KNOW IF THE GUIDE BOOKS HAD MISSED SOME KIND OF SCIENTIFIC EXPERIMENT GONE AWRY, OR SOME NIGHT OF THE LIVING CULTURAL OVERTHROW--
BUT LITERALLY EVERY CITIZEN WE SAW WAS DRESSED HEAD-TO-TOE IN BLACK, WITH SHOCKINGLY SKEWED HAIR AND OIL-SPILL-THICK EYE LINER.
THEY MOVED IN A UNIFIED FRONT.
A PROTEST?
AN ATTACK?
A REVOLUTION?

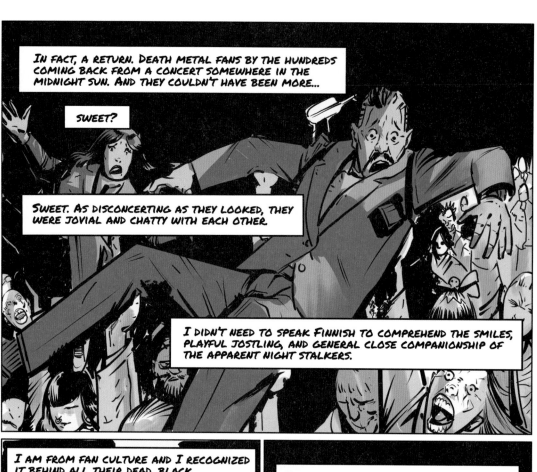

IN FACT, A RETURN. DEATH METAL FANS BY THE HUNDREDS COMING BACK FROM A CONCERT SOMEWHERE IN THE MIDNIGHT SUN. AND THEY COULDN'T HAVE BEEN MORE...

SWEET?

SWEET. AS DISCONCERTING AS THEY LOOKED, THEY WERE JOVIAL AND CHATTY WITH EACH OTHER.

I DIDN'T NEED TO SPEAK FINNISH TO COMPREHEND THE SMILES, PLAYFUL JOSTLING, AND GENERAL CLOSE COMPANIONSHIP OF THE APPARENT NIGHT STALKERS.

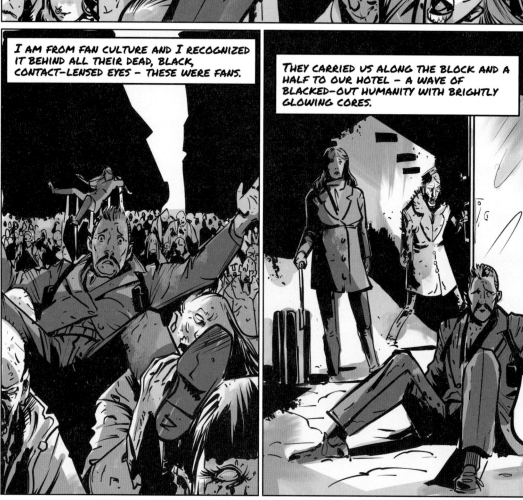

I AM FROM FAN CULTURE AND I RECOGNIZED IT BEHIND ALL THEIR DEAD, BLACK, CONTACT-LENSED EYES – THESE WERE FANS.

THEY CARRIED US ALONG THE BLOCK AND A HALF TO OUR HOTEL – A WAVE OF BLACKED-OUT HUMANITY WITH BRIGHTLY GLOWING CORES.

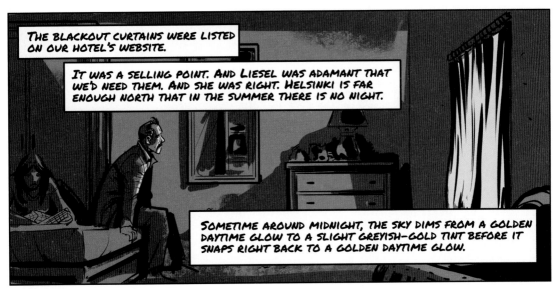

The blackout curtains were listed on our hotel's website.

It was a selling point. And Liesel was adamant that we'd need them. And she was right. Helsinki is far enough north that in the summer there is no night.

Sometime around midnight, the sky dims from a golden daytime glow to a slight greyish-gold tint before it snaps right back to a golden daytime glow.

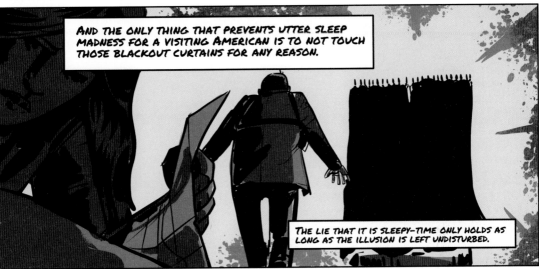

And the only thing that prevents utter sleep madness for a visiting American is to not touch those blackout curtains for any reason.

The lie that it is sleepy-time only holds as long as the illusion is left undisturbed.

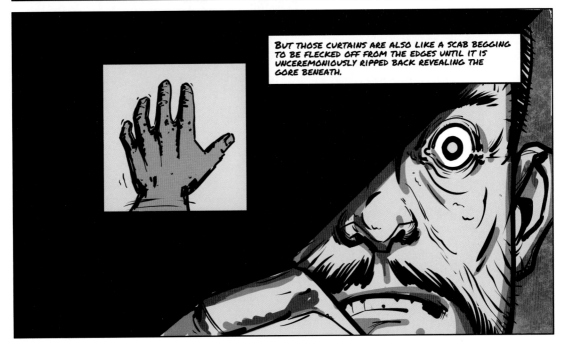

But those curtains are also like a scab begging to be flecked off from the edges until it is unceremoniously ripped back revealing the gore beneath.

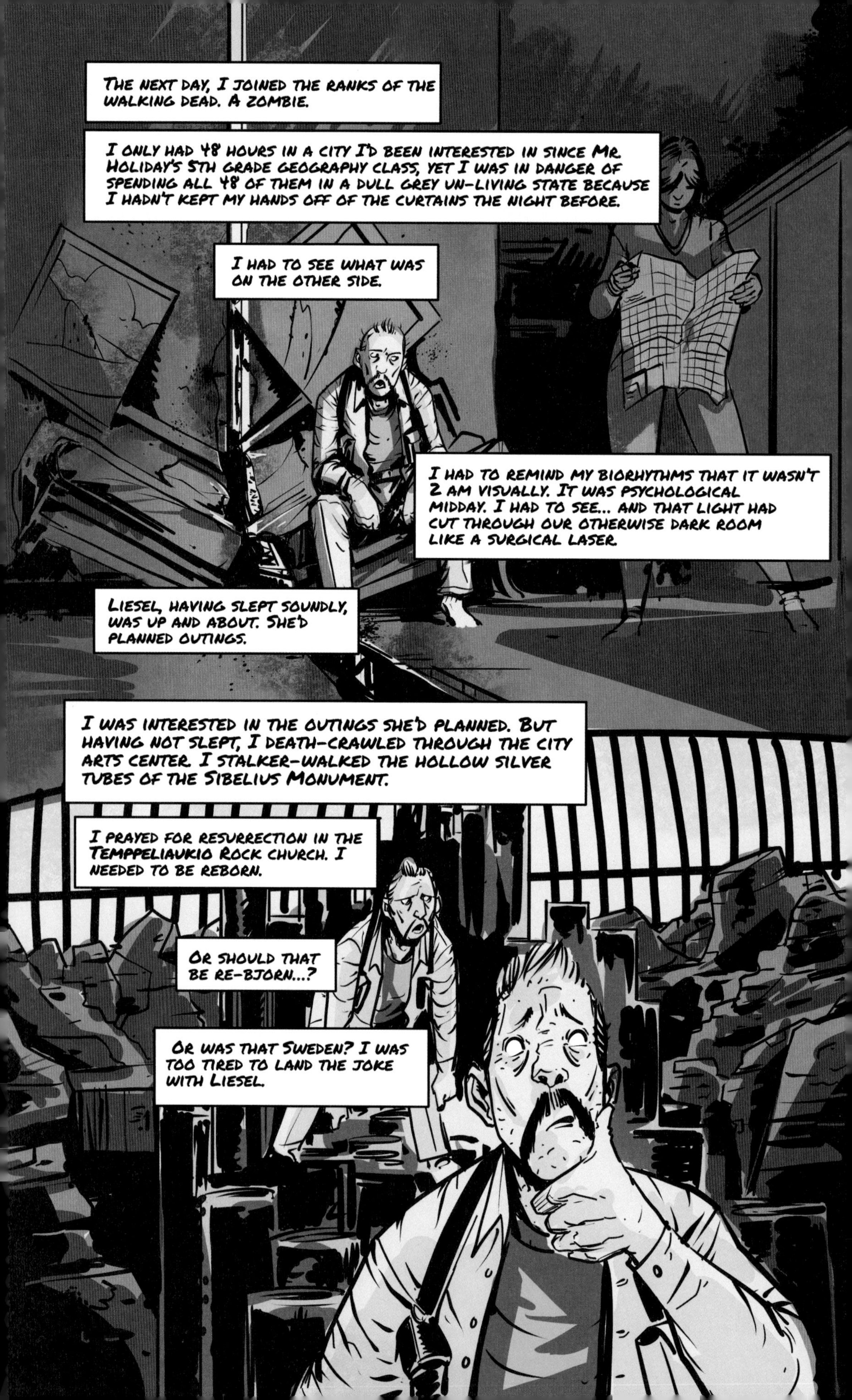
The next day, I joined the ranks of the walking dead. A zombie.
I only had 48 hours in a city I'd been interested in since Mr. Holiday's 5th grade geography class, yet I was in danger of spending all 48 of them in a dull grey un-living state because I hadn't kept my hands off of the curtains the night before.
I had to see what was on the other side.
I had to remind my biorhythms that it wasn't 2 am visually. It was psychological midday. I had to see... and that light had cut through our otherwise dark room like a surgical laser.
Liesel, having slept soundly, was up and about. She'd planned outings.
I was interested in the outings she'd planned. But having not slept, I death-crawled through the city arts center. I stalker-walked the hollow silver tubes of the Sibelius Monument.
I prayed for resurrection in the Temppeliaukio Rock church. I needed to be reborn.
Or should that be re-bjorn...?
Or was that Sweden? I was too tired to land the joke with Liesel.

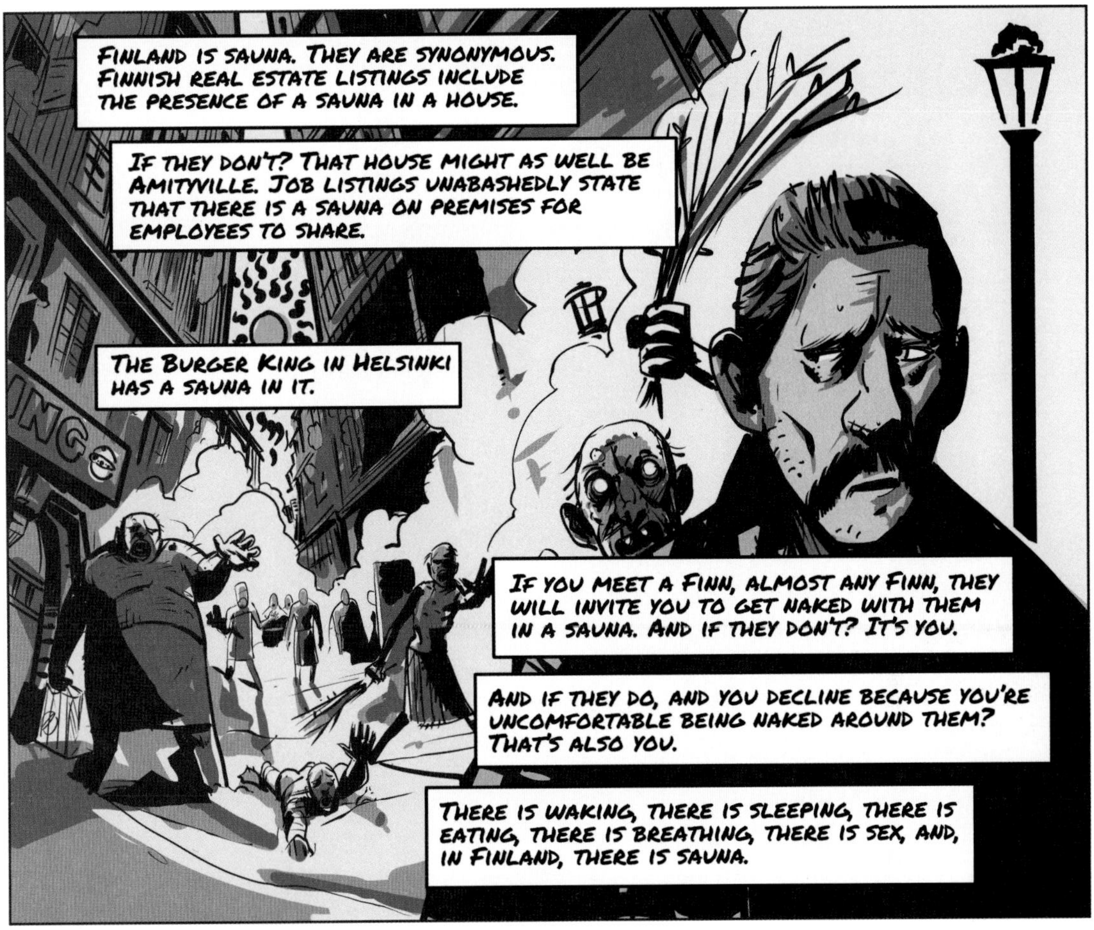
Finland is sauna. They are synonymous. Finnish real estate listings include the presence of a sauna in a house.
If they don't? That house might as well be Amityville. Job listings unabashedly state that there is a sauna on premises for employees to share.
The Burger King in Helsinki has a sauna in it.
If you meet a Finn, almost any Finn, they will invite you to get naked with them in a sauna. And if they don't? It's you.
And if they do, and you decline because you're uncomfortable being naked around them? That's also you.
There is waking, there is sleeping, there is eating, there is breathing, there is sex, and, in Finland, there is sauna.

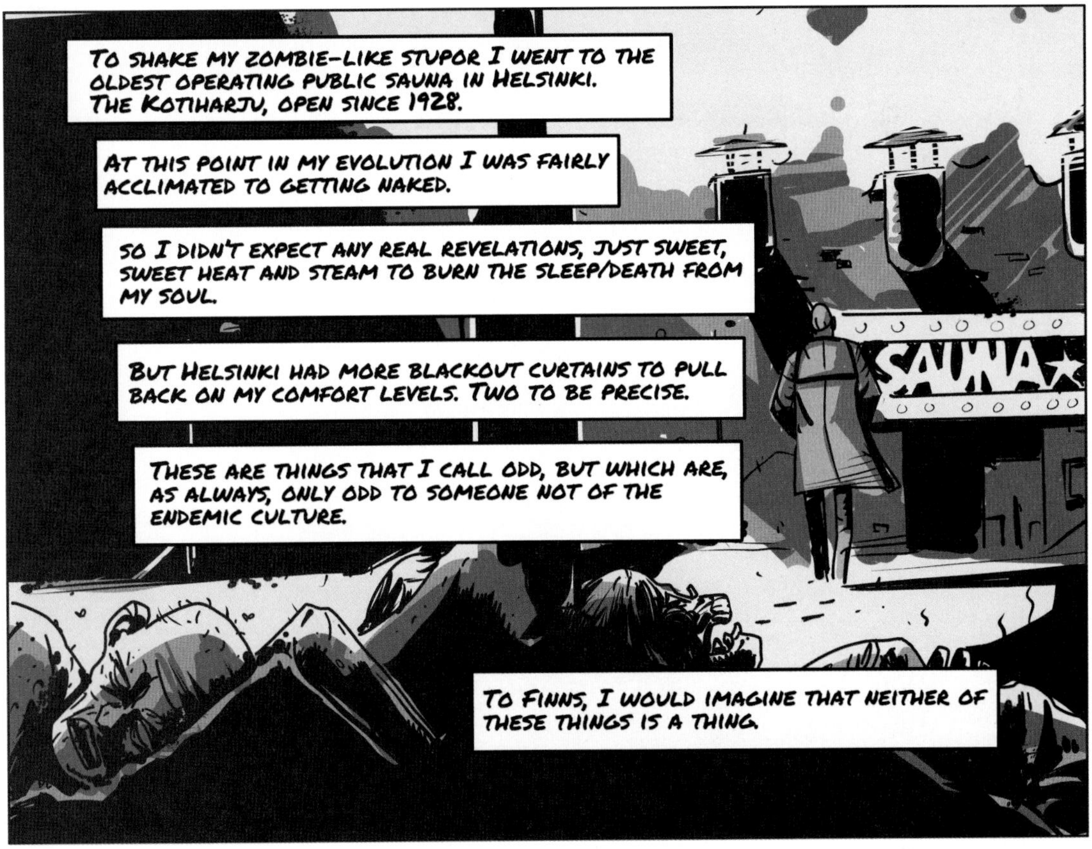
To shake my zombie-like stupor I went to the oldest operating public sauna in Helsinki. The Kotiharju, open since 1928.
At this point in my evolution I was fairly acclimated to getting naked.
so I didn't expect any real revelations, just sweet, sweet heat and steam to burn the sleep/death from my soul.
But Helsinki had more blackout curtains to pull back on my comfort levels. Two to be precise.
These are things that I call odd, but which are, as always, only odd to someone not of the endemic culture.
SAUNA
To Finns, I would imagine that neither of these things is a thing.

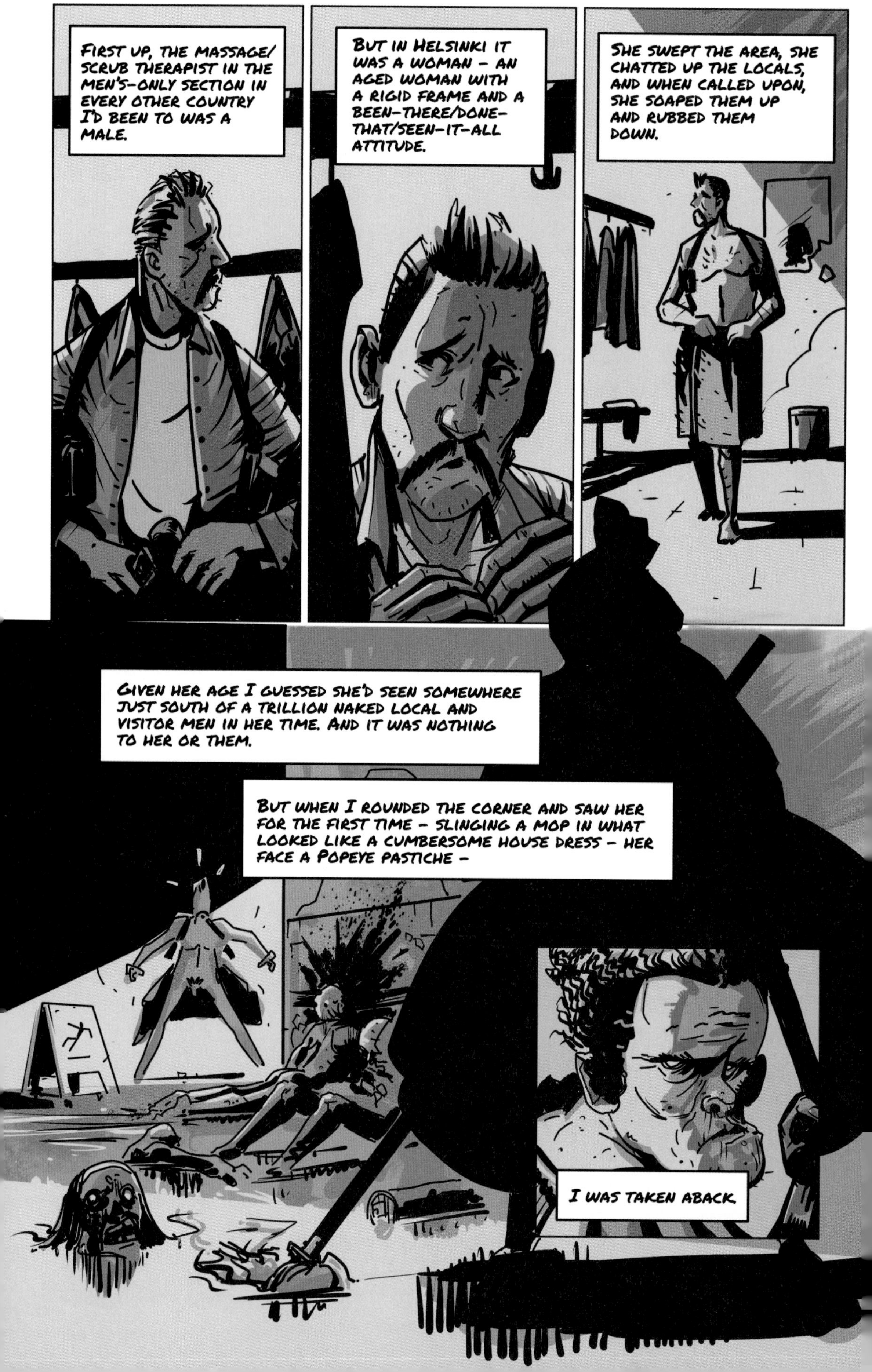
FIRST UP, THE MASSAGE/ SCRUB THERAPIST IN THE MEN'S-ONLY SECTION IN EVERY OTHER COUNTRY I'D BEEN TO WAS A MALE.
BUT IN HELSINKI IT WAS A WOMAN – AN AGED WOMAN WITH A RIGID FRAME AND A BEEN-THERE/DONE-THAT/SEEN-IT-ALL ATTITUDE.
SHE SWEPT THE AREA, SHE CHATTED UP THE LOCALS, AND WHEN CALLED UPON, SHE SOAPED THEM UP AND RUBBED THEM DOWN.
GIVEN HER AGE I GUESSED SHE'D SEEN SOMEWHERE JUST SOUTH OF A TRILLION NAKED LOCAL AND VISITOR MEN IN HER TIME. AND IT WAS NOTHING TO HER OR THEM.
BUT WHEN I ROUNDED THE CORNER AND SAW HER FOR THE FIRST TIME – SLINGING A MOP IN WHAT LOOKED LIKE A CUMBERSOME HOUSE DRESS – HER FACE A POPEYE PASTICHE –
I WAS TAKEN ABACK.

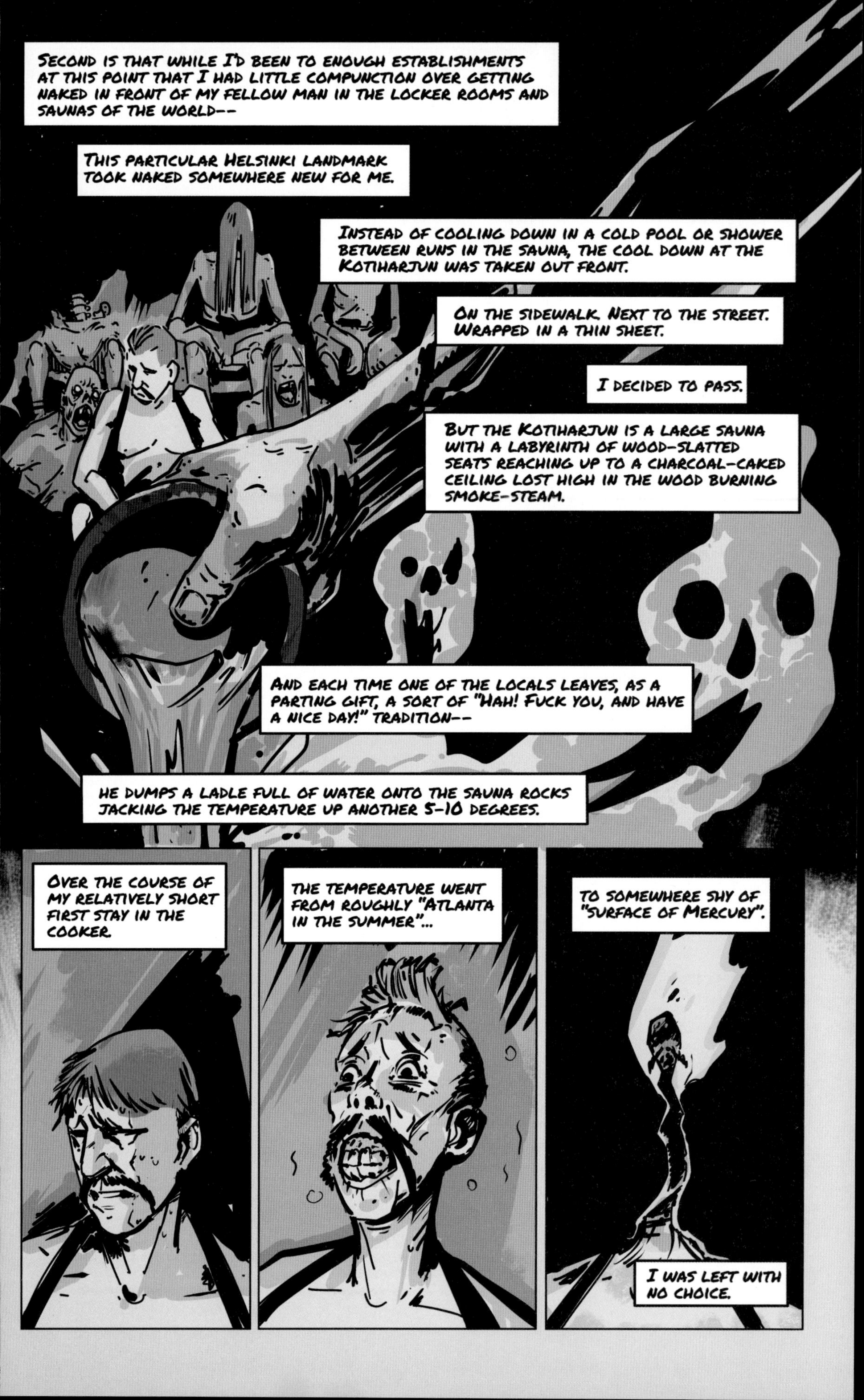

SECOND IS THAT WHILE I'D BEEN TO ENOUGH ESTABLISHMENTS AT THIS POINT THAT I HAD LITTLE COMPUNCTION OVER GETTING NAKED IN FRONT OF MY FELLOW MAN IN THE LOCKER ROOMS AND SAUNAS OF THE WORLD--

THIS PARTICULAR HELSINKI LANDMARK TOOK NAKED SOMEWHERE NEW FOR ME.

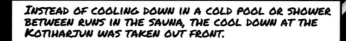

INSTEAD OF COOLING DOWN IN A COLD POOL OR SHOWER BETWEEN RUNS IN THE SAUNA, THE COOL DOWN AT THE KOTIHARJUN WAS TAKEN OUT FRONT.

ON THE SIDEWALK. NEXT TO THE STREET. WRAPPED IN A THIN SHEET.

I DECIDED TO PASS.

BUT THE KOTIHARJUN IS A LARGE SAUNA WITH A LABYRINTH OF WOOD-SLATTED SEATS REACHING UP TO A CHARCOAL-CAKED CEILING LOST HIGH IN THE WOOD BURNING SMOKE-STEAM.

AND EACH TIME ONE OF THE LOCALS LEAVES, AS A PARTING GIFT, A SORT OF "HAH! FUCK YOU, AND HAVE A NICE DAY!" TRADITION--

HE DUMPS A LADLE FULL OF WATER ONTO THE SAUNA ROCKS JACKING THE TEMPERATURE UP ANOTHER 5-10 DEGREES.

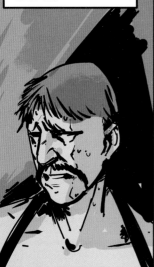

OVER THE COURSE OF MY RELATIVELY SHORT FIRST STAY IN THE COOKER

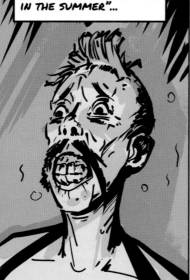

THE TEMPERATURE WENT FROM ROUGHLY "ATLANTA IN THE SUMMER"...

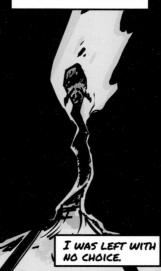

TO SOMEWHERE SHY OF "SURFACE OF MERCURY".

I WAS LEFT WITH NO CHOICE.

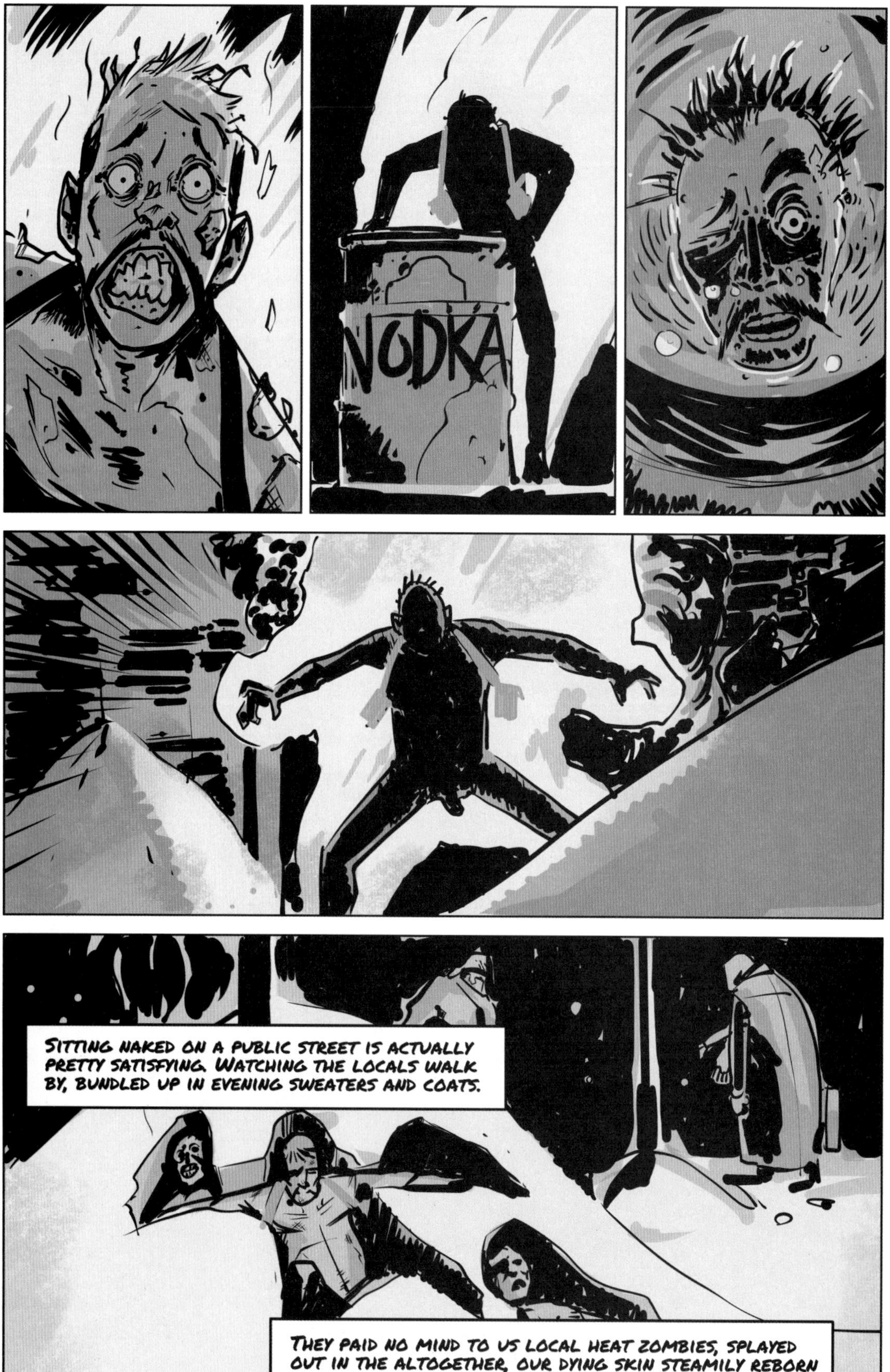
VODKA
SITTING NAKED ON A PUBLIC STREET IS ACTUALLY PRETTY SATISFYING. WATCHING THE LOCALS WALK BY, BUNDLED UP IN EVENING SWEATERS AND COATS.
THEY PAID NO MIND TO US LOCAL HEAT ZOMBIES, SPLAYED OUT IN THE ALTOGETHER, OUR DYING SKIN STEAMILY REBORN IN THE NEVER-SETTING SUN.

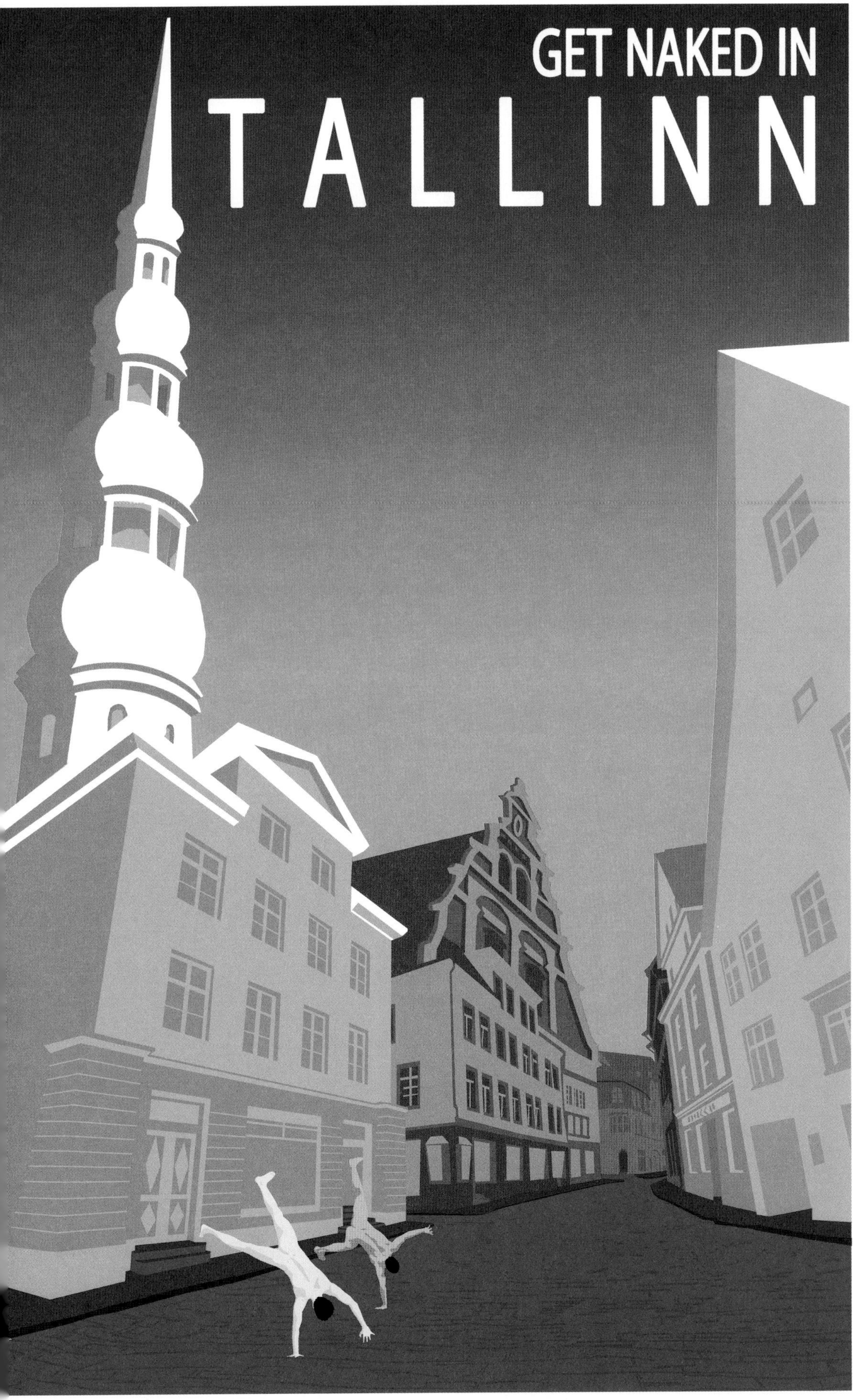
GET NAKED IN
TALLINN

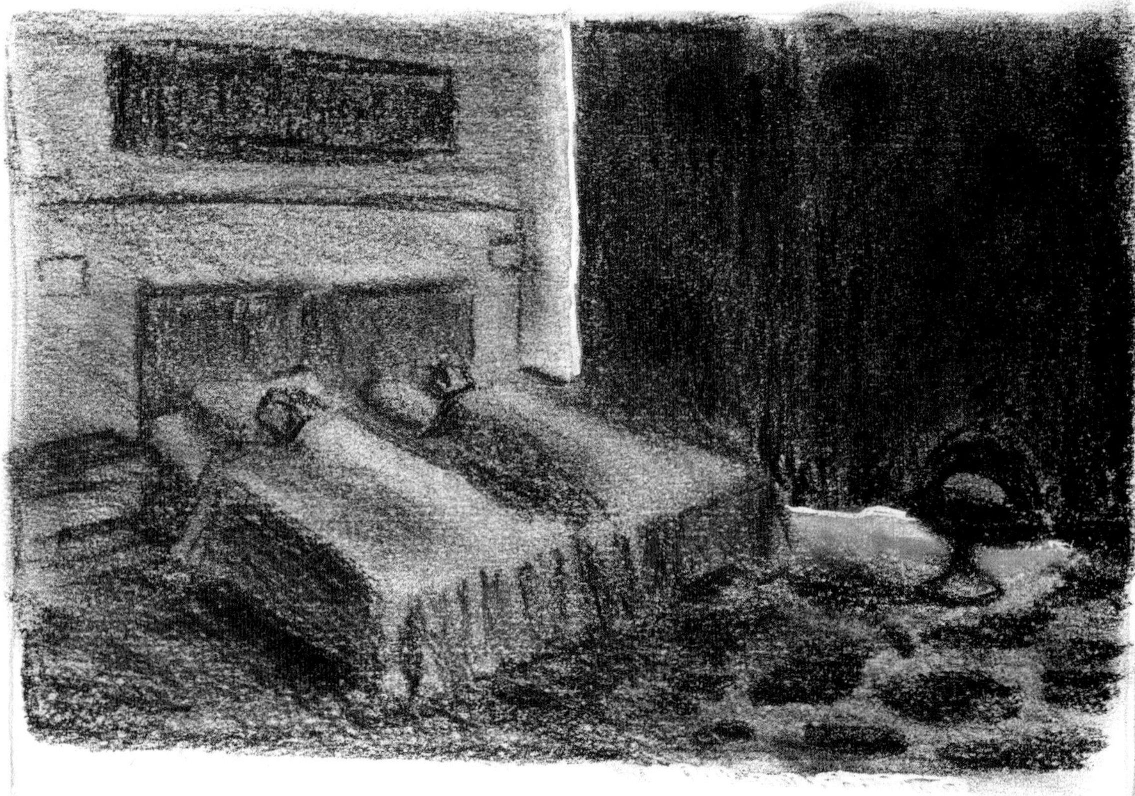

THE BLACKOUT CURTAINS LEAKED LIGHT. THE CURTAINS THEMSELVES WERE LIKE THE MEDICAL APRON A DENTIST DRAPES OVER YOUR TESTICLES TO KEEP THE SPERM SWIMMING WHEN YOU GET AN X-RAY OF YOUR MOLARS. BUT THE ENGINEERING STOPPED AT THE PERIPHERY OF THE WINDOW AND LIGHT CAME AROUND THE EDGES LIKE A TV SCREEN THAT HASN'T FINISHED SHUTTING OFF ALL THE WAY.

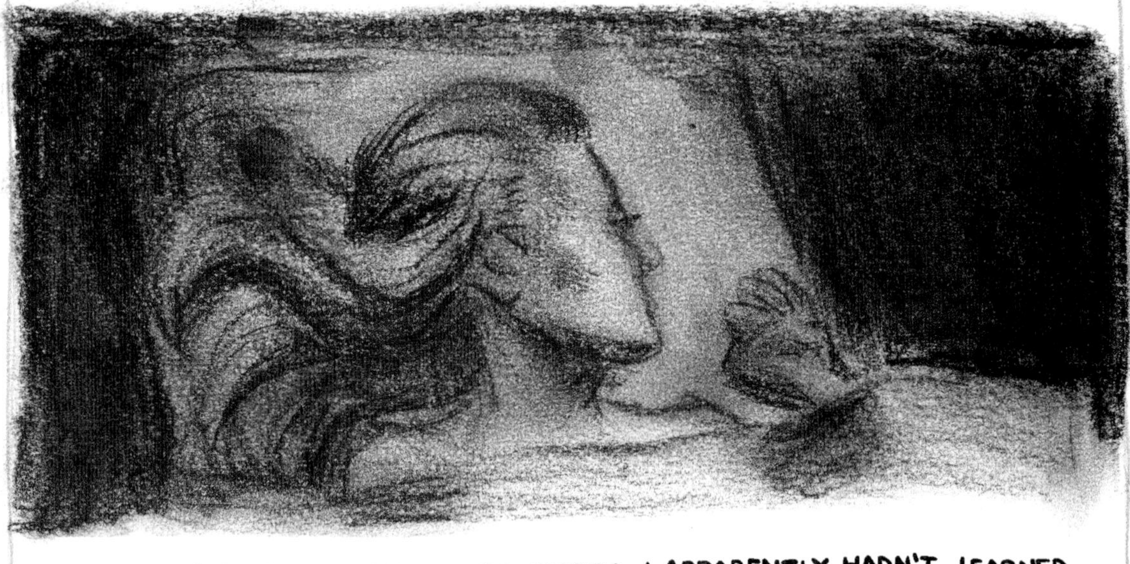

THE DRAPES LEFT A JARRING PENUMBRA. I APPARENTLY HADN'T LEARNED MY LESSON FROM FINLAND, AND DRAGGED MY NAKED ASS OUT OF OUR HOTEL BED IN TALLINN, ESTONIA TO DO SOMETHING I SHOULD NEVER HAVE DONE. I PULLED BACK THE CURTAIN SLIGHTLY TO PEER OUT.

AT FOUR IN THE MORNING THE DOCKSIDE WAS ABUZZ. MOST OF THE ACTIVITY LOOKED TO BE LONGSHOREMEN DOING EARLY PREP ON INCOMING SHIPS - FISH, CARGO, FERRIES FULL OF CARS.

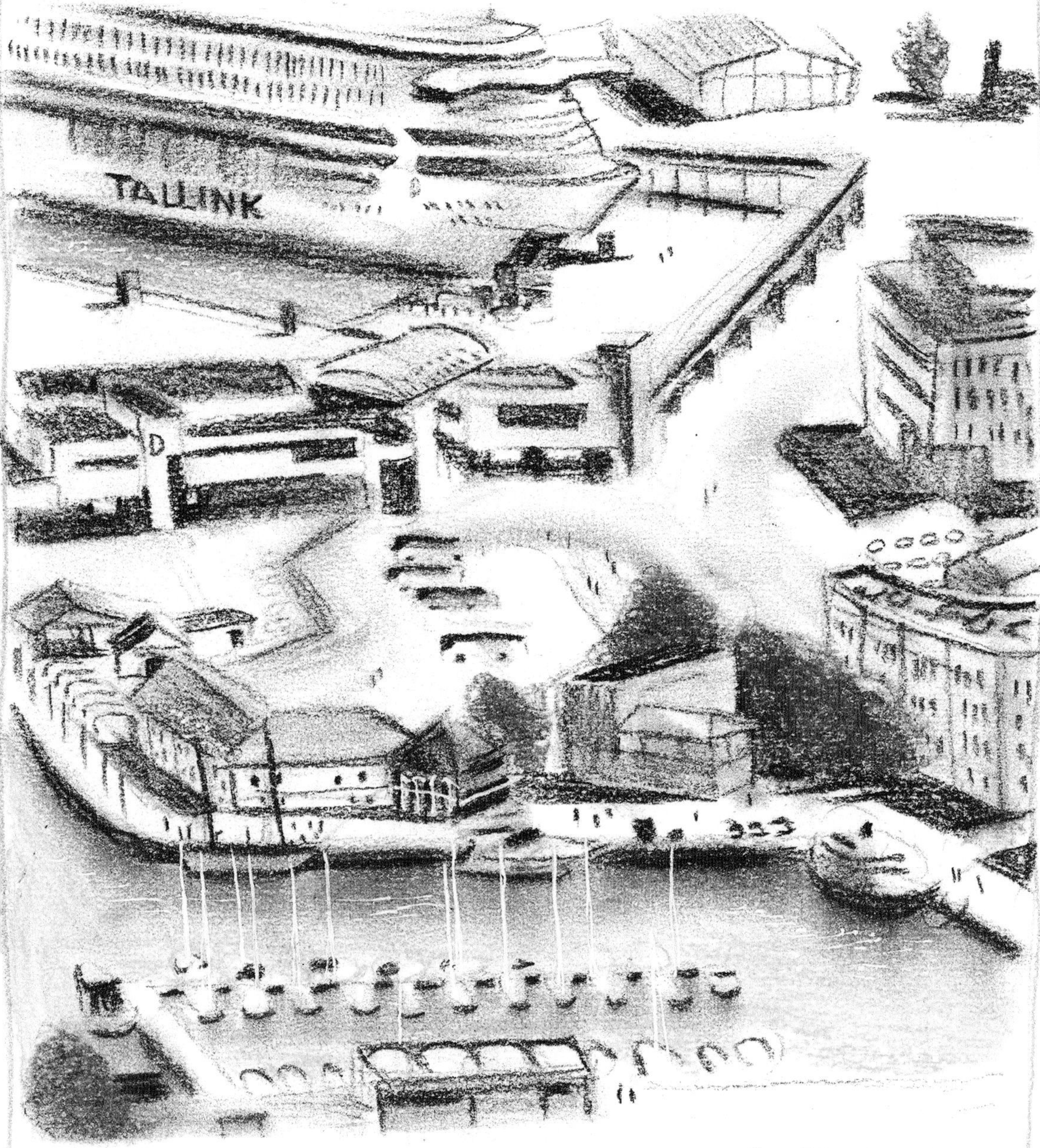
TALLINK

BUT THERE WERE ALSO PLENTY OF "SLEEPWALKERS" - PEOPLE WHO, LIKE ME, WERE CONFUSED BY THE FULL SUN RADIATING IN THE NIGHT SKY. THEY WERE SMOKING, DANCING, DRINKING, HANGING LOOSE IN SOME SOMNAMBULIST SLEEP HANGOVER THAT LASTED HALF A YEAR UNTIL A SIX-MONTH-SLUMBER TOOK OVER AND BALANCED OUT THEIR BIORHYTHMIC CALENDARS.

"...WHAT ARE YOU DOING?" LIESEL WOKE UP. UNDERSTANDABLY - THAT RAZOR-THIN SLIT OF THE PEELED - BACK CURTAIN CUT A LASER—SHARP BAND OF PURE LIGHT ACROSS THE CENTER OF OUR HOTEL ROOM.

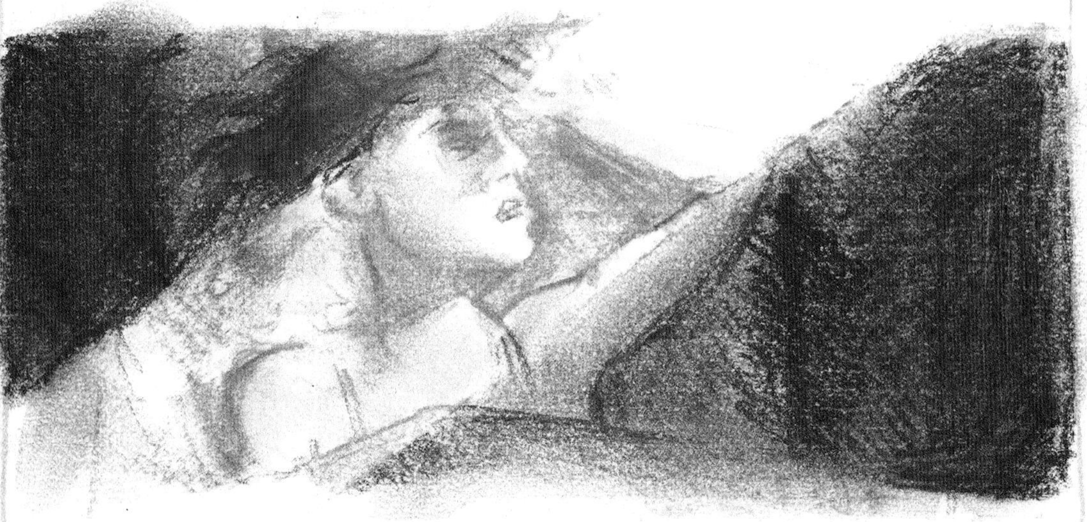

"IT'S BRIGHT OUTSIDE. EVEN AT 4AM." SHE ROLLED OVER WITH A MILD EXASPERATION. "I'M PRETTY SURE WE KNEW THAT. COME BACK TO BED." I DID, BUT THE JIG WAS UP. THESE WERE FALSE SHADOWS. THIS WAS A CONSPIRED "NIGHT". I STAYED AWAKE UNTIL THE CLOCK IN THE ROOM CAUGHT UP WITH THE AMOUNT OF ILLUMINATION OUTSIDE OF IT.

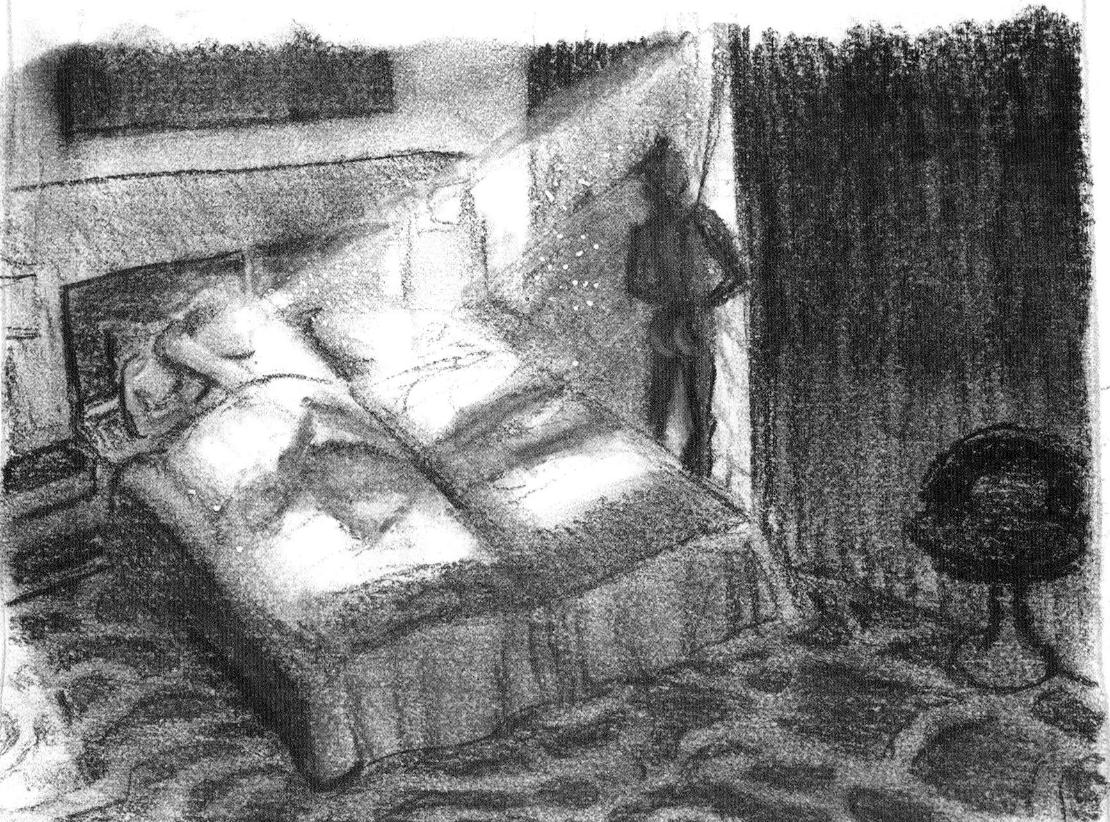

WITH ONLY ONE FULL DAY TO EXPLORE ESTONIA, WE SPLIT THE TIME WE HAD IN HALF. THE MORNING BELONGED TO TOOMPEA, THE ANCIENT CASTLE AND BREATHTAKING MEDIEVAL OLD TOWN ATOP THE CENTRAL HILL OVERLOOKING THE REST OF THE CITY. LIVING IN AN AMERICAN METROPOLIS WHERE THE OLDEST STANDING STRUCTURE IS AN ADOBE HOUSE FROM THE VERY LATE 1800S, IT'S EASY TO BE SWEPT AWAY IN THE ROMANCE OF "UPPER TOWN", A CITY BUILT 500 YEARS BEFORE THAT.

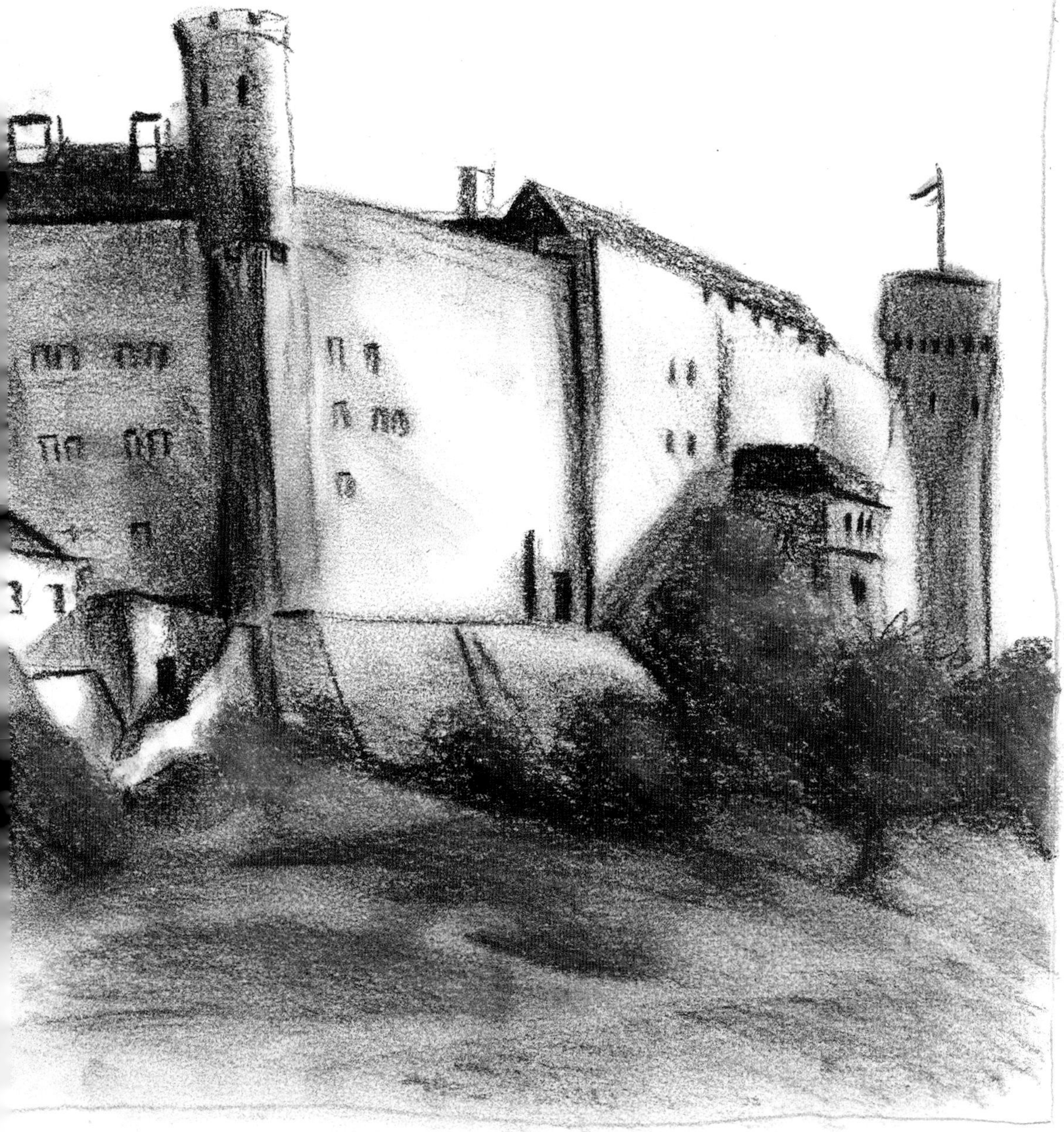

AS WE CLIMBED THE NARROW STAIRS OF ST. OLAF'S CHURCH – A STEEP INCLINE WITH NO SAFETY FEATURES WHATSOEVER AND AN AGGRESSIVE REMINDER THAT PUBLIC SAFETY WAS AN INVENTION OF THE LATE 1900s – I FELT LIKE A FRAUD – LIKE MY COUNTRY'S HISTORY WAS A PALE SHADE OF WHAT THE ESTONIANS MUST FEEL. I FELT WINDED – THE TOWER WAS STEEP. I ALSO FELT EXHAUSTED.

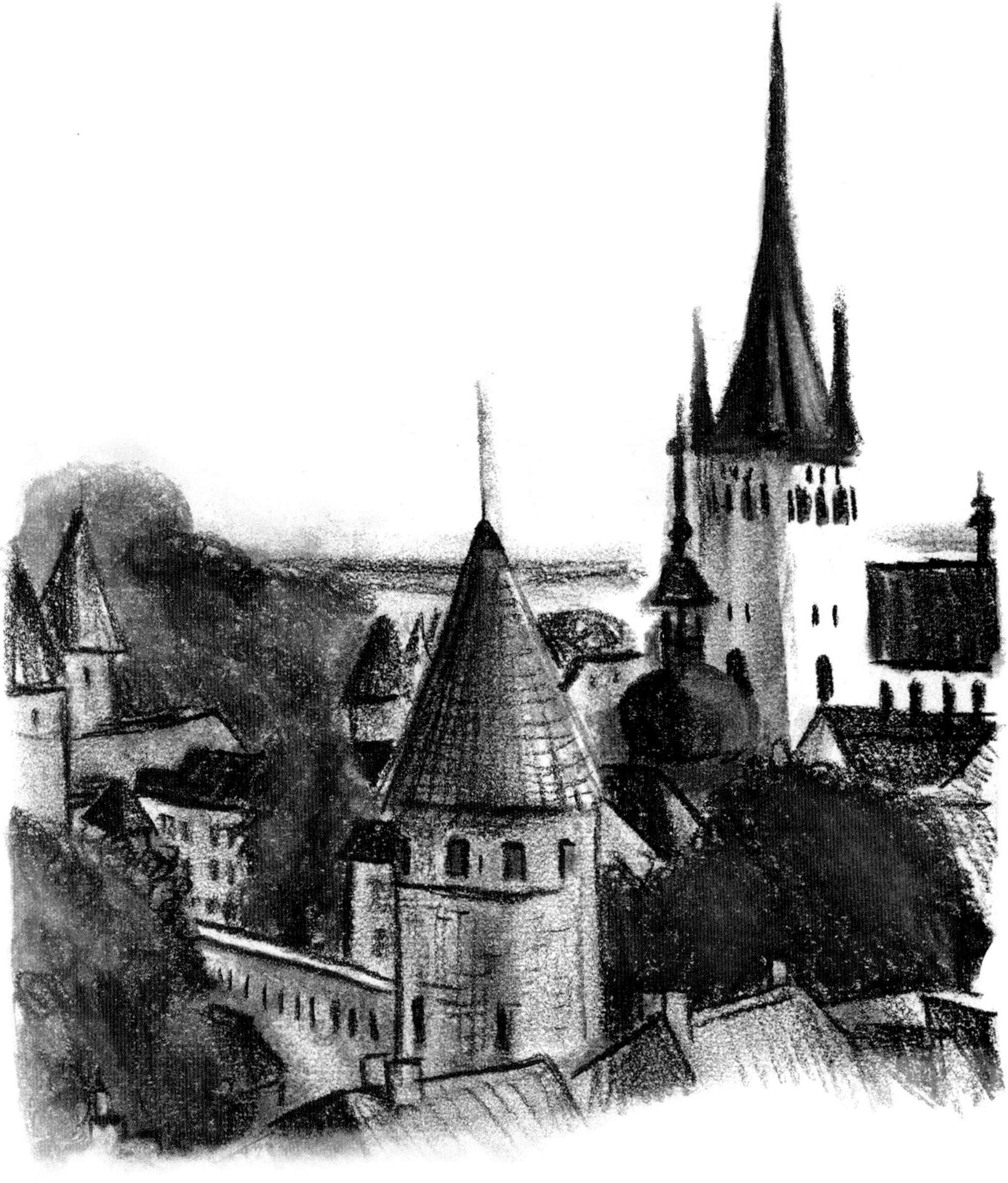

MY LACK OF SLEEP WAS CATCHING UP TO ME. I WANTED TO HEAD BACK TO THE HOTEL SPA AND SLEEP IN THE STEAM ROOM OR, YOU KNOW, JUST SLEEP.

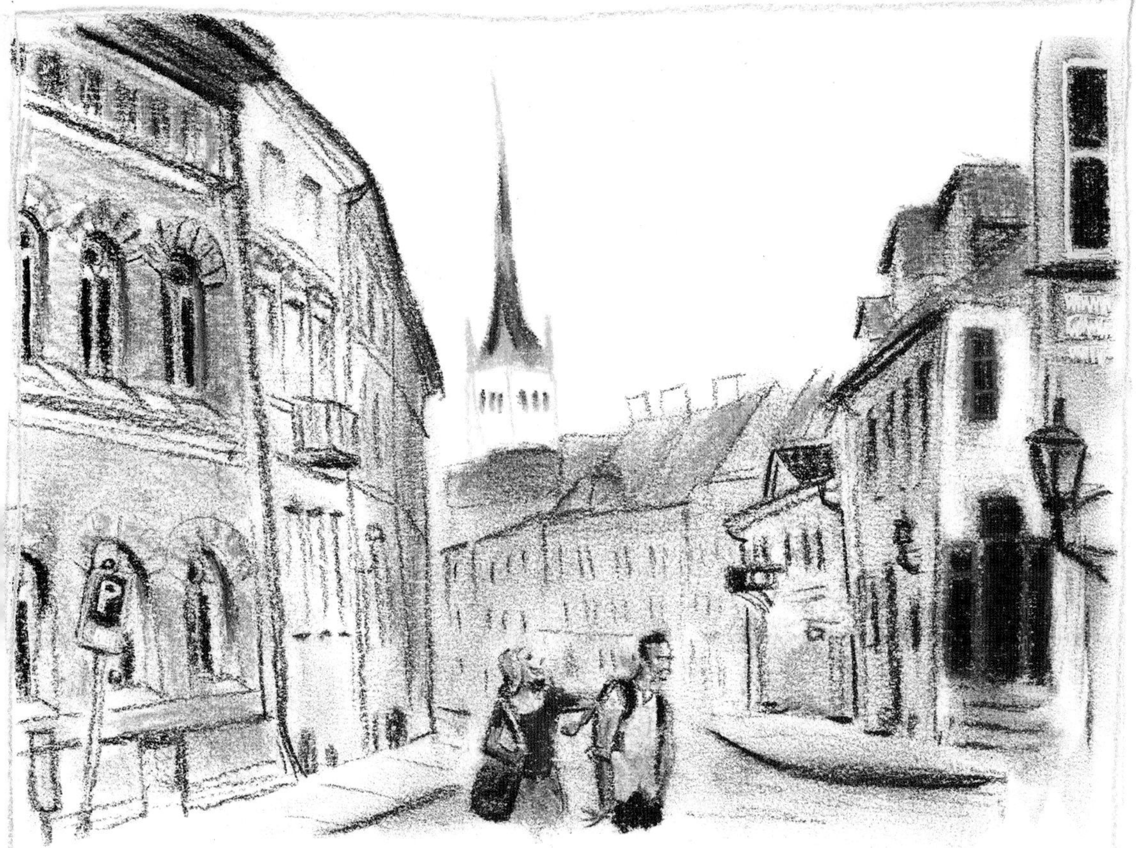

LIESEL REMINDED ME THAT WE STILL HAD HALF A CITY TO SEE AND HALF A DAY TO DO IT IN. "PLUS THOSE EXTRA EIGHT HOURS OF DAYLIGHT FORMERLY KNOWN AS NIGHTTIME," I ADDED TO LITTLE MORE THAN A SHARP ELBOW OF DISAPPROVAL.
"WHAT IF WE DIDN'T WALK?" SHE TEASED.

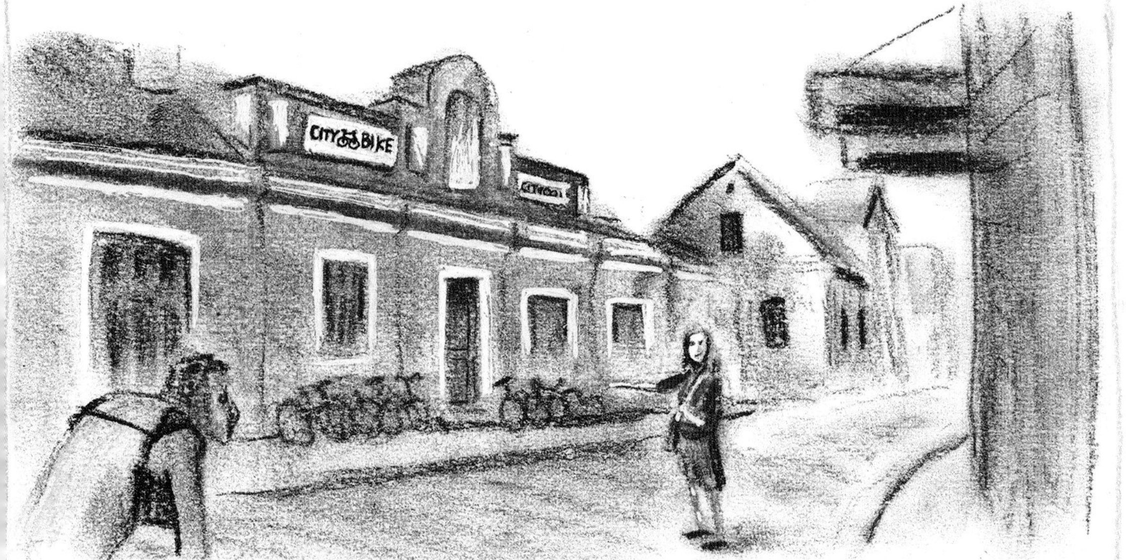
CITY BIKE

I LIKED THE IDEA OF TOURING THE FLATLANDS IN THE BACK OF A CAB. UNFORTUNATELY, IT WAS CLEAR THAT LIESEL STILL HAD HUMAN LOCOMOTION IN MIND WHEN I CAUGHT UP WITH HER AT A BIKE RENTAL STAND.
I DID NOT WANT TO RIDE A BIKE.

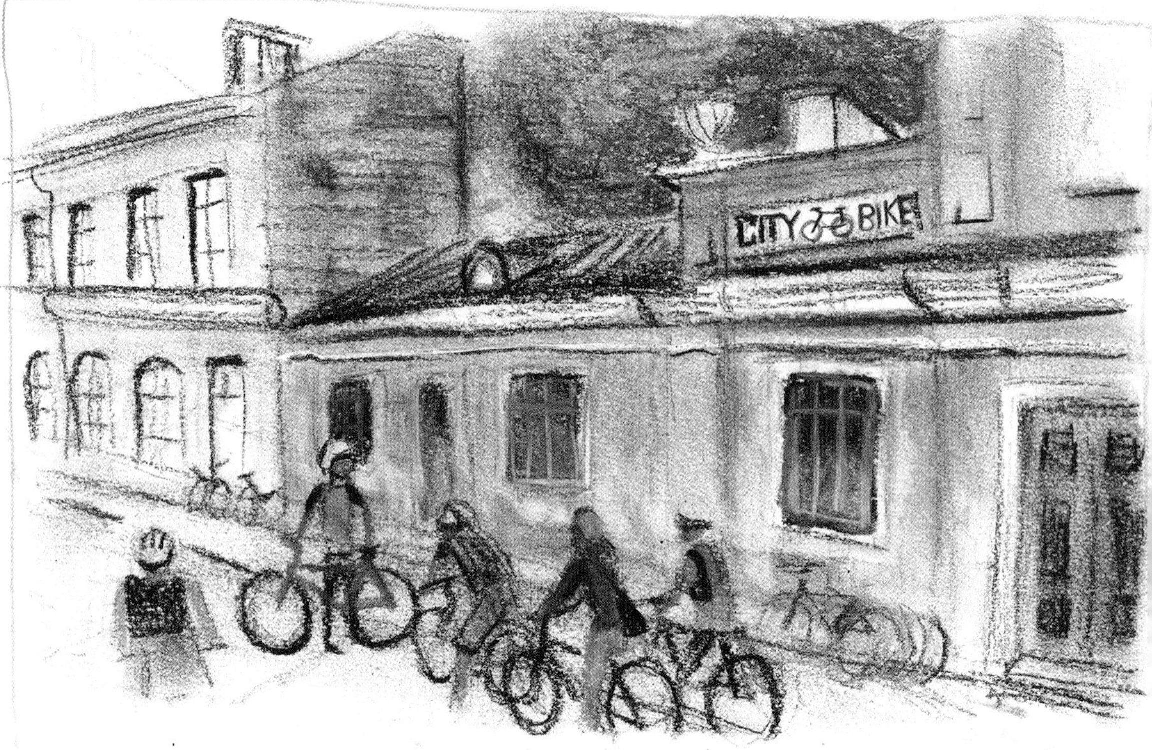
CITY BIKE

AND SHE HADN'T JUST RENTED BIKES, SHE'D ALSO RENTED A BOY — WHICH ISN'T AS UNSEEMLY AS IT SOUNDS. THE BIKE RENTAL WAS A GUIDED TOUR COMPANY.

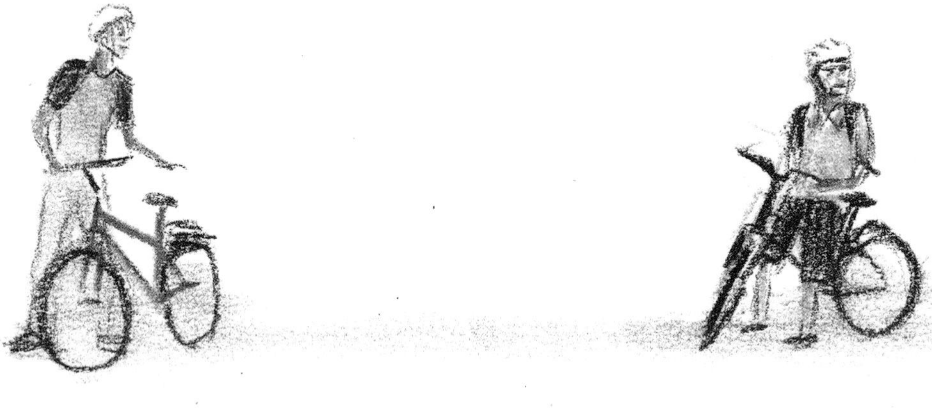

I DID NOT WANT A GUIDED TOUR FROM A VERY YOUNG GUIDE WITH NO SENSE OF THE HISTORY OF THE PLACE.

TOO BAD. WE TOOK OFF ON A PAVED PATH UNDER THE LEADERSHIP OF ERIK, WHO MIGHT HAVE BEEN 23, MIGHT HAVE BEEN 17. HIS ENGLISH WAS AWKWARD, BUT STILL GOOD ENOUGH TO GET HIS POINT ACROSS AND VASTLY BETTER THAN ANY LANGUAGE I'VE EVER TRIED TO LEARN.

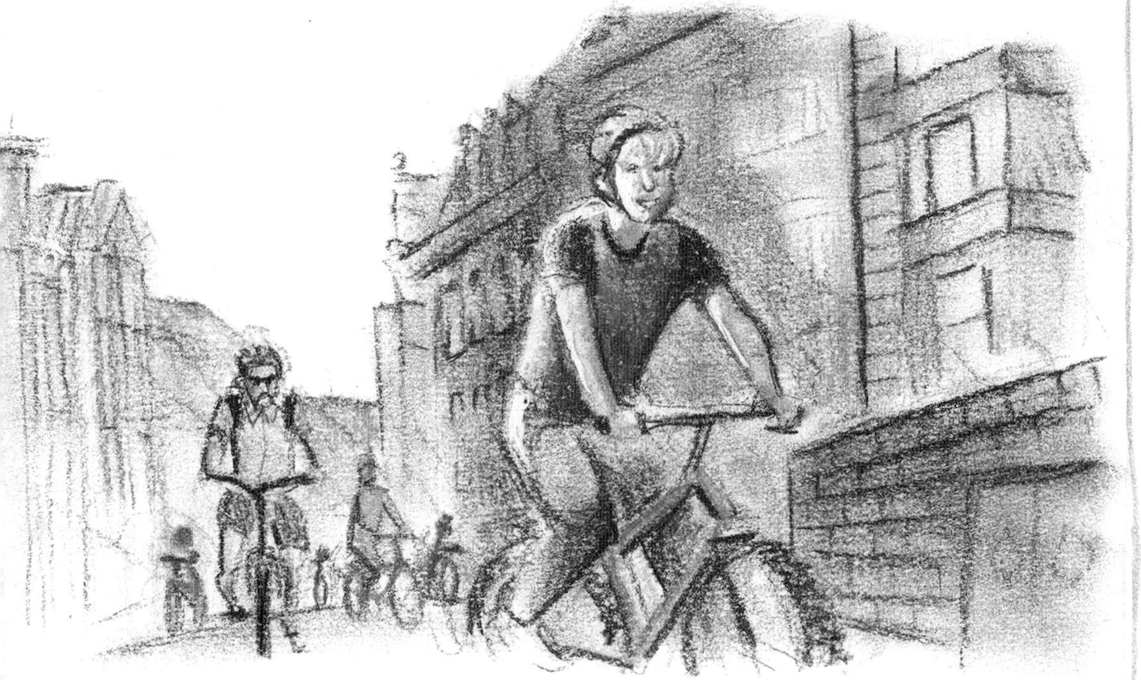

HE RODE FAST AND STOPPED INTERMITTENTLY TO TALK ABOUT THIS STATUE OR THAT PARK. I WAS HOPING MY INCREASINGLY FREQUENT YAWNS WEREN'T INSULTING HIM, BUT I WAS CLOSE TO FALLING ASLEEP ON THE BIKE EACH TIME WE STOPPED.

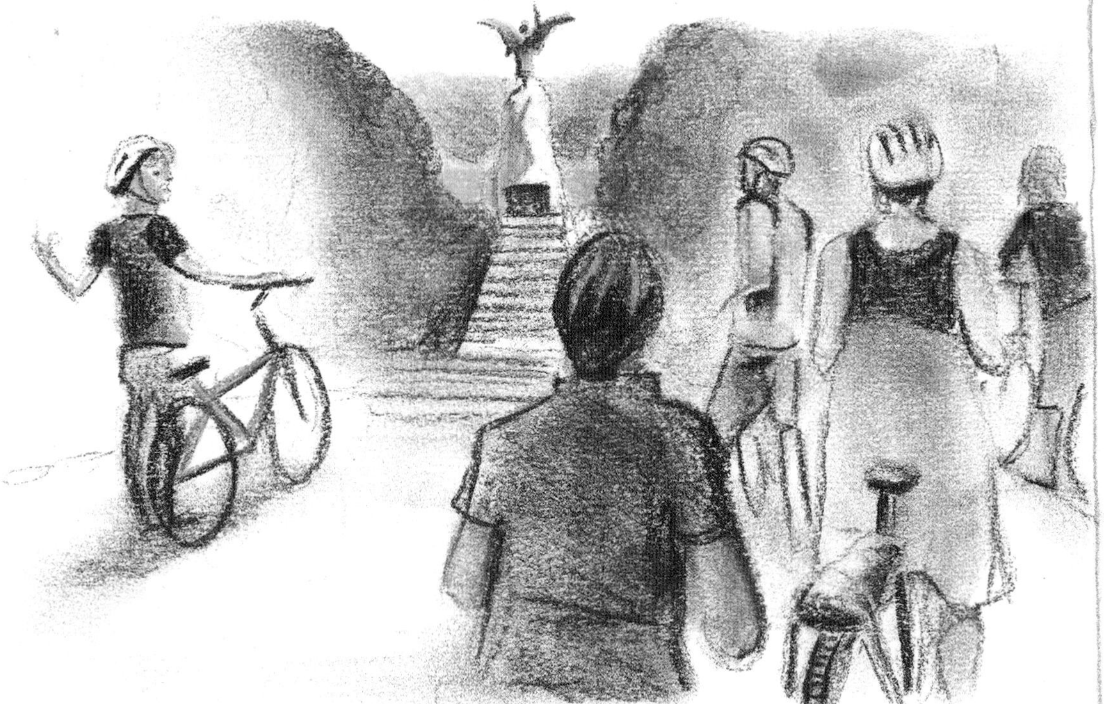

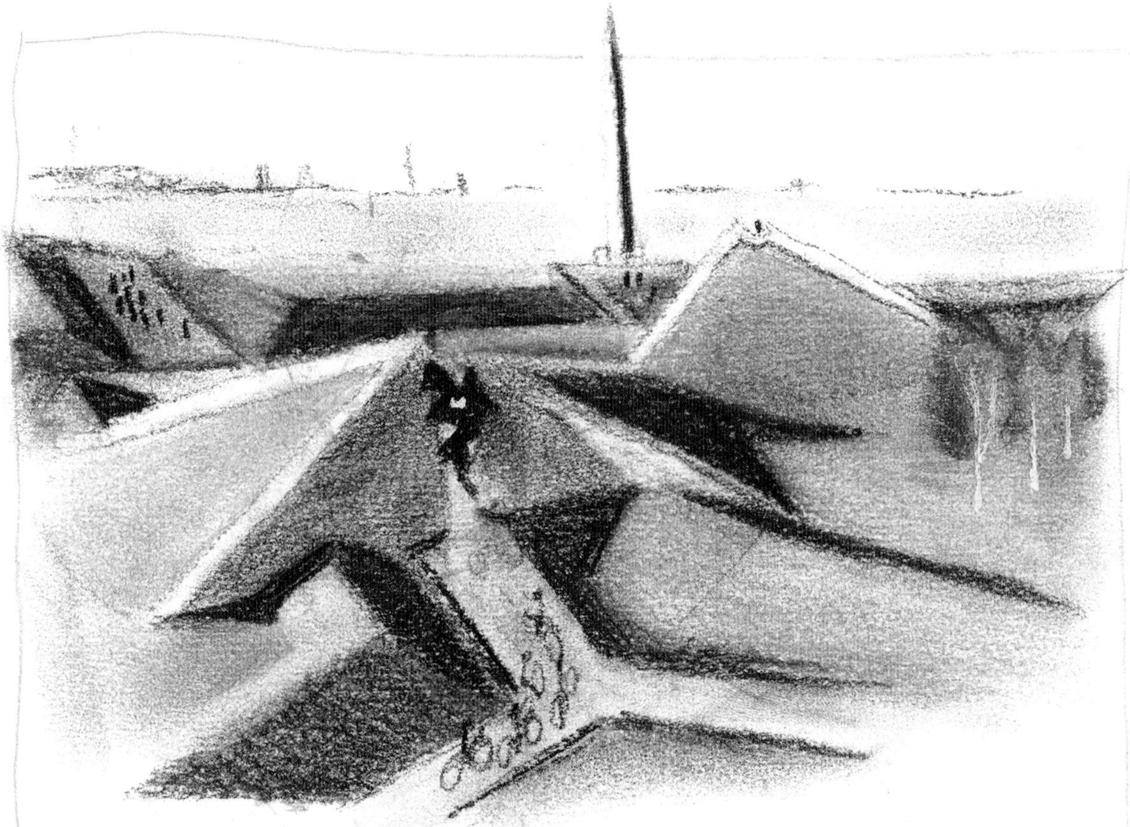

BY THE TIME WE GOT TO THE RUSSIAN WAR MEMORIAL I WAS PANICKED - DOING THE MATH OF HOW FAR WE HAD COME AND HOW FAR BACK IT NOW WAS TO SWEET SLUMBER. THE SUN STAYED IN THE SAME SPOT IN THE SKY CASTING CIRCULAR SHADOWS THAT MOVED BUT NEVER SET.

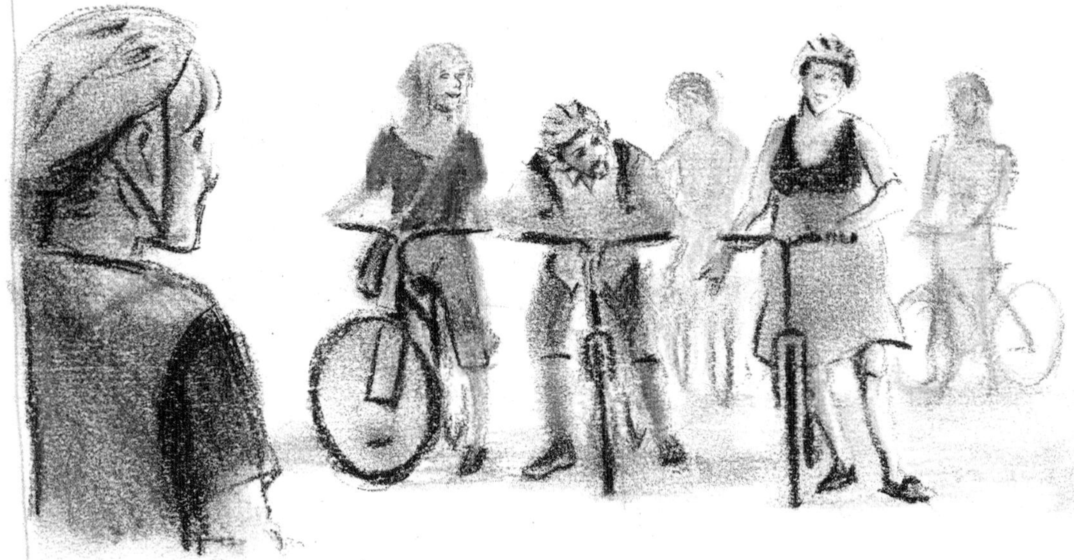

THEN A QUESTION FROM ONE OF THE OTHER CYCLISTS - A FRENCH WOMAN - CUT THROUGH MY INCREASINGLY FREQUENT YAWNS: "WHY WOULD YOU HAVE A MONUMENT FOR THE RUSSIANS? DIDN'T THEY OCCUPY YOUR COUNTRY?"

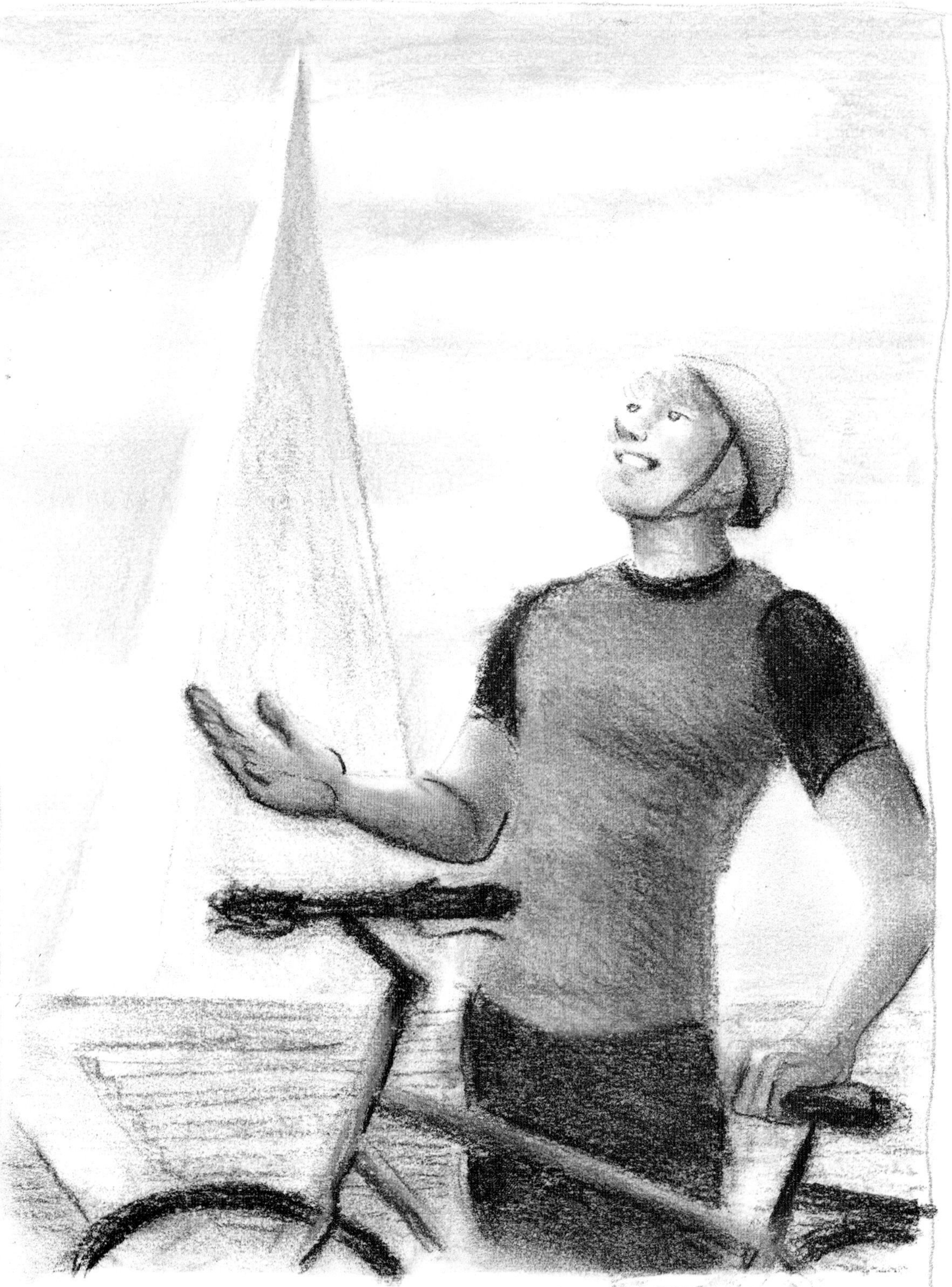

AND ERIK TRANSFORMED. HIS YOUTHFUL SIMPLICITY WAS IMMEDIATELY DISPLACED BY A SERIOUS, EXUBERANT PATRIOTISM.
"UM, YES. THIS MONUMENT IS NOT FOR RUSSIA, BUT BUILT BY RUSSIA WHILE HERE. IT IS HONORING THEIR SOLDIERS WHO FOUGHT AGAINST US. LATER THEY ADD MORE FOR SECOND WORLD WAR, BOTH MUCH OLDER HISTORY."

I FOLLOWED UP, MY IGNORANCE COMPOUNDED MY EXHAUSTION: "YOU THINK OF WORLD WAR 2 AS 'OLDER HISTORY'? I THOUGHT THE CASTLE WAS FROM THE 1200S?"

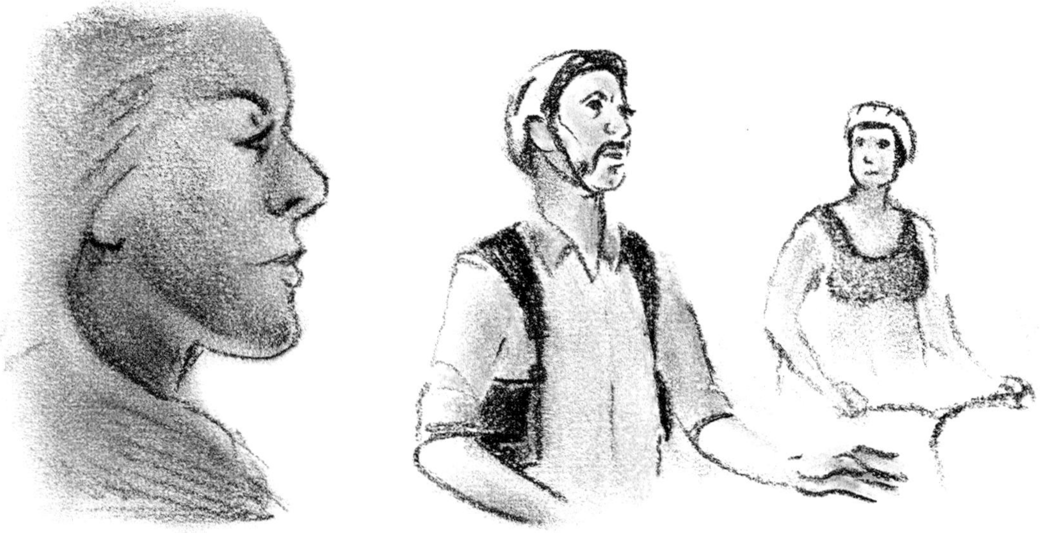

ERIK SMILED, "YES, IT'S TRUE. BUT ESTONIA HAS ONLY HAD OUR FREEDOM FOR 19 YEARS. WE MADE OUR INDEPENDENCE FROM THE SOVIET UNION IN 1991 WHEN I WAS FOUR YEARS OLD ONLY. WE CHERISH WHAT WE HAVE AND WE REMEMBER EACH TIME FROM OUR PAST WHERE WE DIDN'T."

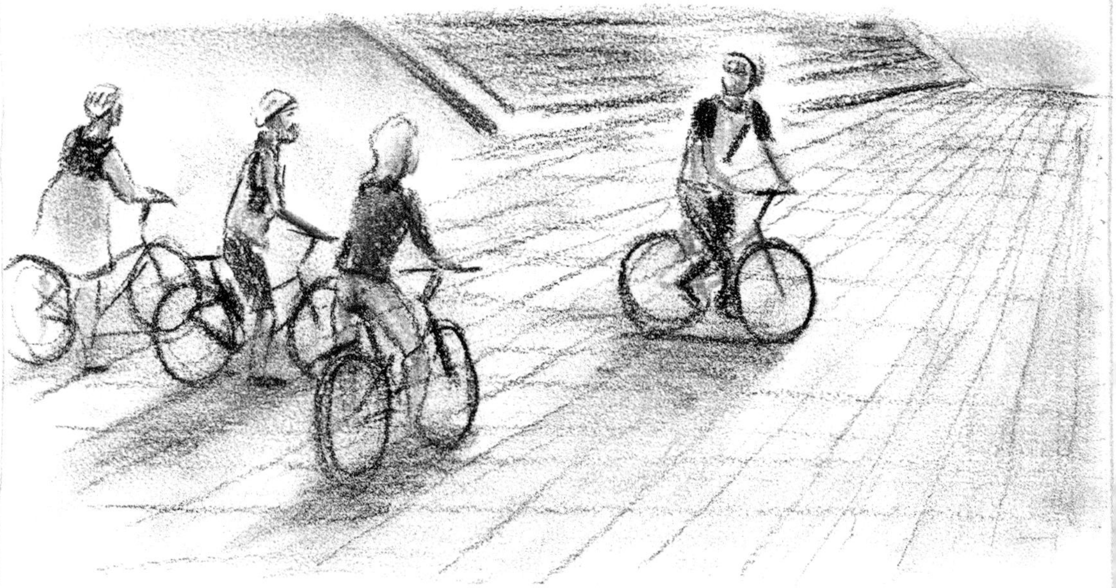

"BUT... WE SHOULD KEEP RIDING TO GET THE GROUP BACK IN TIME AND THERE ARE STILL THINGS TO SEE LIKE THE LAKE AND THE MUSIC CENTER."

ESTONIA WAS A COUNTRY IN COSTUME. IT WAS DRESSED UP AS A HUNDREDS-OF-YEARS-OLD DEMOCRACY, BUT IT TURNED OUT IT WAS BARELY OF VOTING AGE IN THE U.S.A. AND STILL NOT OF DRINKING AGE IN SOME STATES.

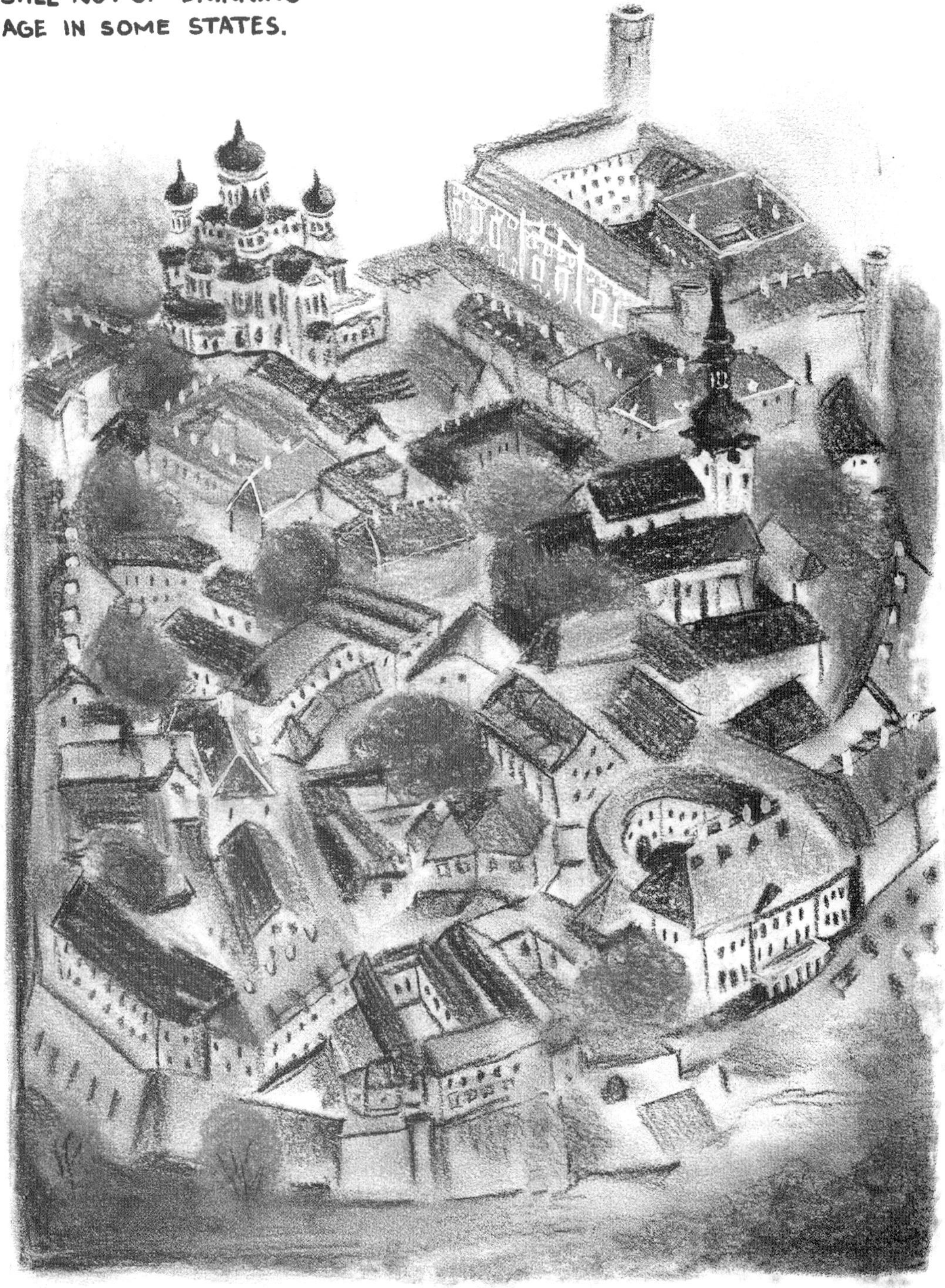

IT GAVE THE VISUAL APPEARANCE OF A BEEN-THERE/DONE-THAT-LONG-AGO NATION, BUT WAS STILL A JUBILANT-BUT-NERVOUS NEWBORN ON THE WORLD STAGE. AND ERIK, YOUNG THOUGH HE WAS, WAS INTENT ON MAKING A GOOD IMPRESSION.

RIDING BACK, I SAW THE COUNTRY IN A DRAMATICALLY
DIFFERENT PENUMBRA — A SOBERING DEMOGRAPHIC SCHISM.
ANYONE OVER THIRTY CARRIED WITH THEM A SPECIFIC
URBAN DNA — THEY HAD LIVED UNDER A LESS OPEN, LESS
DEMOCRATIZED POLITICAL SYSTEM.

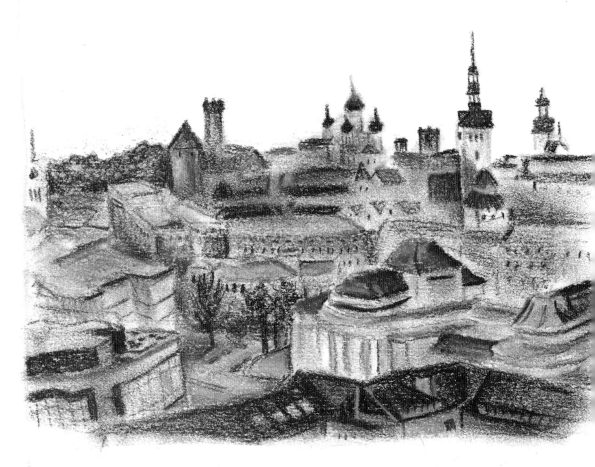

THEY HAD LIVED BEHIND BLACKOUT CURTAINS — OF THE IRON
VARIETY. AND NOW THEY WERE AWASH IN AN UNACCUSTOMED
FREEDOM — LEARNING TO SWIM ITS CURRENTS — THE AIR HAD
CHANGED AROUND THEM IN THEIR LIFETIME.

AND THEN THERE WERE THE ERIKS OF THIS PLACE, WHO
MOVED WITH THE SWAGGER OF NEWFOUND FREEDOM.

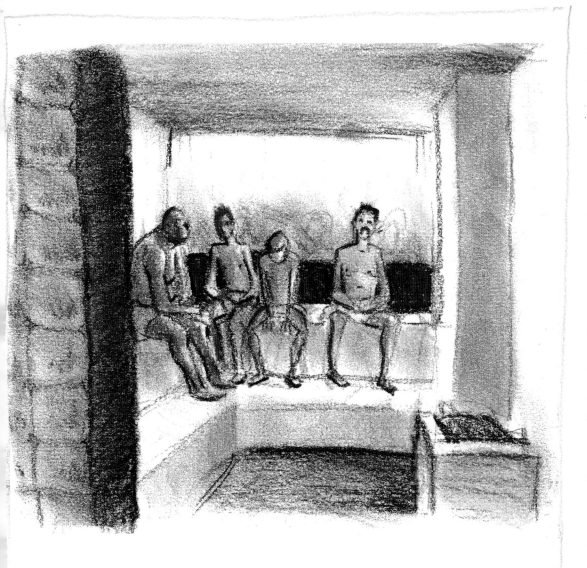

BACK AT OUR HOTEL, LIESEL AND I MADE OUR WAY TO THE LARGE
ATTACHED WATERPARK AND SPA. I SWAM LAPS NEXT TO GNARLED
OLDER ESTONIANS WHO LIVED LONG ENOUGH TO SEE THEIR CITY
REEMERGE ON THE WORLD STAGE. HOTELS, RESTAURANTS, SPAS.

IN THE SAUNA AFTER, NAKED AGAIN, MY EXHAUSTION DEMANDING
I CEDE TO IT, I HAD TO MOVE OVER TO MAKE WAY FOR A FATHER
AND HIS TWO SONS. THE FATHER, MY AGE, HAD LIVED HIS TEENAGE
YEARS UNDER THE REPRESSIVE CURTAIN. HIS TWO BOYS, ONE 19
ONE 14, WERE LIVING UNDER A DIFFERENT SUN. THEY WERE OF ERIK'S
GENERATION, BORN IN A FREE SOCIETY AND WOULD, HOPEFULLY,
NEVER FALL UNDER ANYONE'S SHADOW.

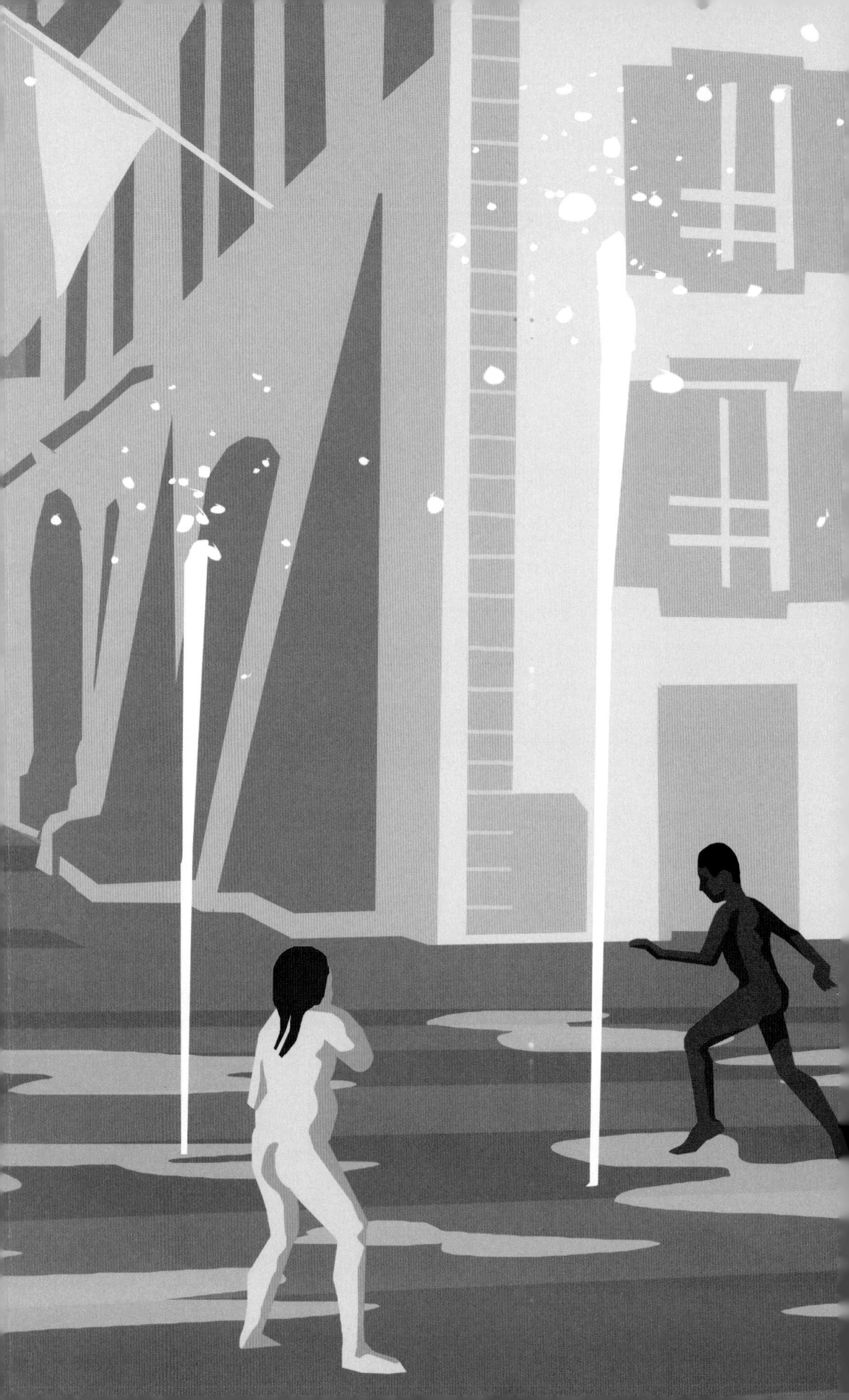

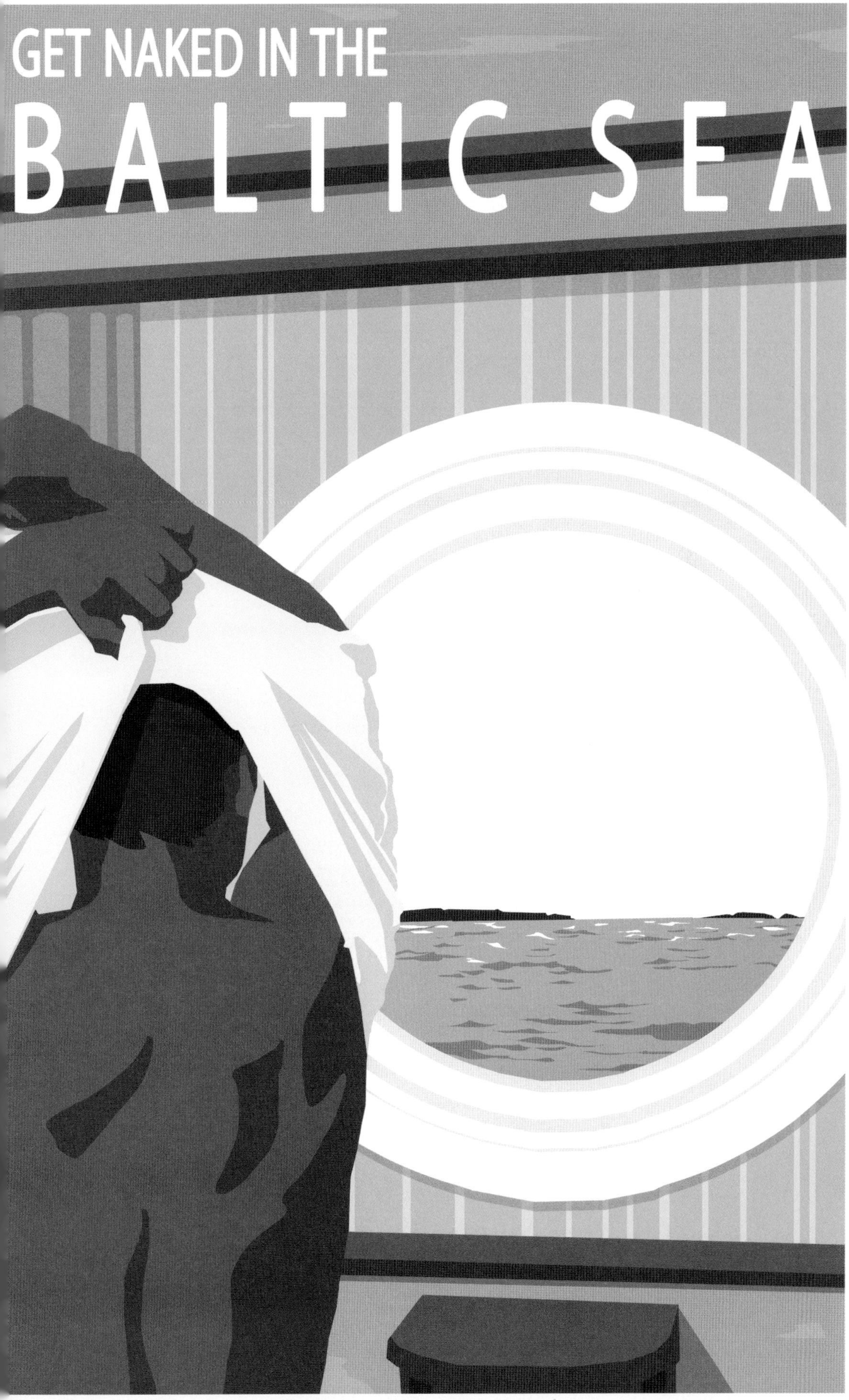
GET NAKED IN THE
BALTIC SEA

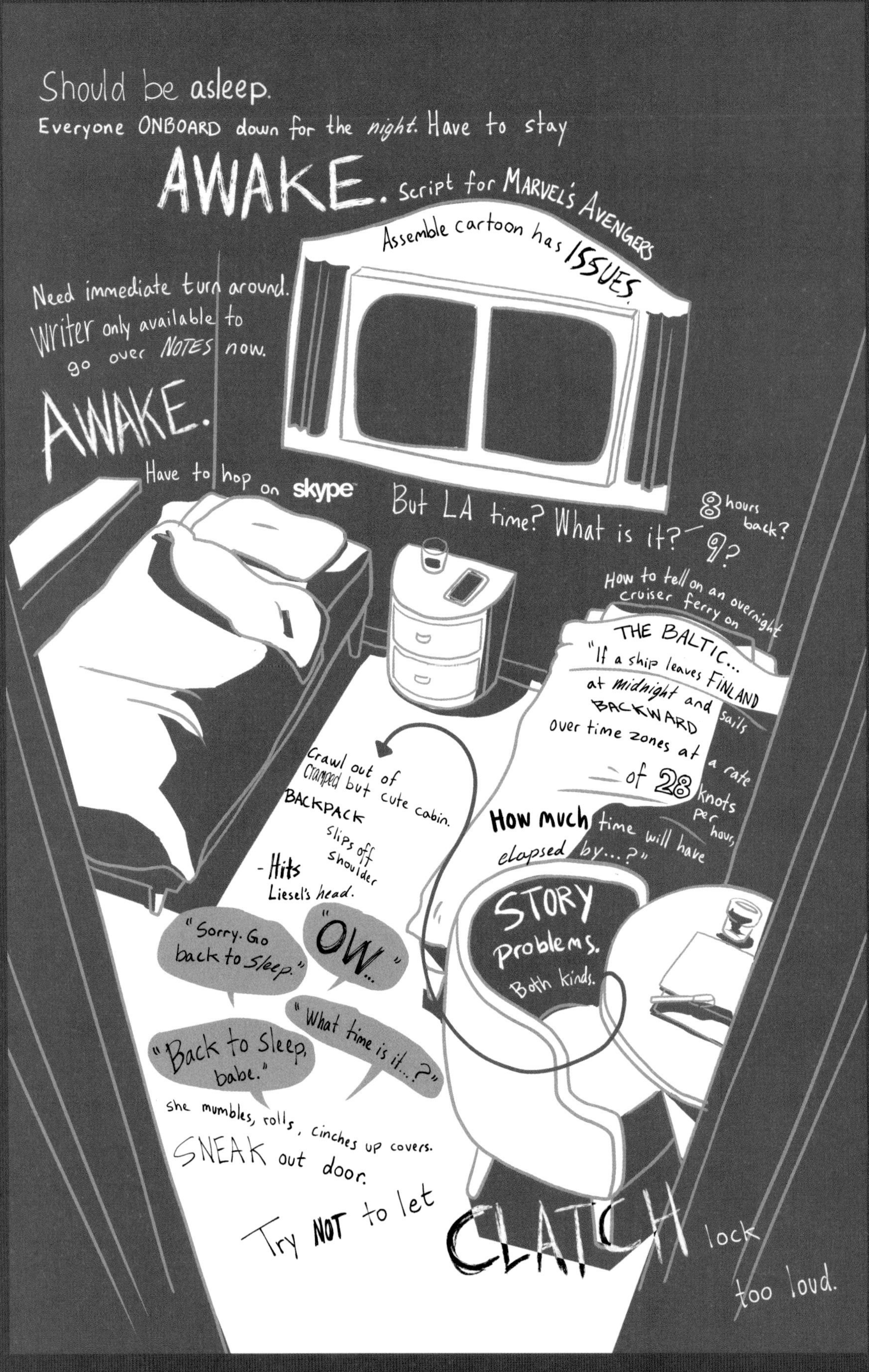
Should be asleep.
Everyone ONBOARD down for the night. Have to stay
AWAKE. Script for MARVEL'S AVENGERS
Assemble cartoon has ISSUES.
Need immediate turn around. Writer only available to go over NOTES now.
AWAKE.
Have to hop on skype
But LA time? What is it? 8 hours back? 9?
How to tell on an overnight cruiser ferry on THE BALTIC...
"If a ship leaves FINLAND at midnight and sails BACKWARD over time zones at a rate of 28 knots per hour, HOW MUCH time will have elapsed by...?"
Crawl out of cramped but cute cabin.
BACKPACK slips off shoulder
-Hits Liesel's head.
"Sorry. Go back to sleep."
"OW..."
"What time is it...?"
"Back to sleep, babe."
she mumbles, rolls, cinches up covers.
SNEAK out door.
STORY problems. Both kinds.
Try NOT to let
CLATCH lock
too loud.

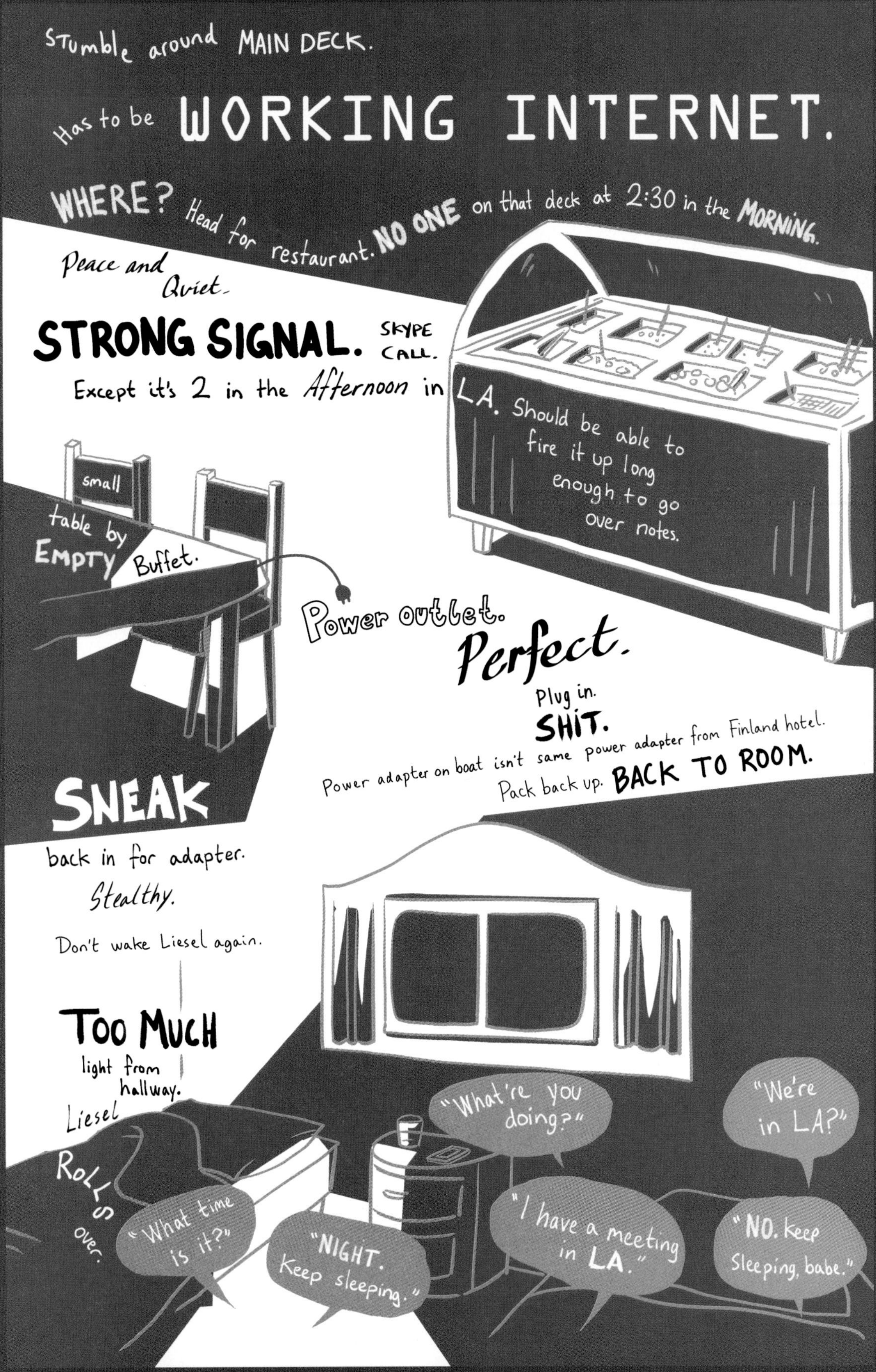

Stumble around MAIN DECK.
Has to be WORKING INTERNET.
WHERE? Head for restaurant. NO ONE on that deck at 2:30 in the MORNING.
Peace and Quiet.
STRONG SIGNAL. SKYPE CALL.
Except it's 2 in the Afternoon in L.A. Should be able to fire it up long enough to go over notes.
small table by EMPTY Buffet.
Power outlet.
Perfect.
Plug in.
SHIT.
Power adapter on boat isn't same power adapter from Finland hotel.
Pack back up. BACK TO ROOM.
SNEAK back in for adapter.
Stealthy.
Don't wake Liesel again.
TOO MUCH light from hallway.
Liesel ROLLS over.
"What time is it?"
"NIGHT. Keep sleeping."
"What're you doing?"
"I have a meeting in LA."
"We're in LA?"
"NO. Keep Sleeping, babe."

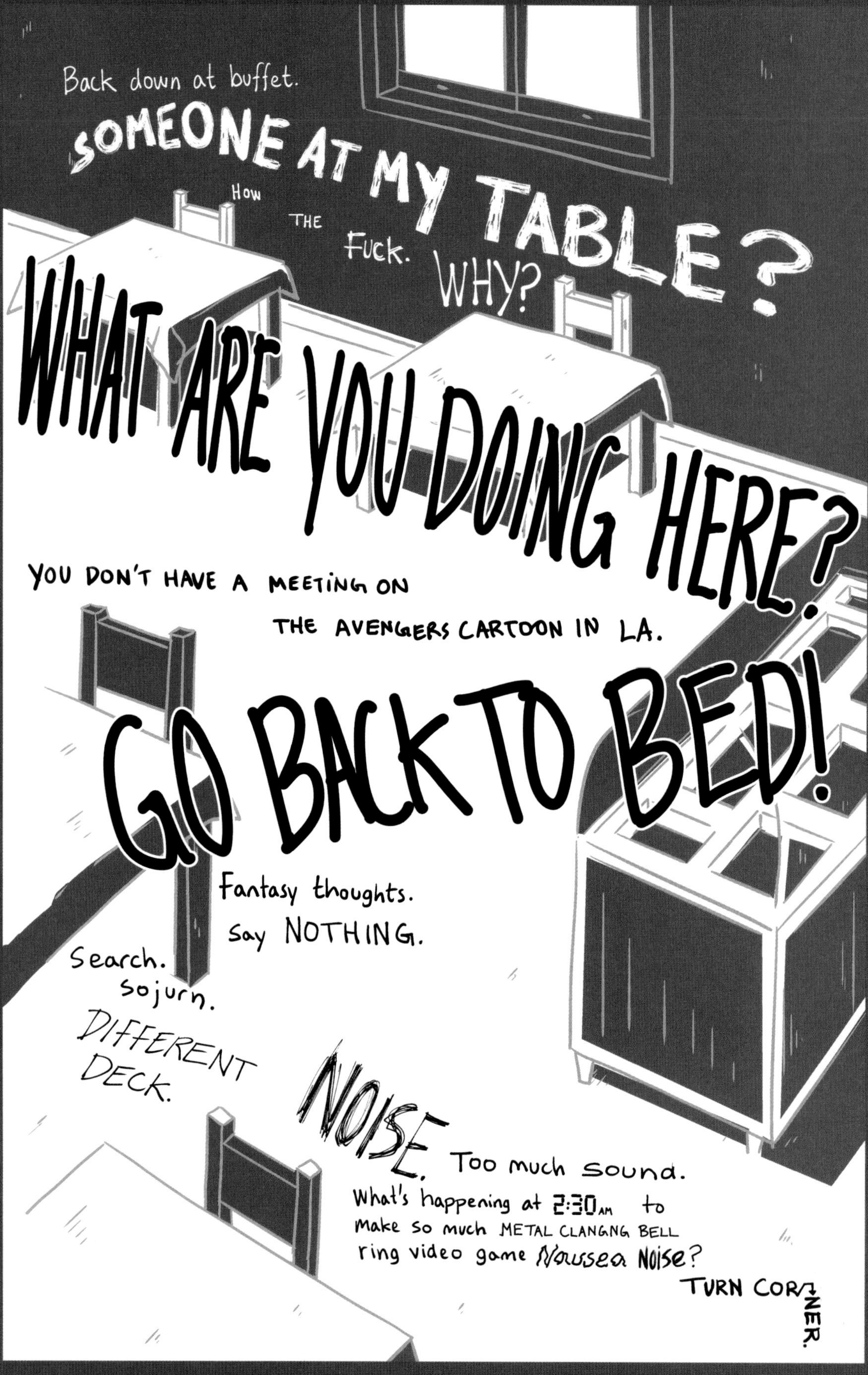
Back down at buffet.
SOMEONE AT MY TABLE?
How THE Fuck. WHY?
WHAT ARE YOU DOING HERE?
YOU DON'T HAVE A MEETING ON THE AVENGERS CARTOON IN LA.
GO BACK TO BED!
Fantasy thoughts. Say NOTHING.
Search. sojurn.
DIFFERENT DECK.
NOISE. Too much sound.
What's happening at 2:30AM to make so much METAL CLANGING BELL ring video game Nausea NOISE?
TURN CORNER.

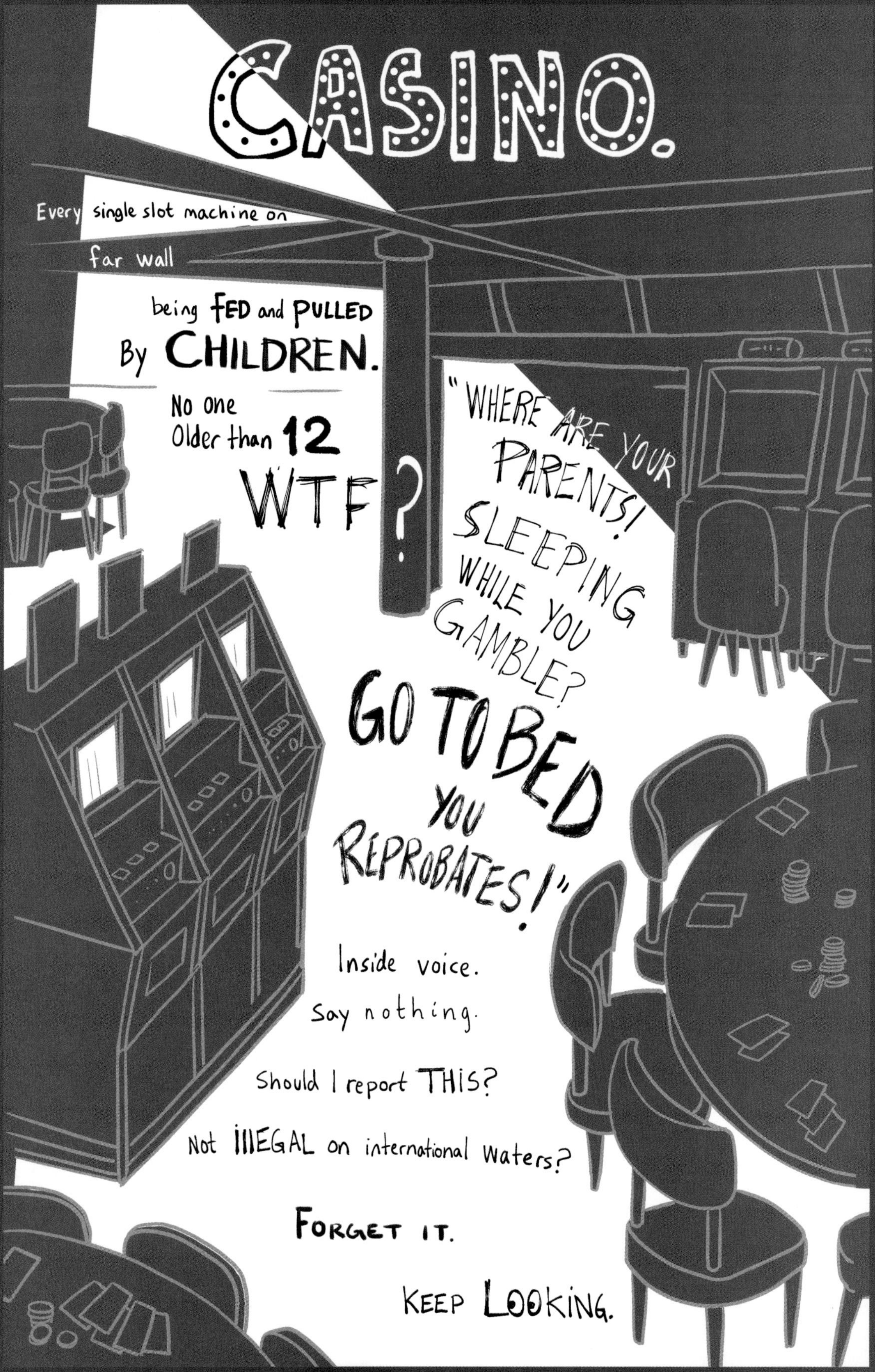
CASINO.
Every single slot machine on
far wall
being FED and PULLED
By CHILDREN.
No one
Older than 12
WTF?
"WHERE ARE YOUR PARENTS!
SLEEPING WHILE YOU GAMBLE?
GO TO BED
YOU
REPROBATES!"
Inside voice.
Say nothing.
Should I report THIS?
Not ILLEGAL on international waters?
FORGET IT.
KEEP LOOKING.

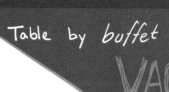

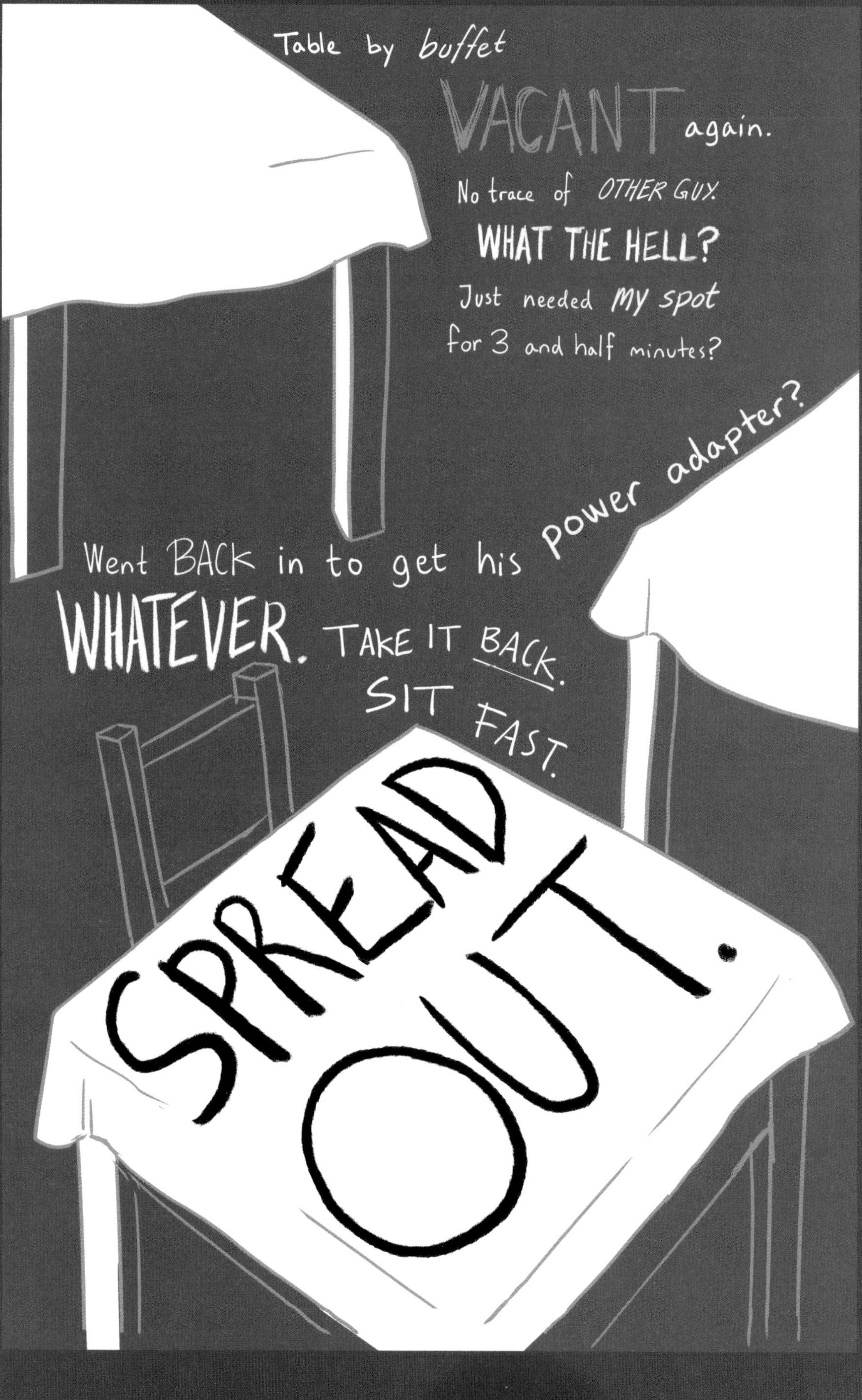

Table by *buffet*

VACANT again.

No trace of OTHER GUY.

WHAT THE HELL?

Just needed MY spot
for 3 and half minutes?

Went BACK in to get his power adapter?

WHATEVER. TAKE IT BACK.
SIT FAST.

SPREAD OUT.

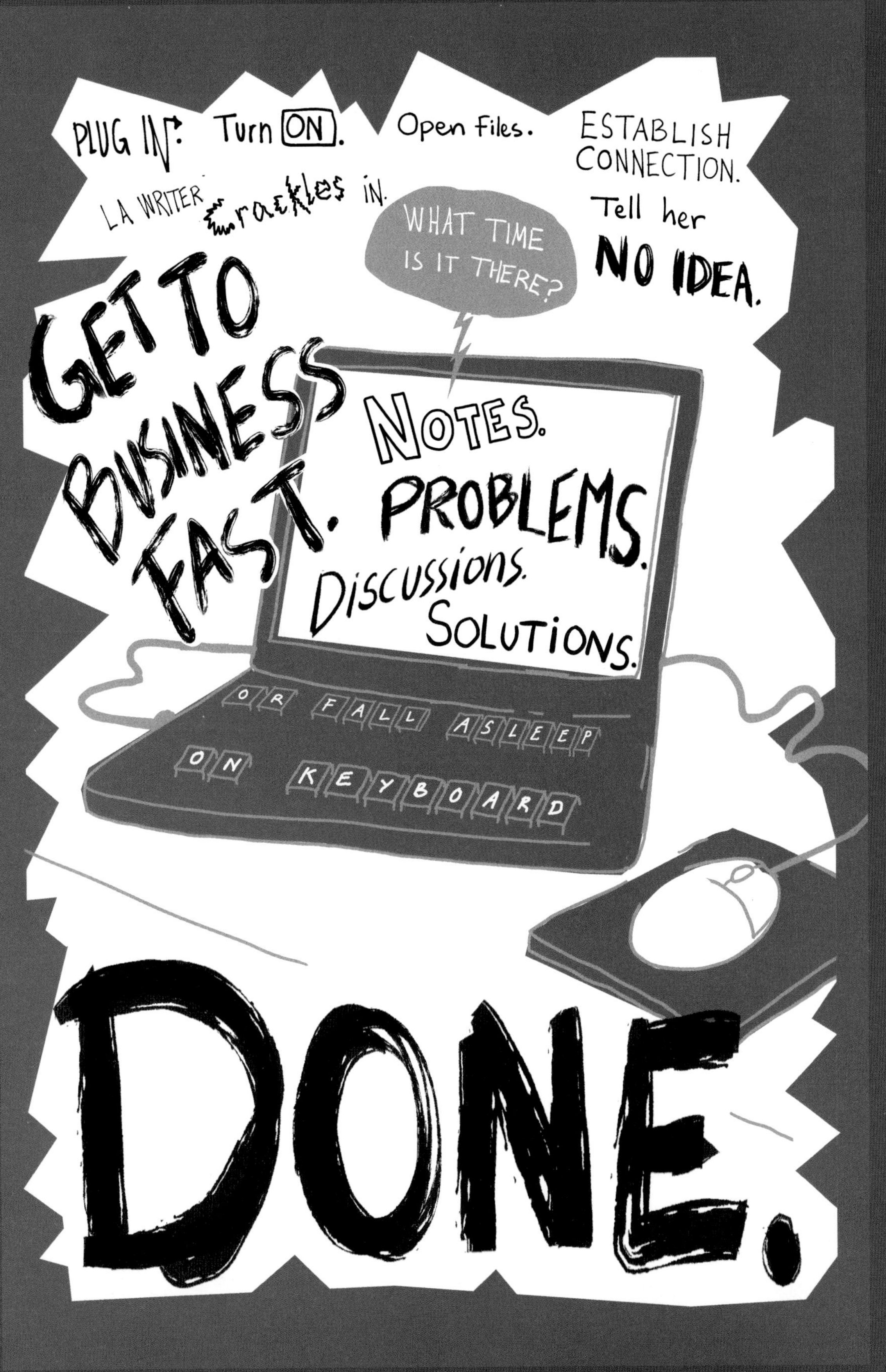

PLUG IN. Turn ON. Open files. ESTABLISH CONNECTION.
LA WRITER crackles in.
WHAT TIME IS IT THERE?
Tell her NO IDEA.
GET TO BUSINESS FAST.
NOTES. PROBLEMS. Discussions. SOLUTIONS.
OR FALL ASLEEP ON KEYBOARD
DONE.

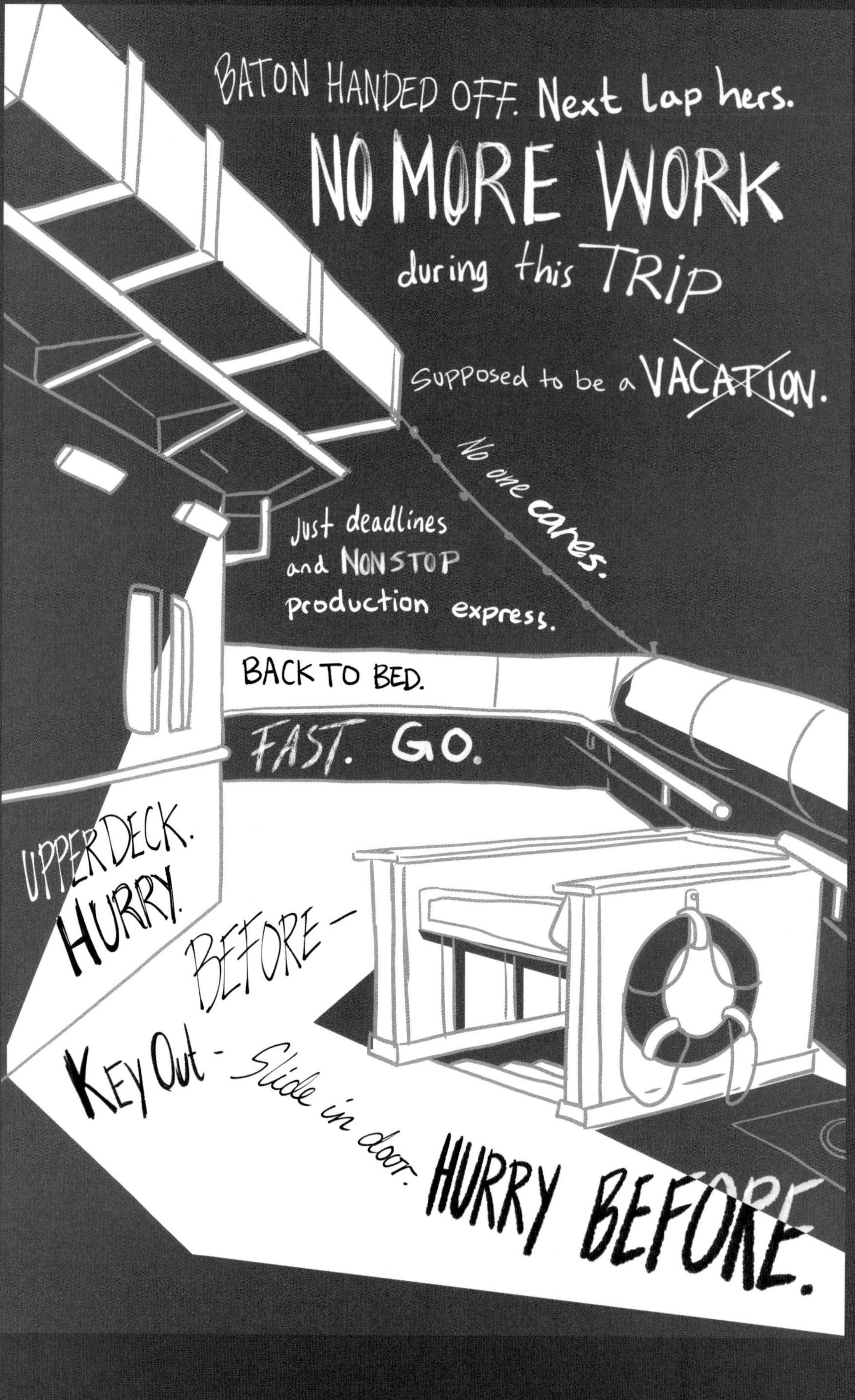

BATON HANDED OFF. Next lap hers.
NO MORE WORK
during this TRIP
Supposed to be a VACATION.
No one cares.
Just deadlines
and NONSTOP
production express.
BACK TO BED.
FAST. GO.
UPPERDECK.
HURRY.
BEFORE-
Key Out - Slide in door.
HURRY BEFORE.

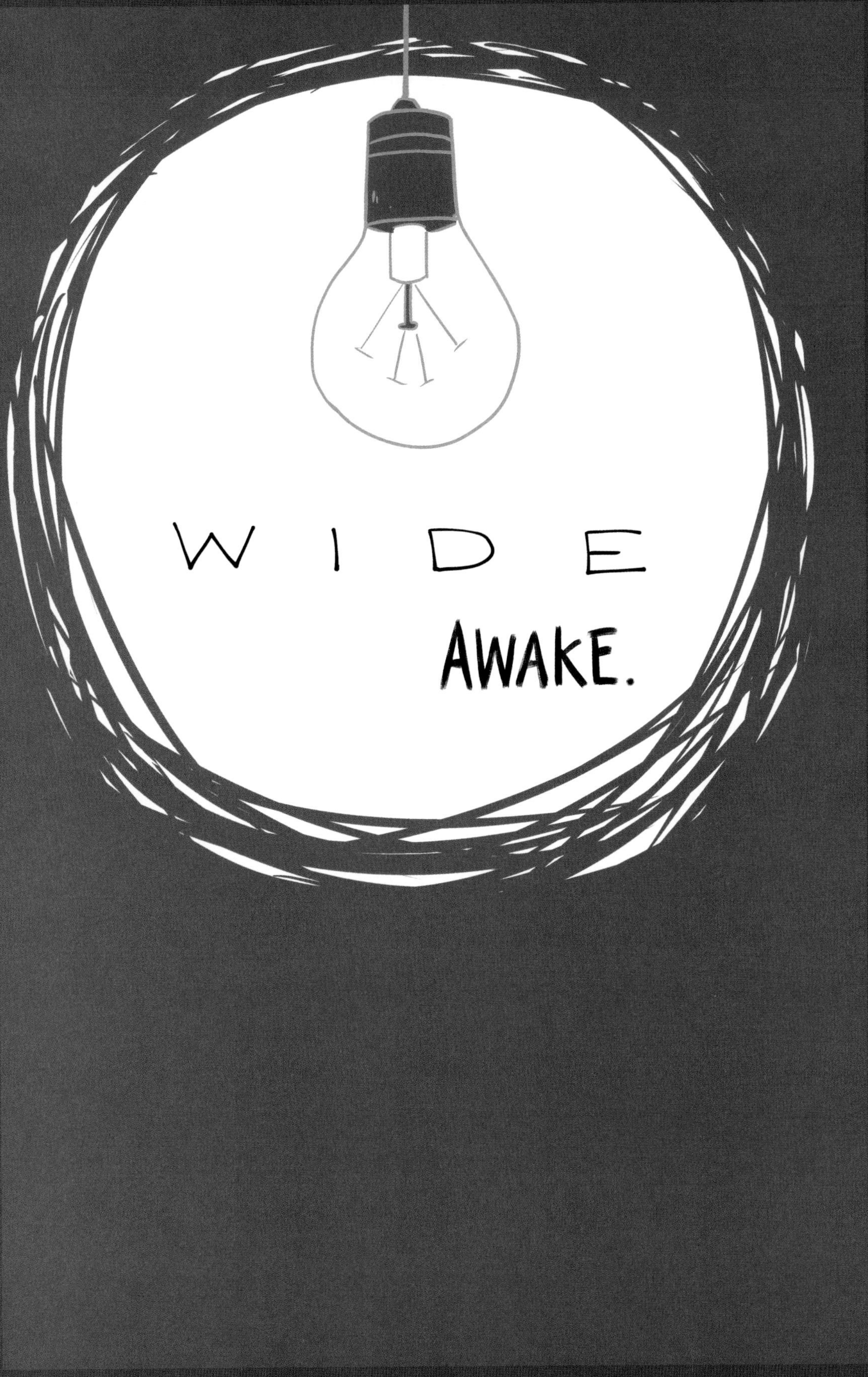
WIDE
AWAKE.

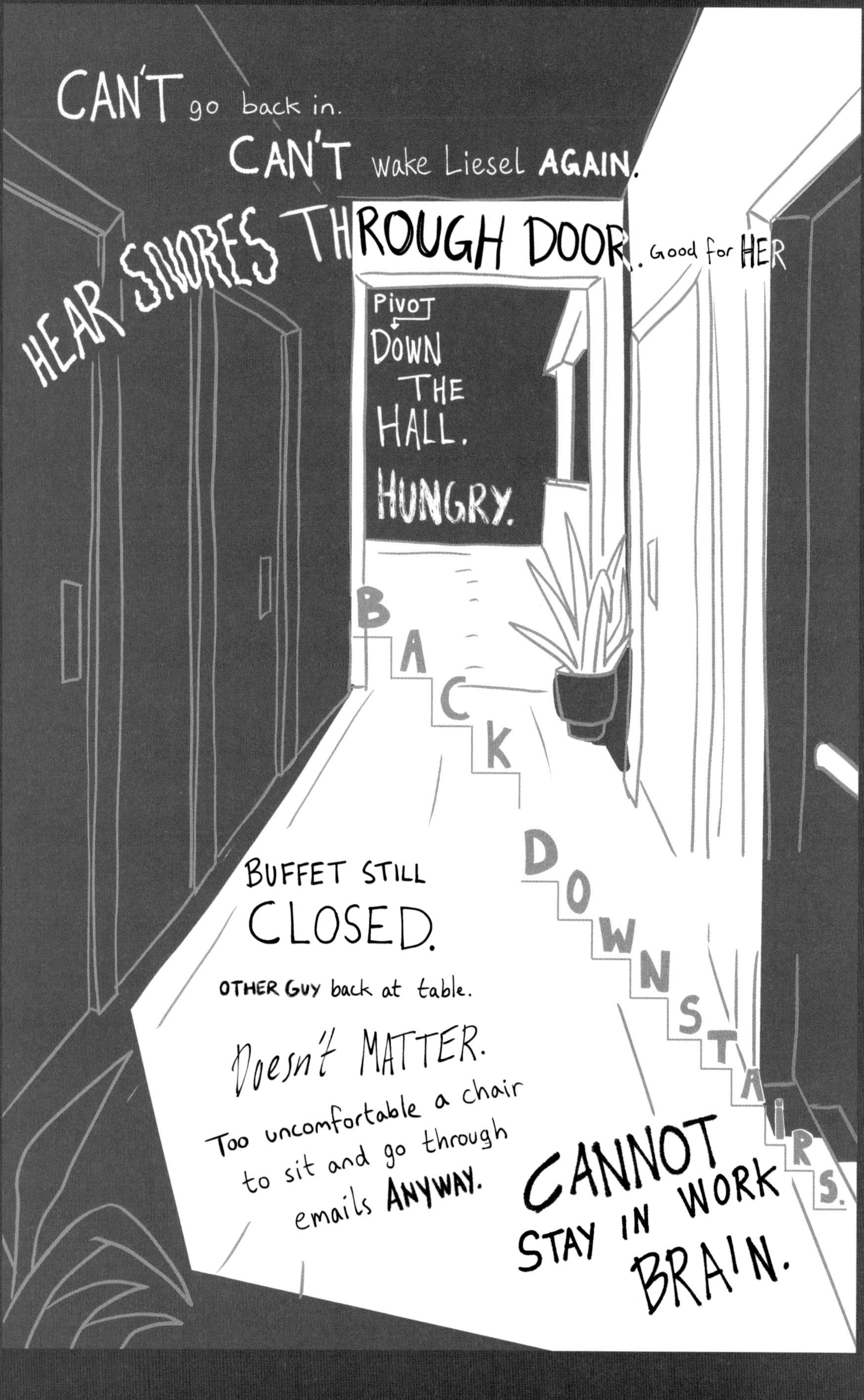
CAN'T go back in.
CAN'T wake Liesel AGAIN.
HEAR SNORES THROUGH DOOR. Good for HER
PIVOT DOWN THE HALL.
HUNGRY.
BACK DOWNSTAIRS.
BUFFET STILL CLOSED.
OTHER GUY back at table.
Doesn't MATTER.
Too uncomfortable a chair to sit and go through emails ANYWAY.
CANNOT STAY IN WORK BRAIN.

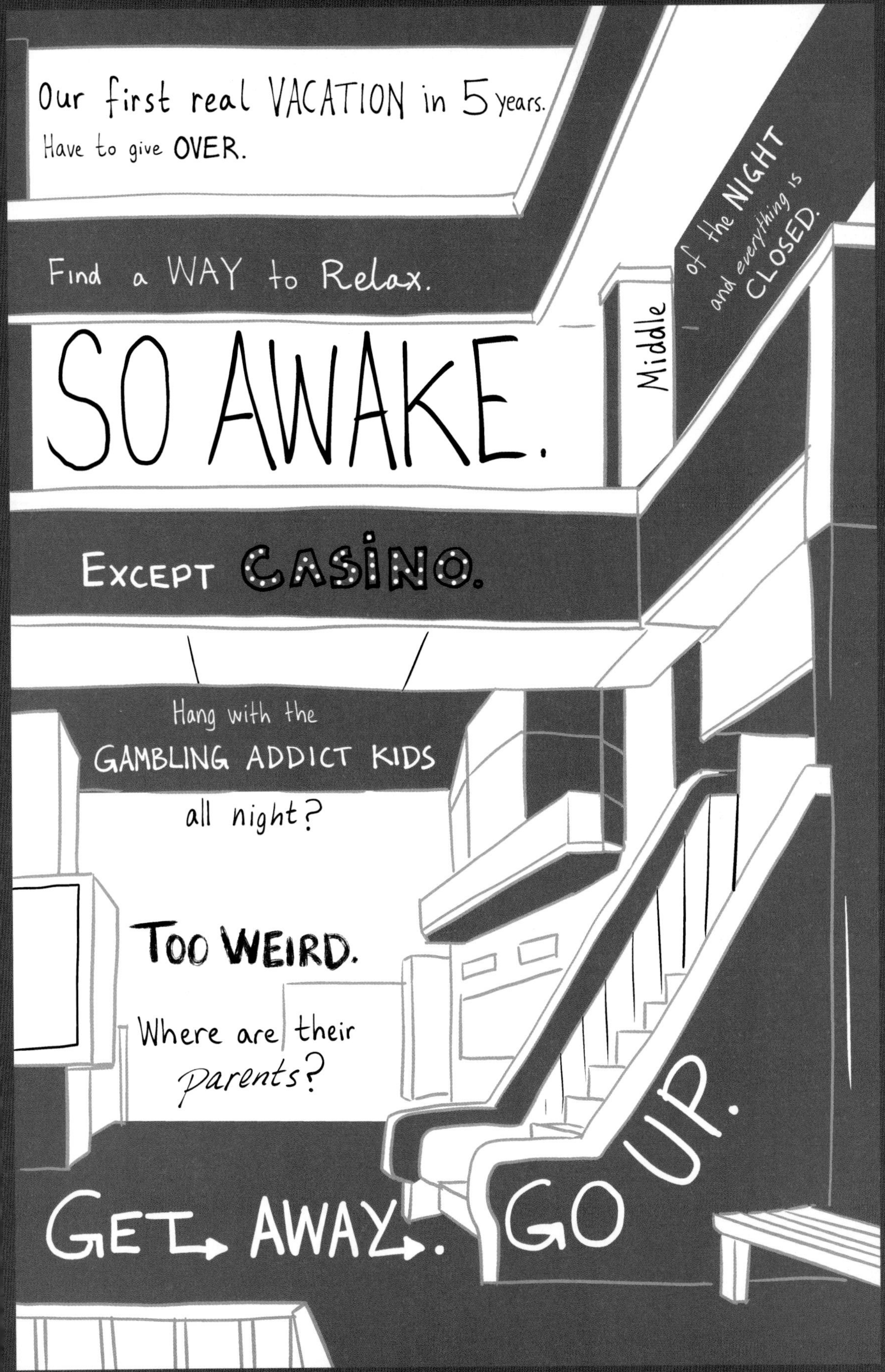
Our first real VACATION in 5 years.
Have to give OVER.
Find a WAY to Relax.
SO AWAKE.
Middle of the NIGHT and everything is CLOSED.
EXCEPT CASINO.
Hang with the GAMBLING ADDICT KIDS all night?
TOO WEIRD.
Where are their parents?
GET AWAY. GO UP.

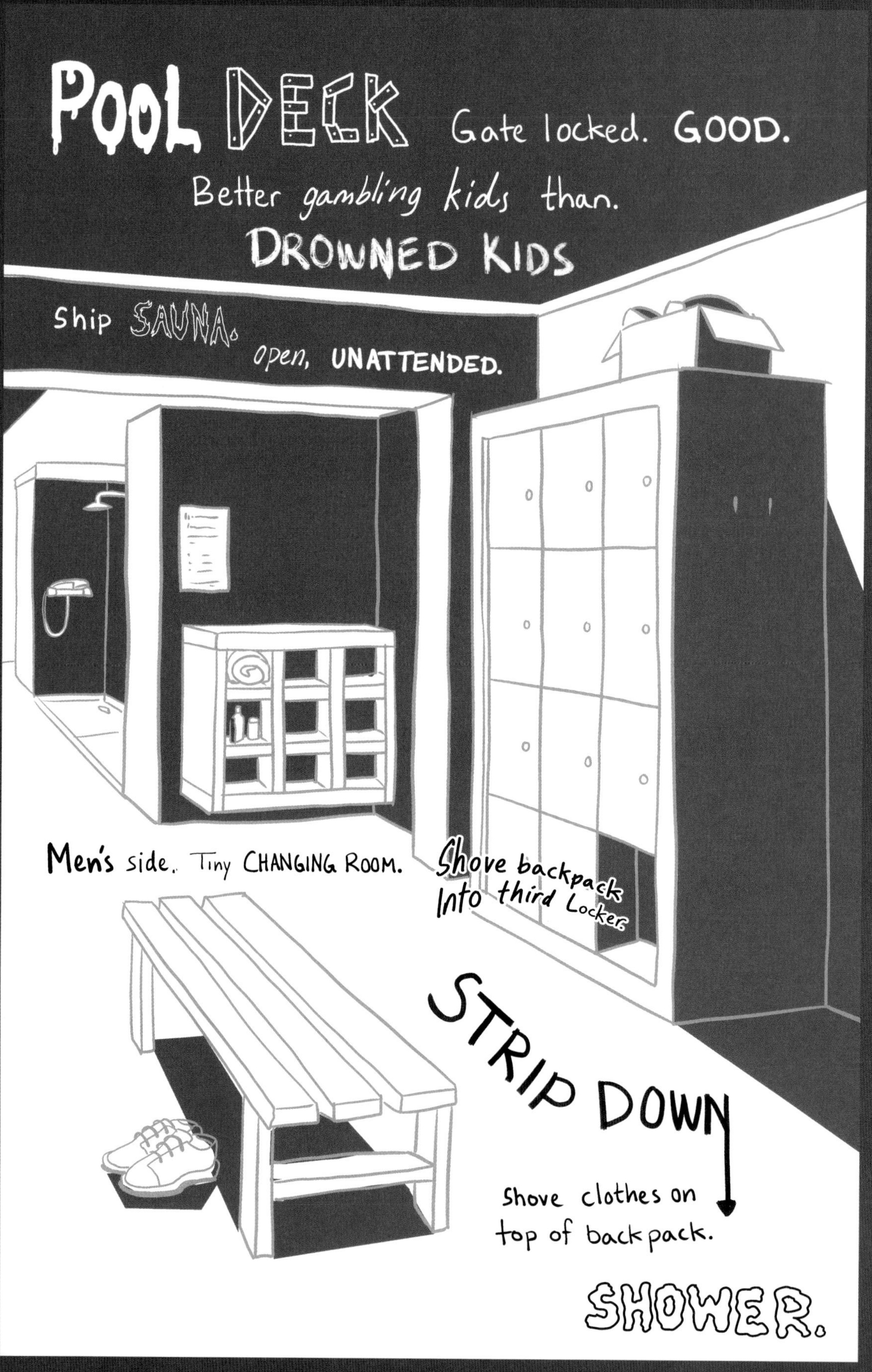

POOL DECK
Gate locked. GOOD.

Better *gambling* kids than.

DROWNED KIDS

Ship SAUNA. open, UNATTENDED.

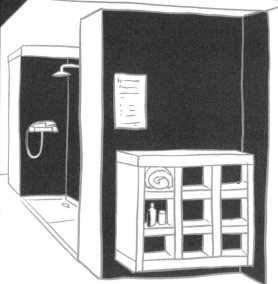
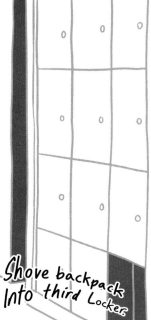

Men's side. Tiny CHANGING ROOM.

Shove backpack Into third Locker

STRIP DOWN

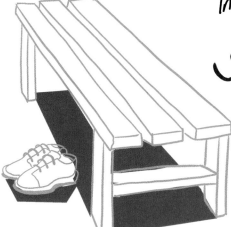

Shove clothes on top of backpack.

SHOWER.

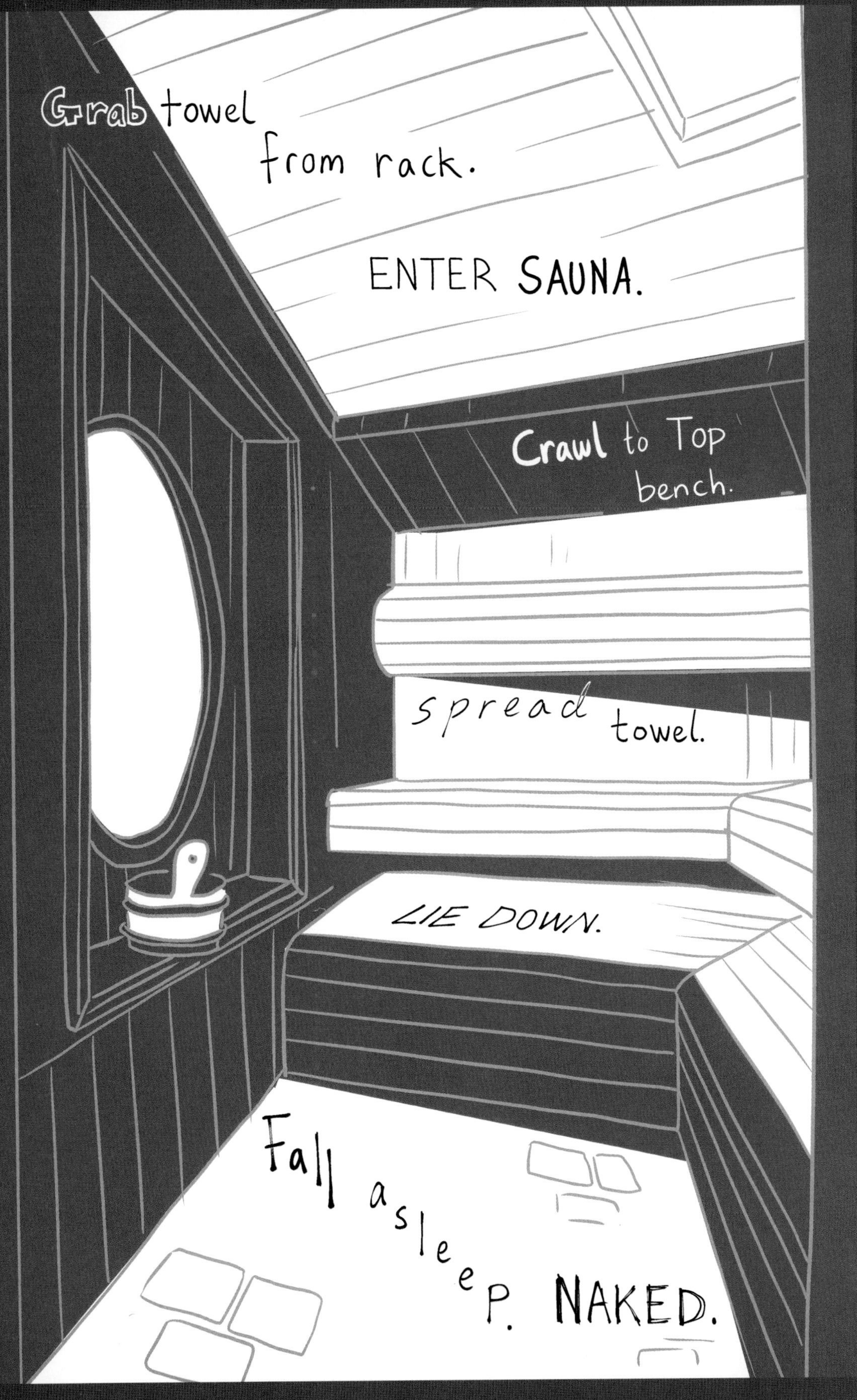
Grab towel from rack.
ENTER SAUNA.
Crawl to Top bench.
spread towel.
LIE DOWN.
Fall asleep. NAKED.

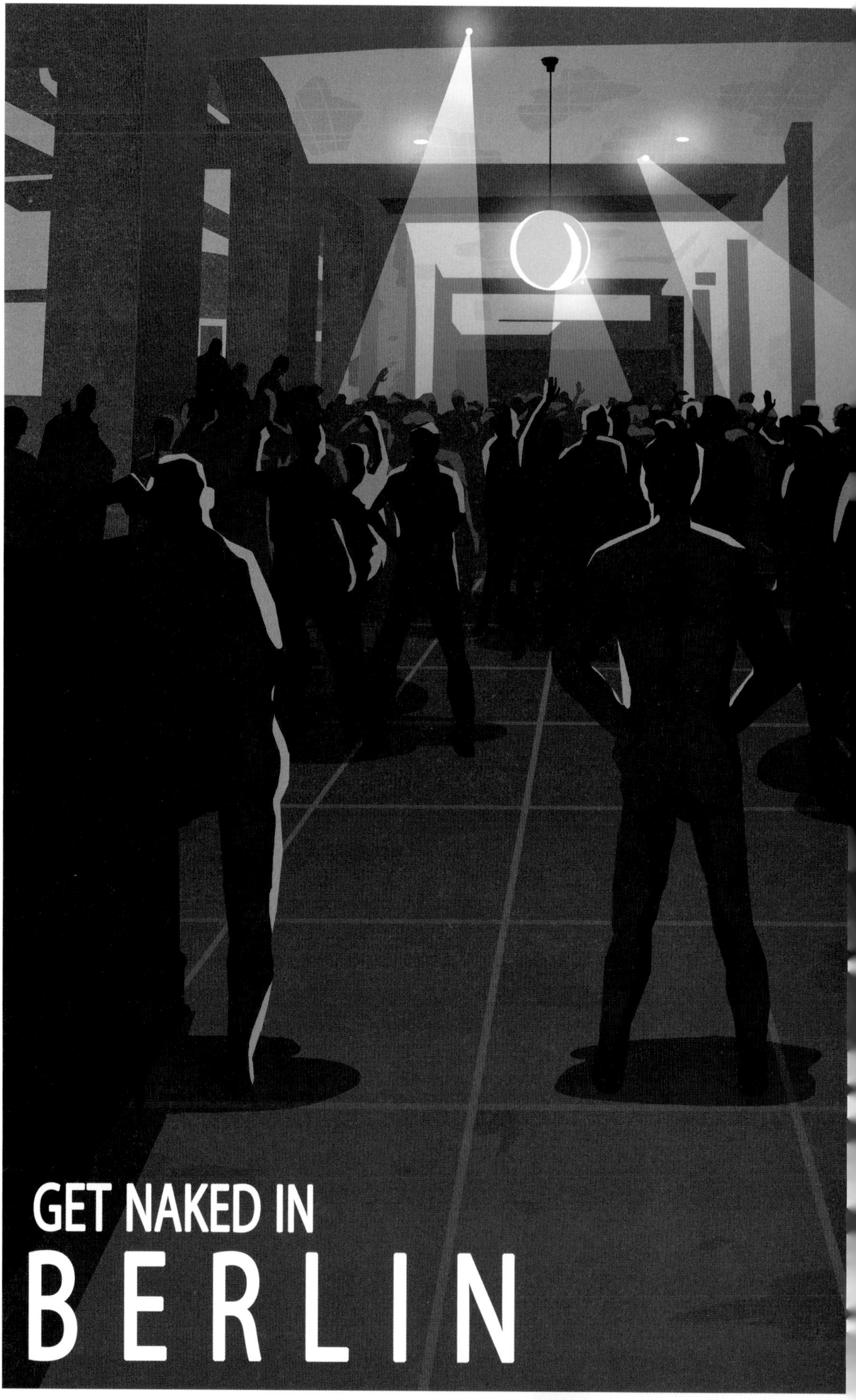
GET NAKED IN
BERLIN

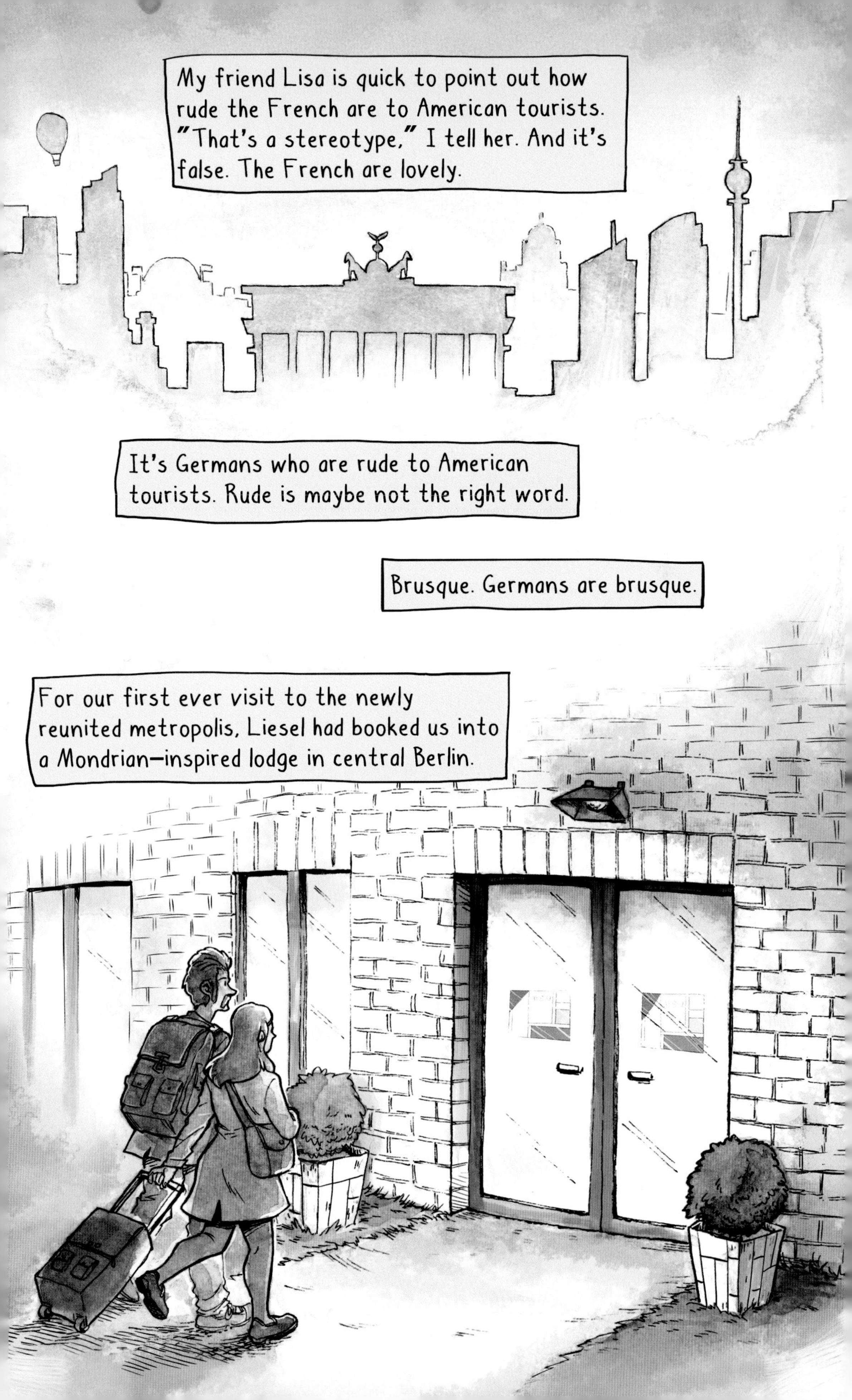
My friend Lisa is quick to point out how rude the French are to American tourists. "That's a stereotype," I tell her. And it's false. The French are lovely.
It's Germans who are rude to American tourists. Rude is maybe not the right word.
Brusque. Germans are brusque.
For our first ever visit to the newly reunited metropolis, Liesel had booked us into a Mondrian-inspired lodge in central Berlin.

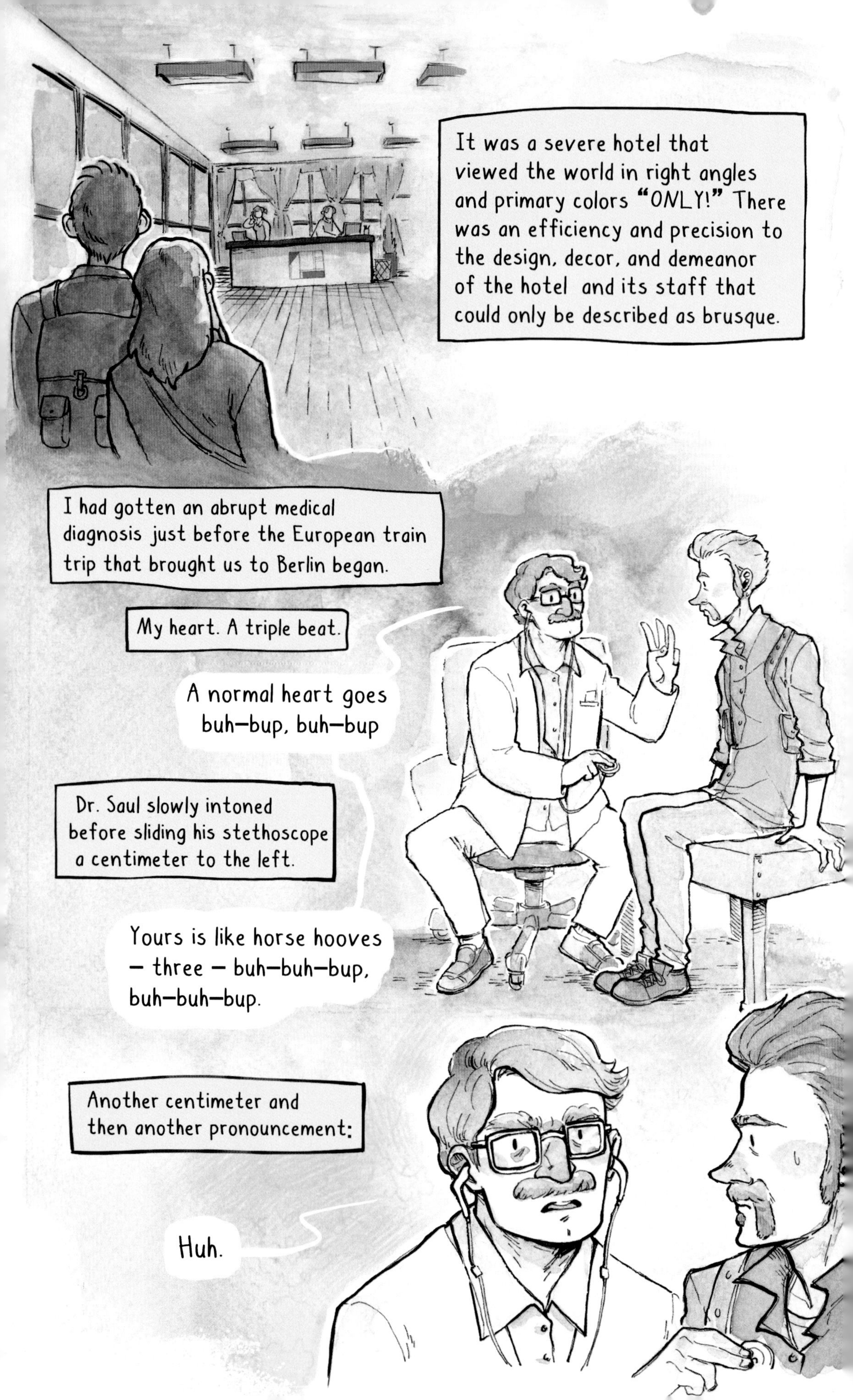
It was a severe hotel that viewed the world in right angles and primary colors "ONLY!" There was an efficiency and precision to the design, decor, and demeanor of the hotel and its staff that could only be described as brusque.
I had gotten an abrupt medical diagnosis just before the European train trip that brought us to Berlin began.
My heart. A triple beat.
A normal heart goes buh–bup, buh–bup
Dr. Saul slowly intoned before sliding his stethoscope a centimeter to the left.
Yours is like horse hooves – three – buh–buh–bup, buh–buh–bup.
Another centimeter and then another pronouncement:
Huh.

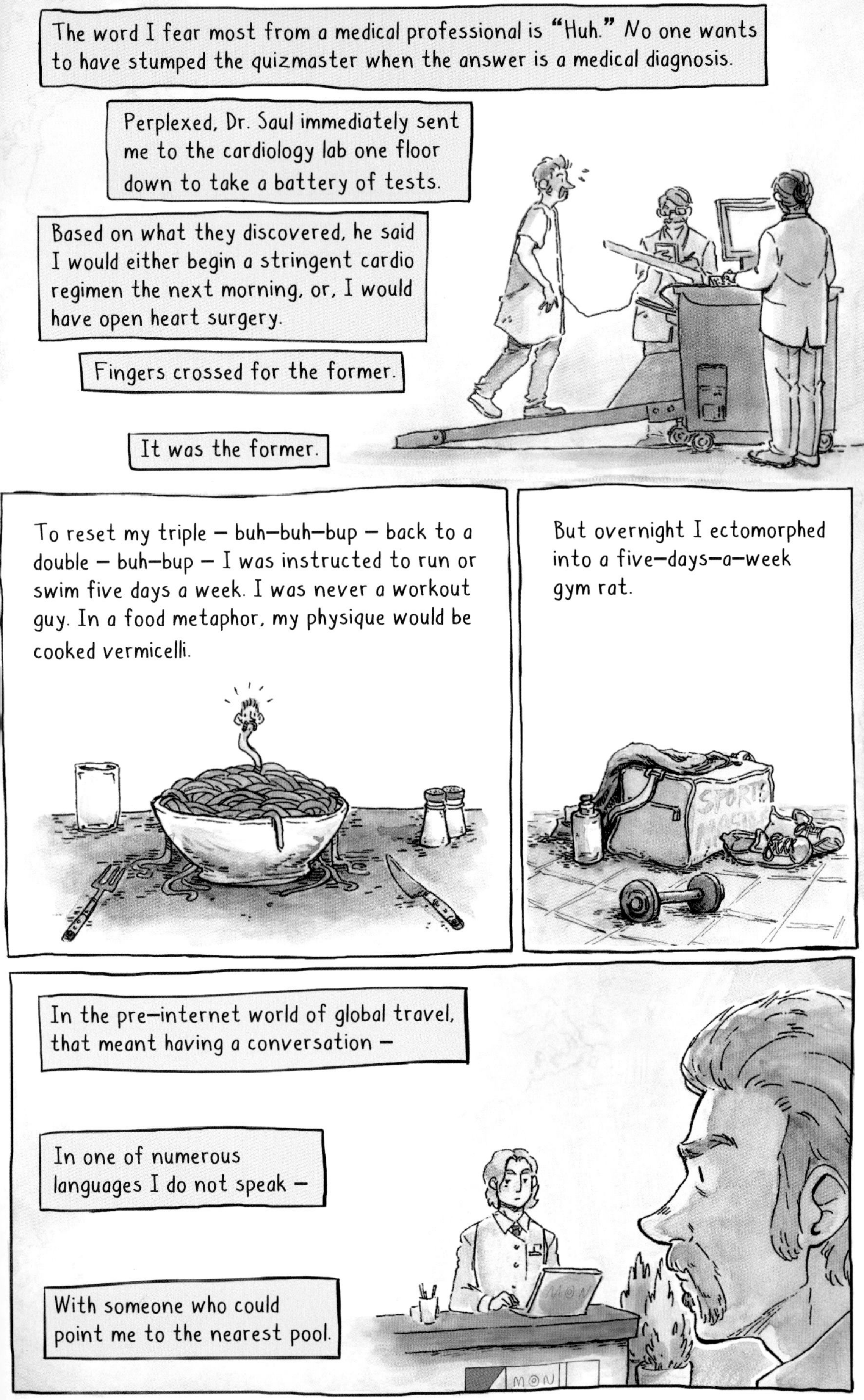
The word I fear most from a medical professional is "Huh." No one wants to have stumped the quizmaster when the answer is a medical diagnosis.
Perplexed, Dr. Saul immediately sent me to the cardiology lab one floor down to take a battery of tests.
Based on what they discovered, he said I would either begin a stringent cardio regimen the next morning, or, I would have open heart surgery.
Fingers crossed for the former.
It was the former.
To reset my triple – buh–buh–bup – back to a double – buh–bup – I was instructed to run or swim five days a week. I was never a workout guy. In a food metaphor, my physique would be cooked vermicelli.
But overnight I ectomorphed into a five–days–a–week gym rat.
In the pre–internet world of global travel, that meant having a conversation –
In one of numerous languages I do not speak –
With someone who could point me to the nearest pool.

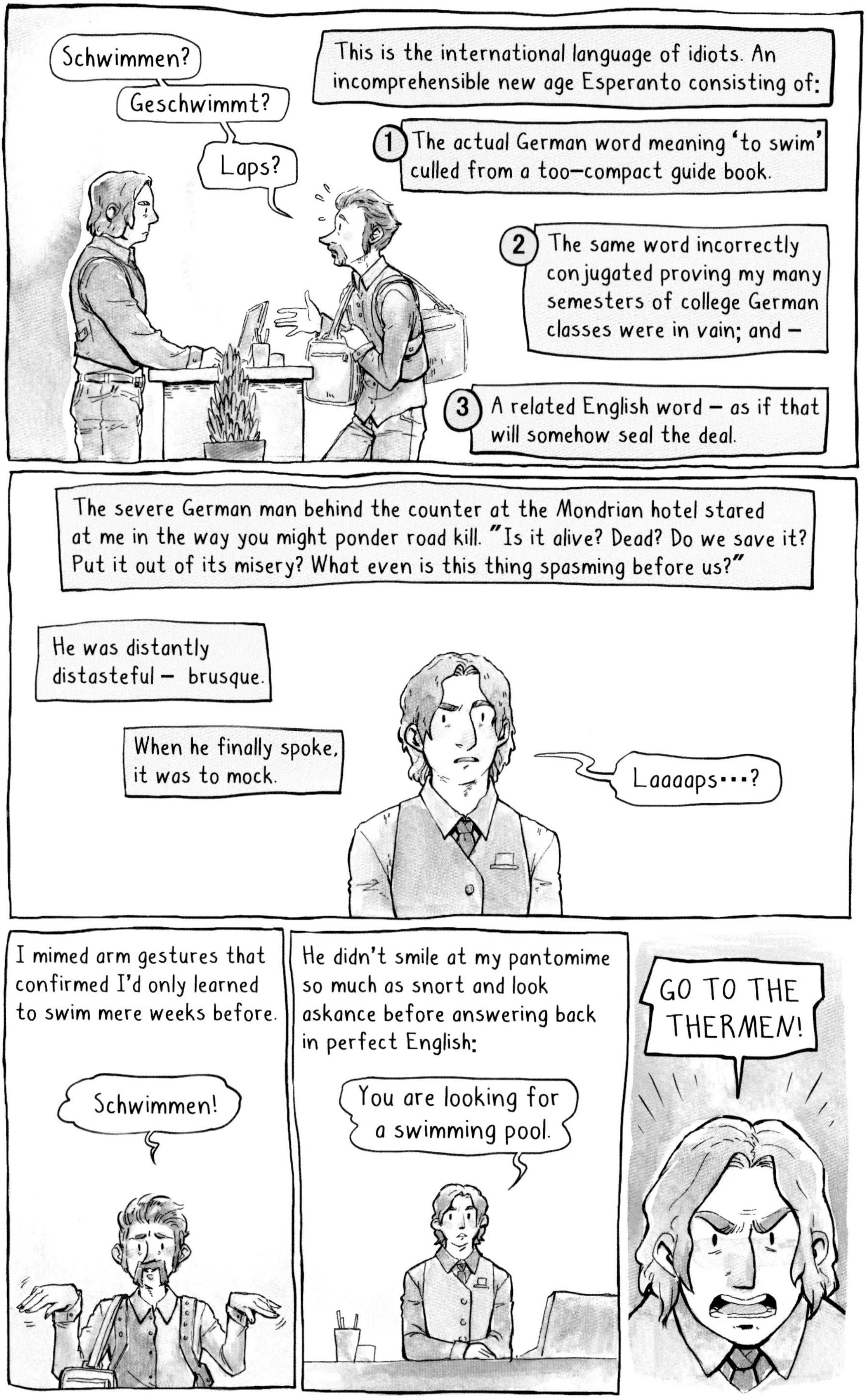
Schwimmen?
Geschwimmt?
Laps?
This is the international language of idiots. An incomprehensible new age Esperanto consisting of:
1 The actual German word meaning 'to swim' culled from a too-compact guide book.
2 The same word incorrectly conjugated proving my many semesters of college German classes were in vain; and –
3 A related English word – as if that will somehow seal the deal.
The severe German man behind the counter at the Mondrian hotel stared at me in the way you might ponder road kill. "Is it alive? Dead? Do we save it? Put it out of its misery? What even is this thing spasming before us?"
He was distantly distasteful – brusque.
When he finally spoke, it was to mock.
Laaaaps...?
I mimed arm gestures that confirmed I'd only learned to swim mere weeks before.
Schwimmen!
He didn't smile at my pantomime so much as snort and look askance before answering back in perfect English:
You are looking for a swimming pool.
GO TO THE THERMEN!

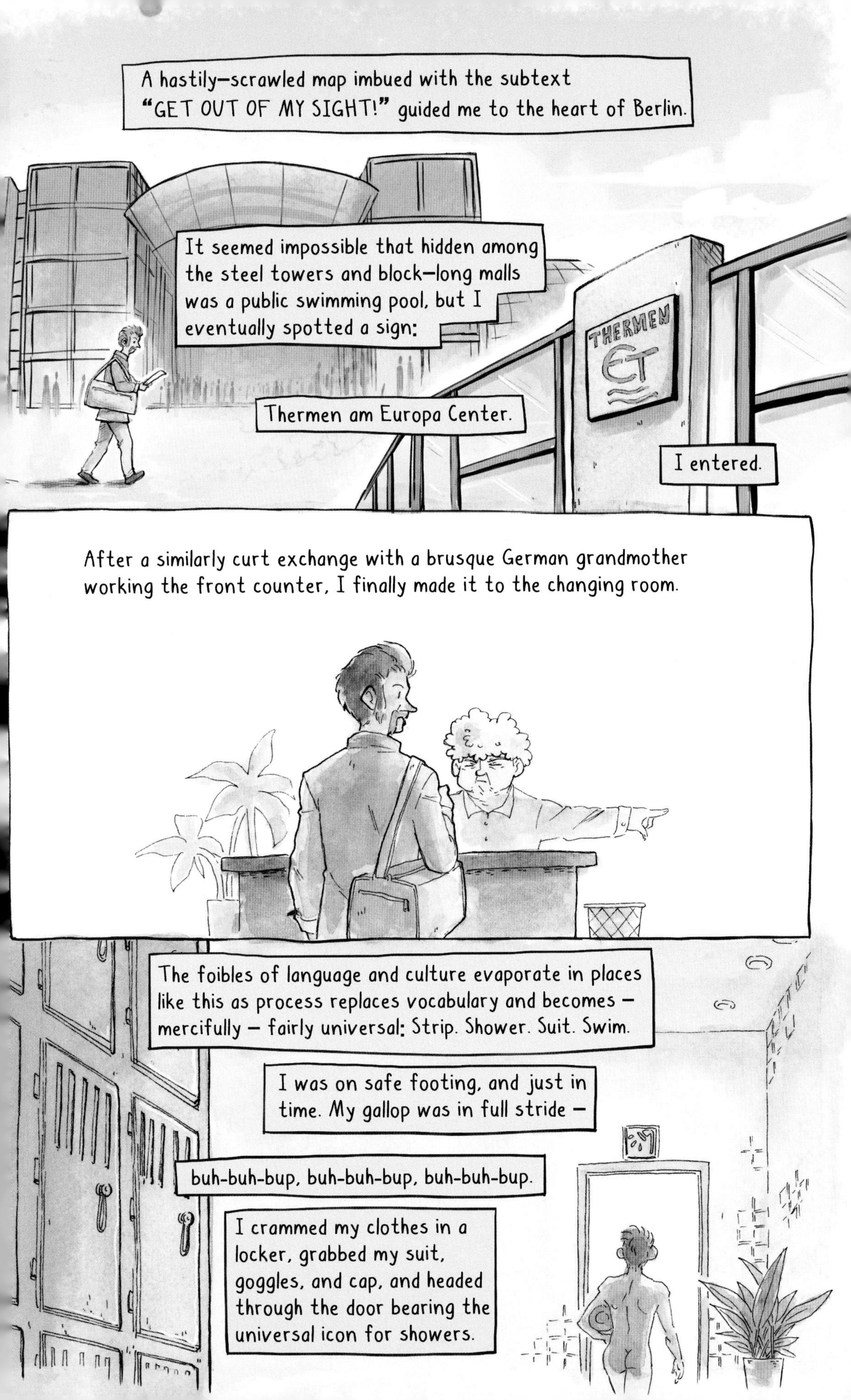
A hastily-scrawled map imbued with the subtext "GET OUT OF MY SIGHT!" guided me to the heart of Berlin.
It seemed impossible that hidden among the steel towers and block-long malls was a public swimming pool, but I eventually spotted a sign:
THERMEN
ET
Thermen am Europa Center.
I entered.
After a similarly curt exchange with a brusque German grandmother working the front counter, I finally made it to the changing room.
The foibles of language and culture evaporate in places like this as process replaces vocabulary and becomes — mercifully — fairly universal: Strip. Shower. Suit. Swim.
I was on safe footing, and just in time. My gallop was in full stride —
buh-buh-bup, buh-buh-bup, buh-buh-bup.
I crammed my clothes in a locker, grabbed my suit, goggles, and cap, and headed through the door bearing the universal icon for showers.

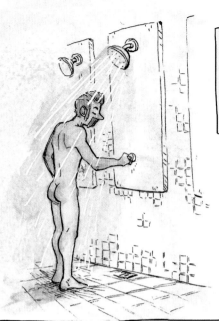

I stepped up to one of the many open-area showers and craned my head under the center of the jet. It felt like the water might shear my hair off at the follicles. It was harsh. It was brutal.

It was German.

I leaned slightly forward and let it slice into the back of my neck. It cut the tension away with surgical precision. I wondered why American showers lacked this excruciatingly wonderful water sadism.

My head bowed in hydro reverence, I noticed someone step up to the open stall beside me. Someone with nicely toned legs.

Meticulously hairless legs.

I knew from German porn that this was a country that obsessively removed body hair, but for a guy to get this smooth he'd have to really invest time, products, and high-powered lasers.

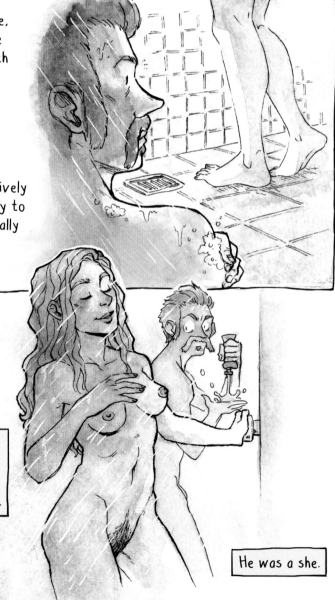

I looked up to grab my swimsuit from the shower handle where I'd hung it.

I was stopped cold by the realization that the hairless guy next to me had no penis and very pronounced breasts.

He was a she.

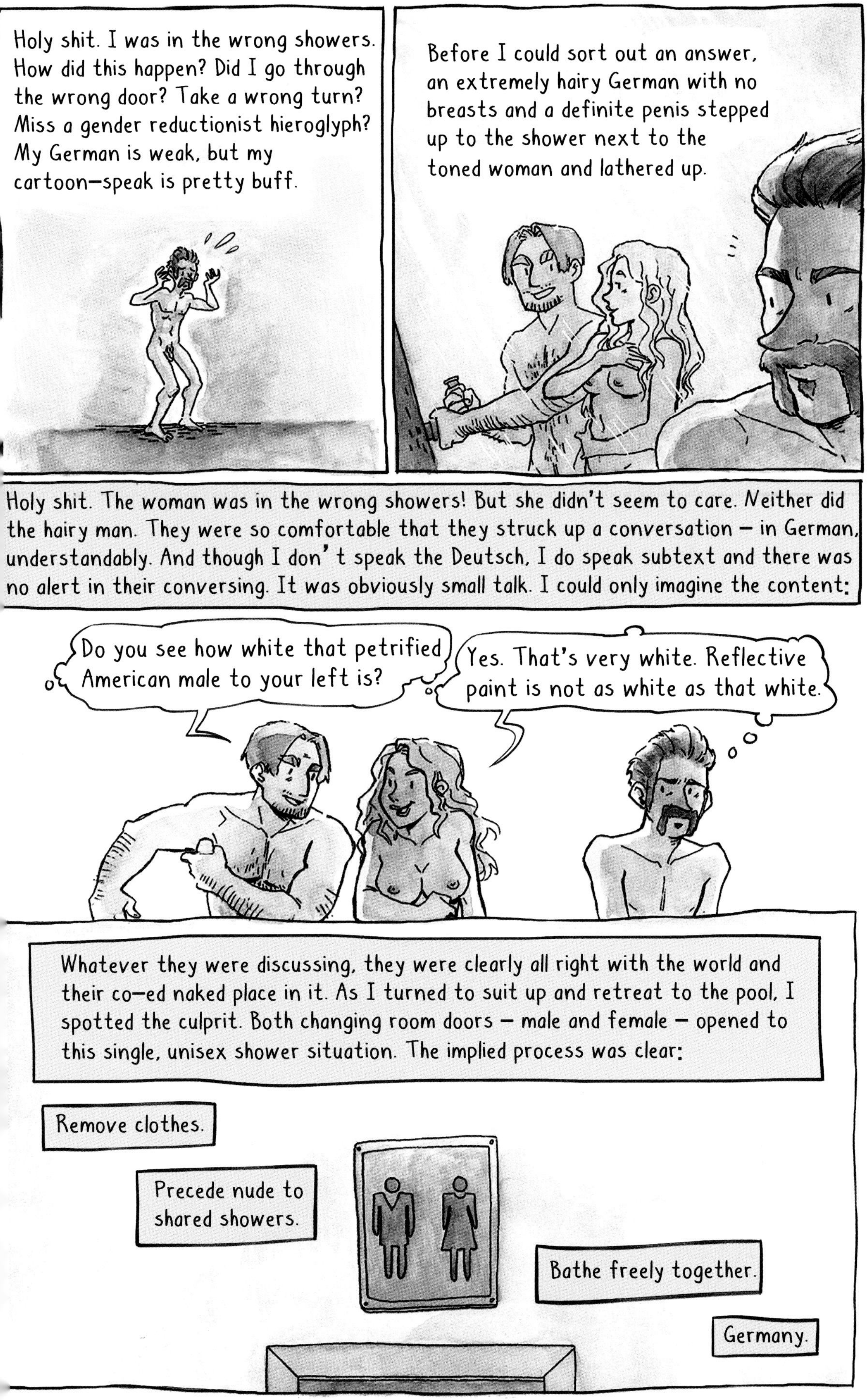

Holy shit. I was in the wrong showers. How did this happen? Did I go through the wrong door? Take a wrong turn? Miss a gender reductionist hieroglyph? My German is weak, but my cartoon—speak is pretty buff.
Before I could sort out an answer, an extremely hairy German with no breasts and a definite penis stepped up to the shower next to the toned woman and lathered up.
Holy shit. The woman was in the wrong showers! But she didn't seem to care. Neither did the hairy man. They were so comfortable that they struck up a conversation – in German, understandably. And though I don't speak the Deutsch, I do speak subtext and there was no alert in their conversing. It was obviously small talk. I could only imagine the content:
Do you see how white that petrified American male to your left is?
Yes. That's very white. Reflective paint is not as white as that white.
Whatever they were discussing, they were clearly all right with the world and their co–ed naked place in it. As I turned to suit up and retreat to the pool, I spotted the culprit. Both changing room doors – male and female – opened to this single, unisex shower situation. The implied process was clear:
Remove clothes.
Precede nude to shared showers.
Bathe freely together.
Germany.

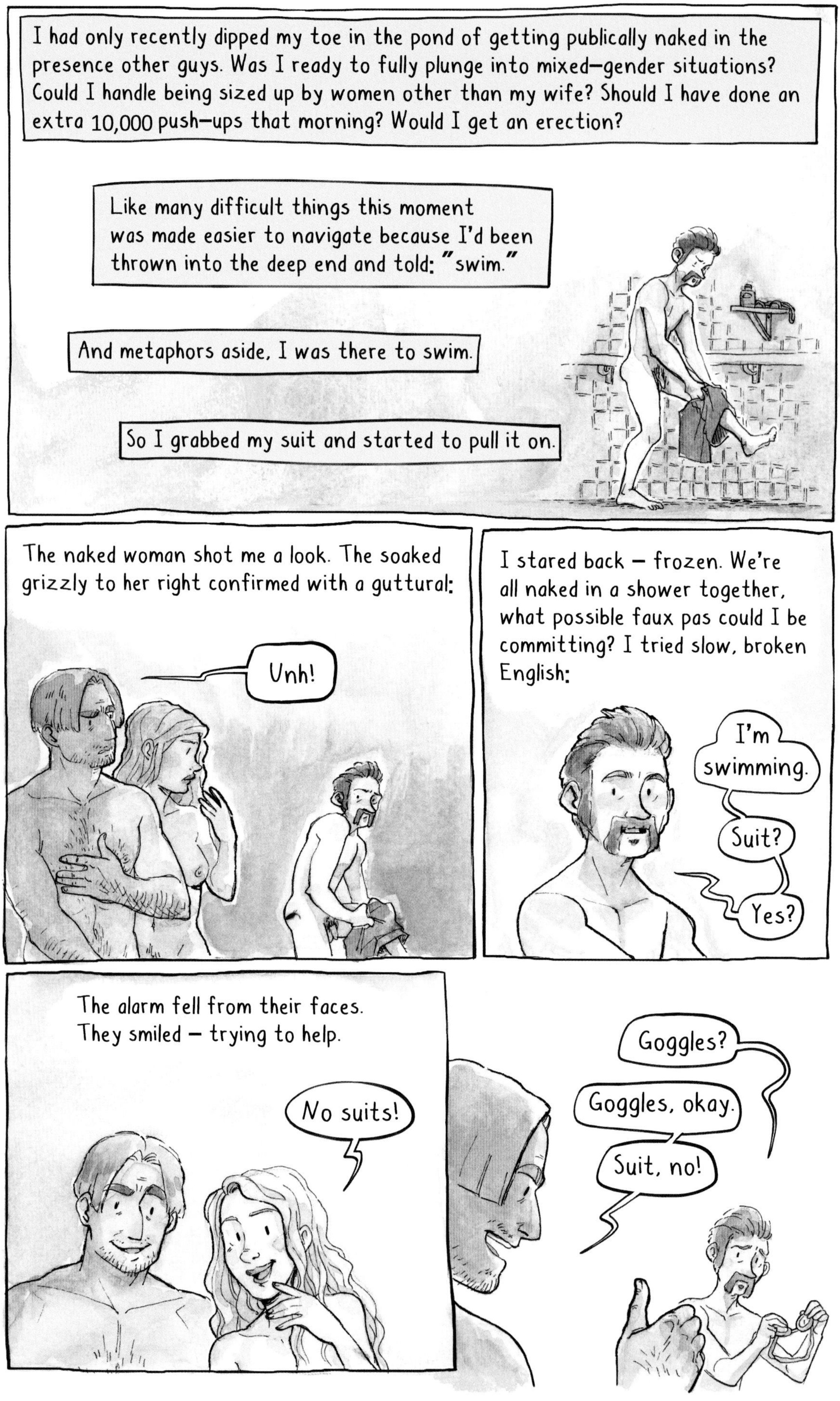
I had only recently dipped my toe in the pond of getting publically naked in the presence other guys. Was I ready to fully plunge into mixed-gender situations? Could I handle being sized up by women other than my wife? Should I have done an extra 10,000 push-ups that morning? Would I get an erection?
Like many difficult things this moment was made easier to navigate because I'd been thrown into the deep end and told: "swim."
And metaphors aside, I was there to swim.
So I grabbed my suit and started to pull it on.
The naked woman shot me a look. The soaked grizzly to her right confirmed with a guttural:
Unh!
I stared back – frozen. We're all naked in a shower together, what possible faux pas could I be committing? I tried slow, broken English:
I'm swimming.
Suit?
Yes?
The alarm fell from their faces. They smiled – trying to help.
No suits!
Goggles?
Goggles, okay.
Suit, no!

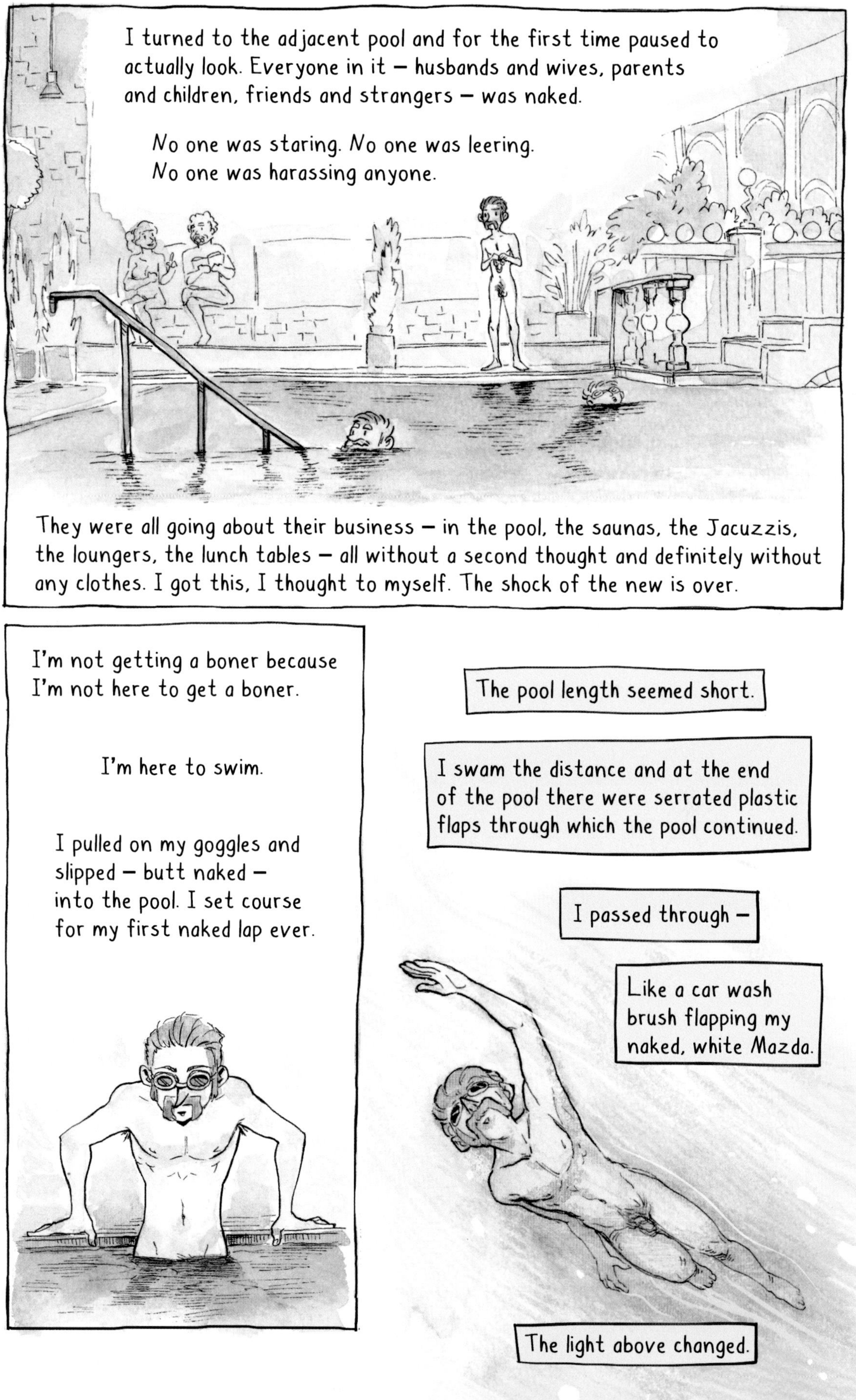
I turned to the adjacent pool and for the first time paused to actually look. Everyone in it — husbands and wives, parents and children, friends and strangers — was naked.
No one was staring. No one was leering. No one was harassing anyone.
They were all going about their business — in the pool, the saunas, the Jacuzzis, the loungers, the lunch tables — all without a second thought and definitely without any clothes. I got this, I thought to myself. The shock of the new is over.
I'm not getting a boner because I'm not here to get a boner.
I'm here to swim.
I pulled on my goggles and slipped — butt naked — into the pool. I set course for my first naked lap ever.
The pool length seemed short.
I swam the distance and at the end of the pool there were serrated plastic flaps through which the pool continued.
I passed through —
Like a car wash brush flapping my naked, white Mazda.
The light above changed.

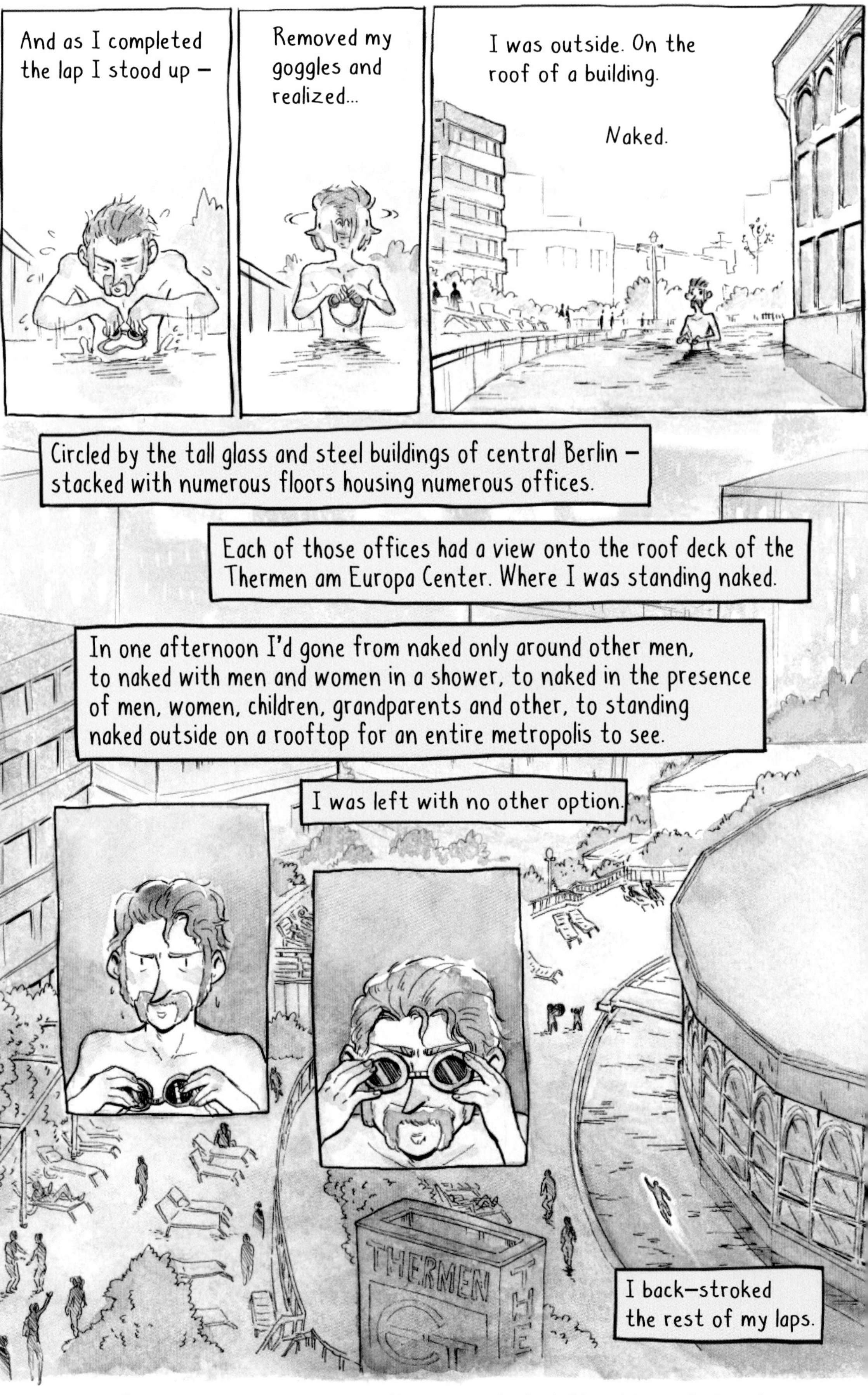
And as I completed the lap I stood up –
Removed my goggles and realized...
I was outside. On the roof of a building.
Naked.
Circled by the tall glass and steel buildings of central Berlin – stacked with numerous floors housing numerous offices.
Each of those offices had a view onto the roof deck of the Thermen am Europa Center. Where I was standing naked.
In one afternoon I'd gone from naked only around other men, to naked with men and women in a shower, to naked in the presence of men, women, children, grandparents and other, to standing naked outside on a rooftop for an entire metropolis to see.
I was left with no other option.
THERMEN
I back-stroked the rest of my laps.

There might be someone on the moon who hadn't gotten a look yet.

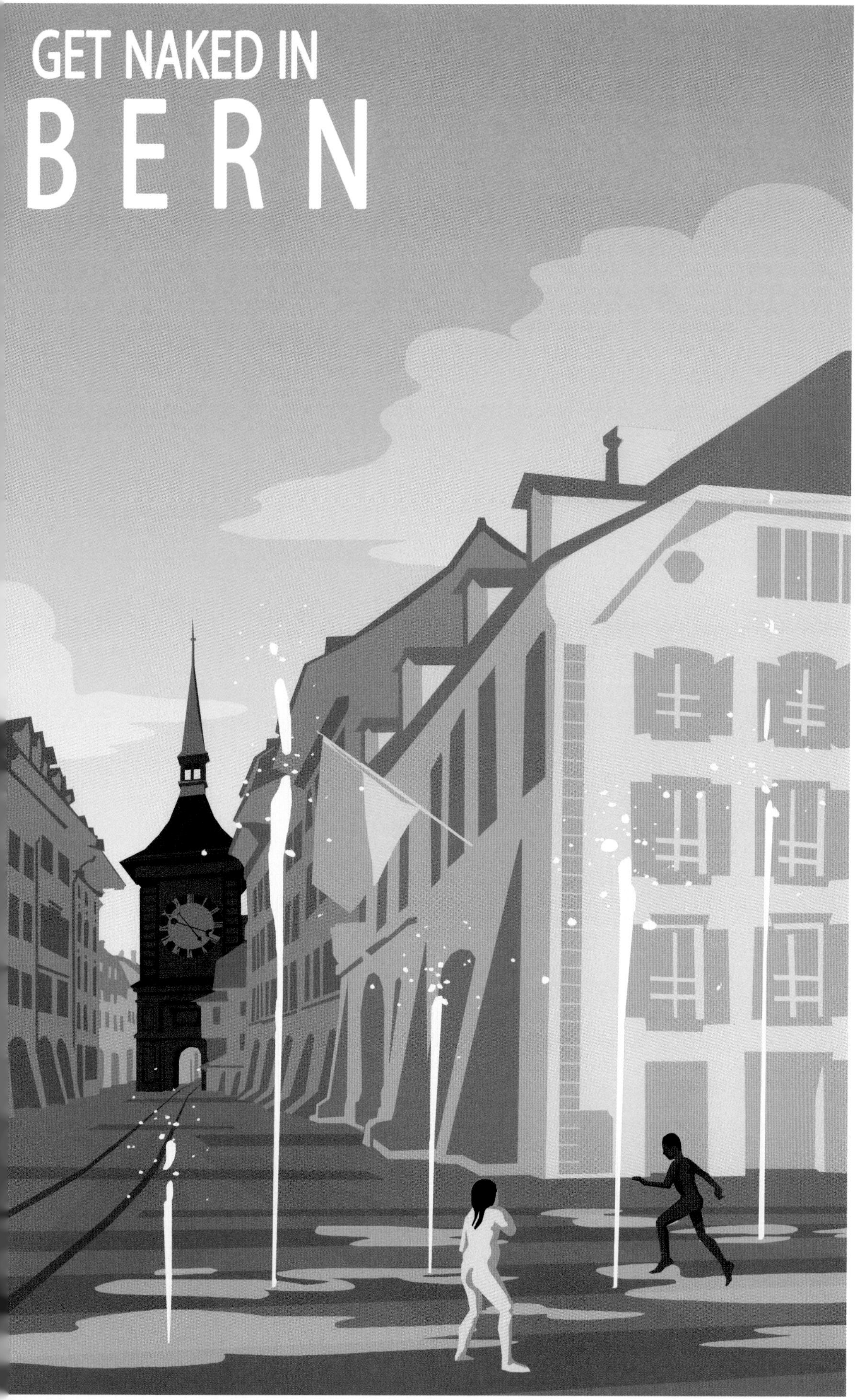
GET NAKED IN
BERN

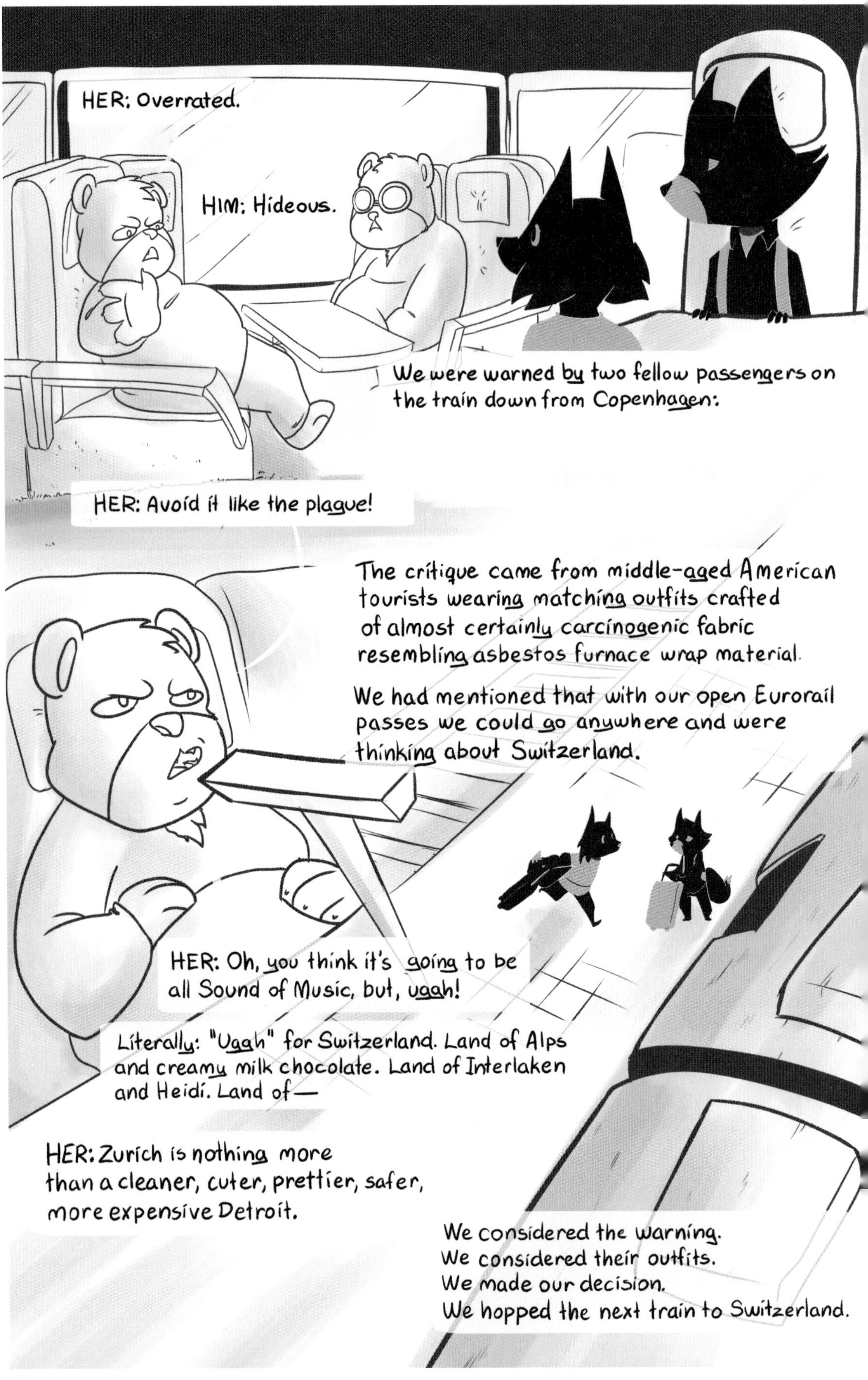
HER: Overrated.
HIM: Hideous.
We were warned by two fellow passengers on the train down from Copenhagen:
HER: Avoid it like the plague!
The critique came from middle-aged American tourists wearing matching outfits crafted of almost certainly carcinogenic fabric resembling asbestos furnace wrap material.
We had mentioned that with our open Eurorail passes we could go anywhere and were thinking about Switzerland.
HER: Oh, you think it's going to be all Sound of Music, but, uggh!
Literally: "Uggh" for Switzerland. Land of Alps and creamy milk chocolate. Land of Interlaken and Heidi. Land of—
HER: Zurich is nothing more than a cleaner, cuter, prettier, safer, more expensive Detroit.
We considered the warning.
We considered their outfits.
We made our decision.
We hopped the next train to Switzerland.

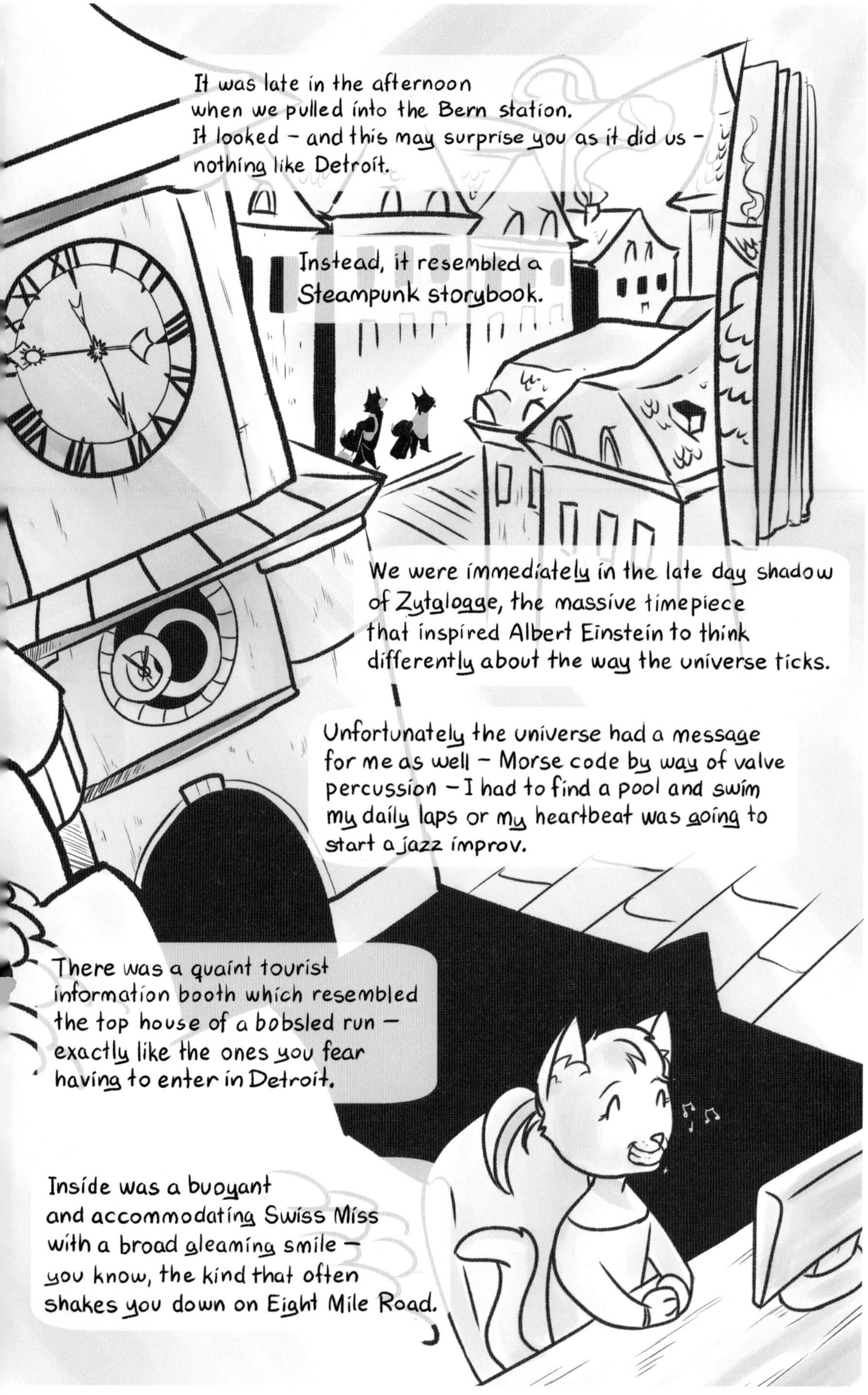
It was late in the afternoon when we pulled into the Bern station. It looked – and this may surprise you as it did us – nothing like Detroit.
Instead, it resembled a Steampunk storybook.
We were immediately in the late day shadow of Zytglogge, the massive timepiece that inspired Albert Einstein to think differently about the way the universe ticks.
Unfortunately the universe had a message for me as well – Morse code by way of valve percussion – I had to find a pool and swim my daily laps or my heartbeat was going to start a jazz improv.
There was a quaint tourist information booth which resembled the top house of a bobsled run – exactly like the ones you fear having to enter in Detroit.
Inside was a buoyant and accommodating Swiss Miss with a broad gleaming smile – you know, the kind that often shakes you down on Eight Mile Road.

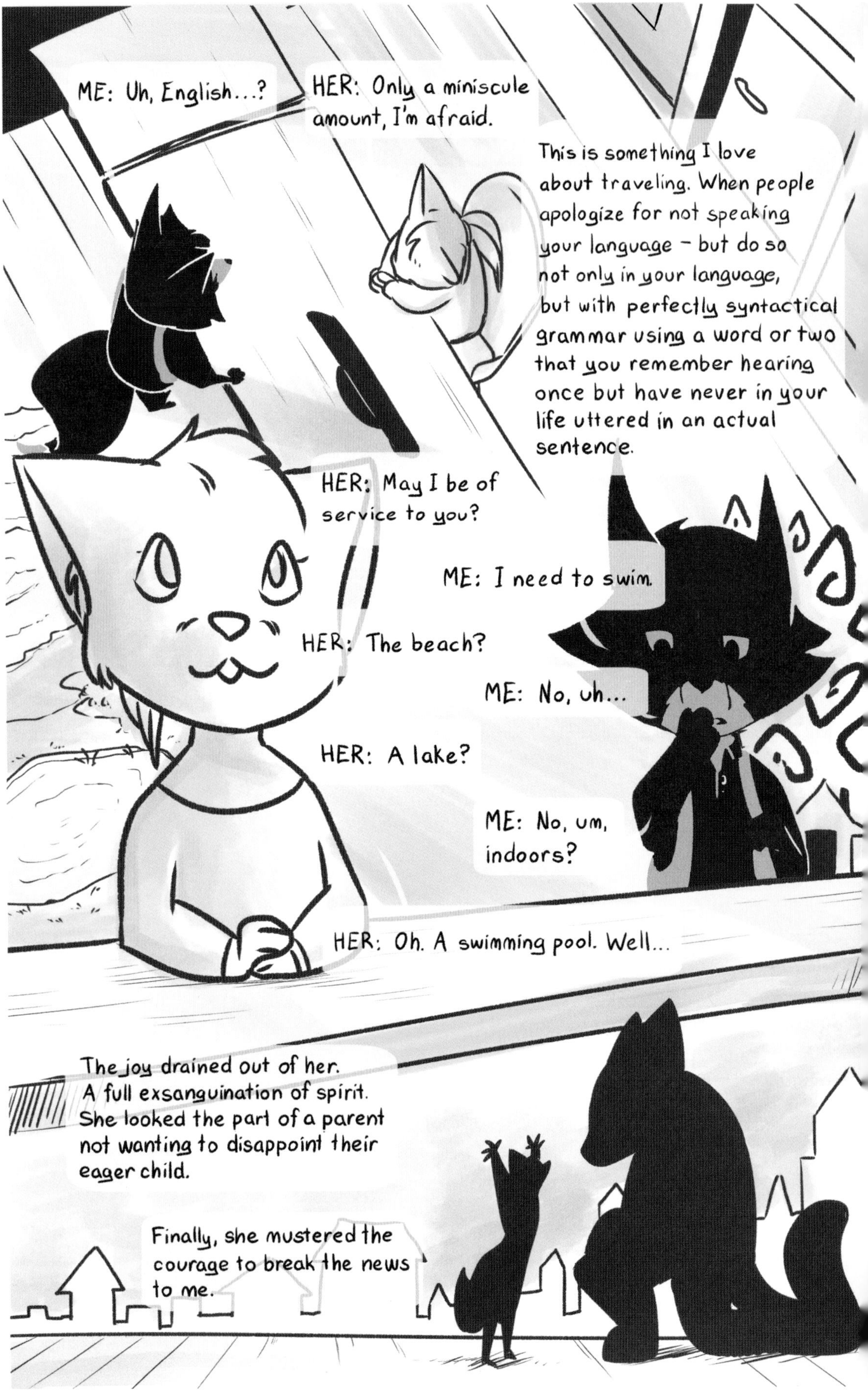
ME: Uh, English...?
HER: Only a miniscule amount, I'm afraid.
This is something I love about traveling. When people apologize for not speaking your language – but do so not only in your language, but with perfectly syntactical grammar using a word or two that you remember hearing once but have never in your life uttered in an actual sentence.
HER: May I be of service to you?
ME: I need to swim.
HER: The beach?
ME: No, uh...
HER: A lake?
ME: No, um, indoors?
HER: Oh. A swimming pool. Well...
The joy drained out of her. A full exsanguination of spirit. She looked the part of a parent not wanting to disappoint their eager child.
Finally, she mustered the courage to break the news to me.

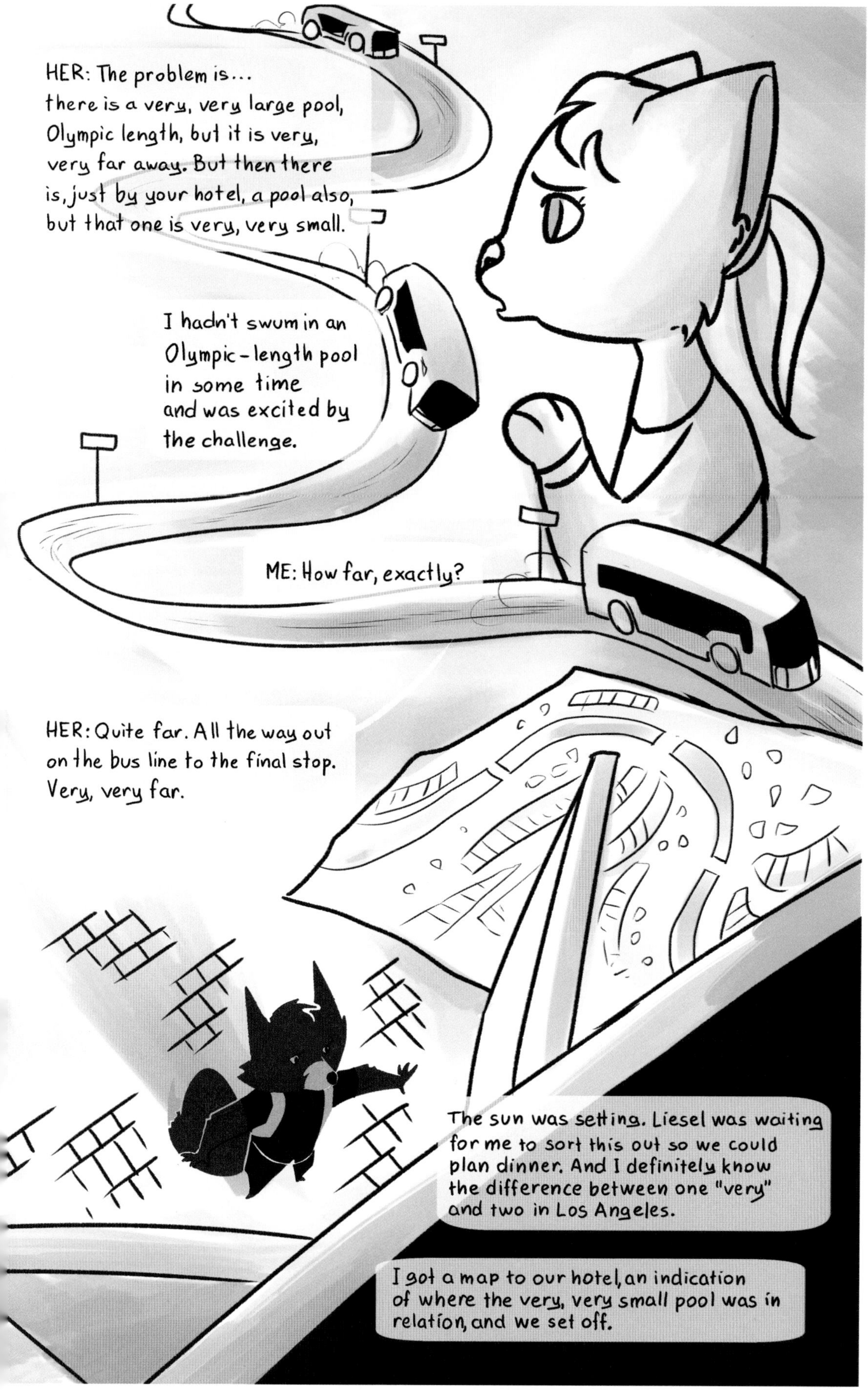
HER: The problem is... there is a very, very large pool, Olympic length, but it is very, very far away. But then there is, just by your hotel, a pool also, but that one is very, very small.
I hadn't swum in an Olympic-length pool in some time and was excited by the challenge.
ME: How far, exactly?
HER: Quite far. All the way out on the bus line to the final stop. Very, very far.
The sun was setting. Liesel was waiting for me to sort this out so we could plan dinner. And I definitely know the difference between one "very" and two in Los Angeles.
I got a map to our hotel, an indication of where the very, very small pool was in relation, and we set off.

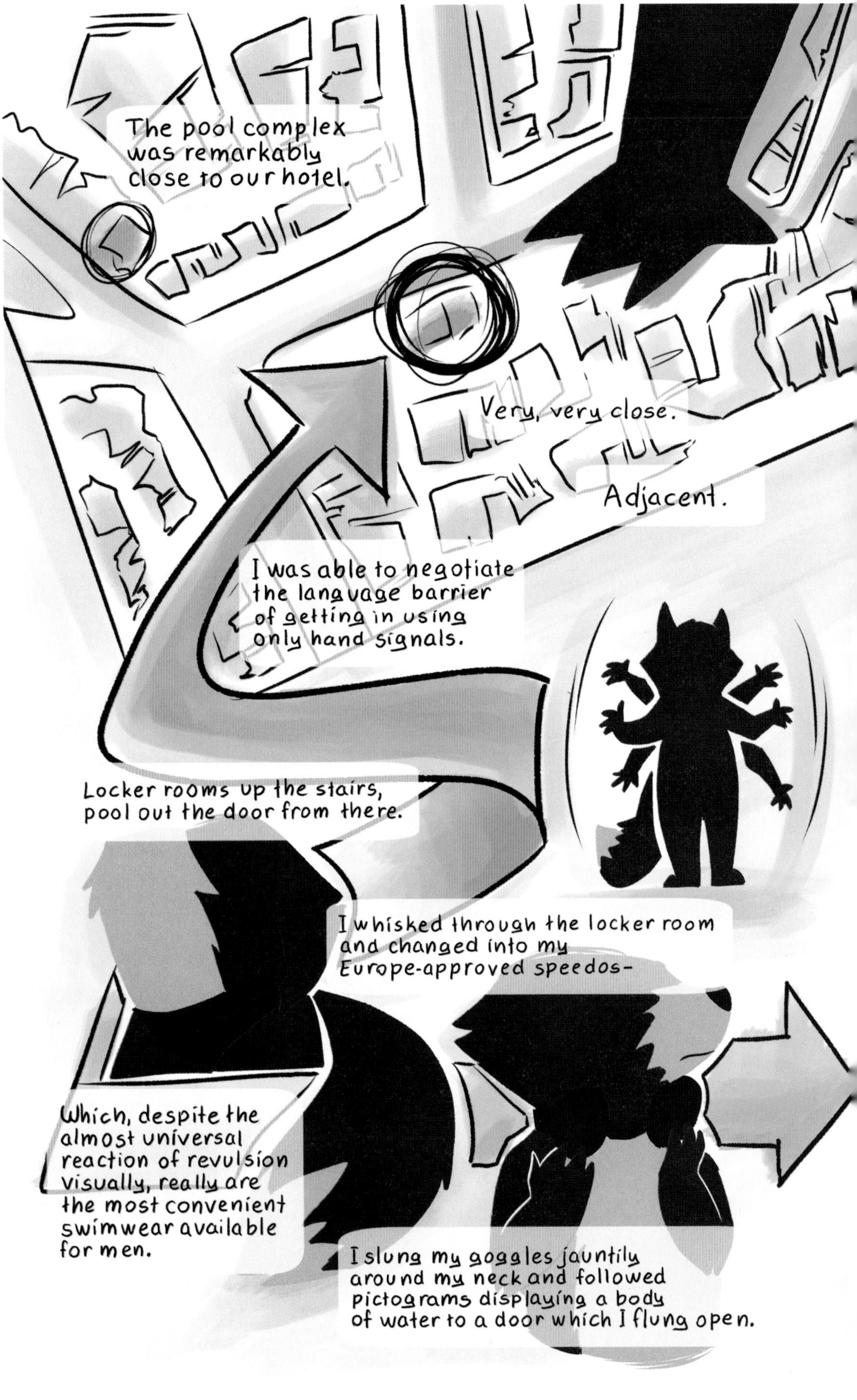

The pool complex was remarkably close to our hotel.
Very, very close.
Adjacent.
I was able to negotiate the language barrier of getting in using only hand signals.
Locker rooms up the stairs, pool out the door from there.
I whisked through the locker room and changed into my Europe-approved speedos-
Which, despite the almost universal reaction of revulsion visually, really are the most convenient swimwear available for men.
I slung my goggles jauntily around my neck and followed pictograms displaying a body of water to a door which I flung open.

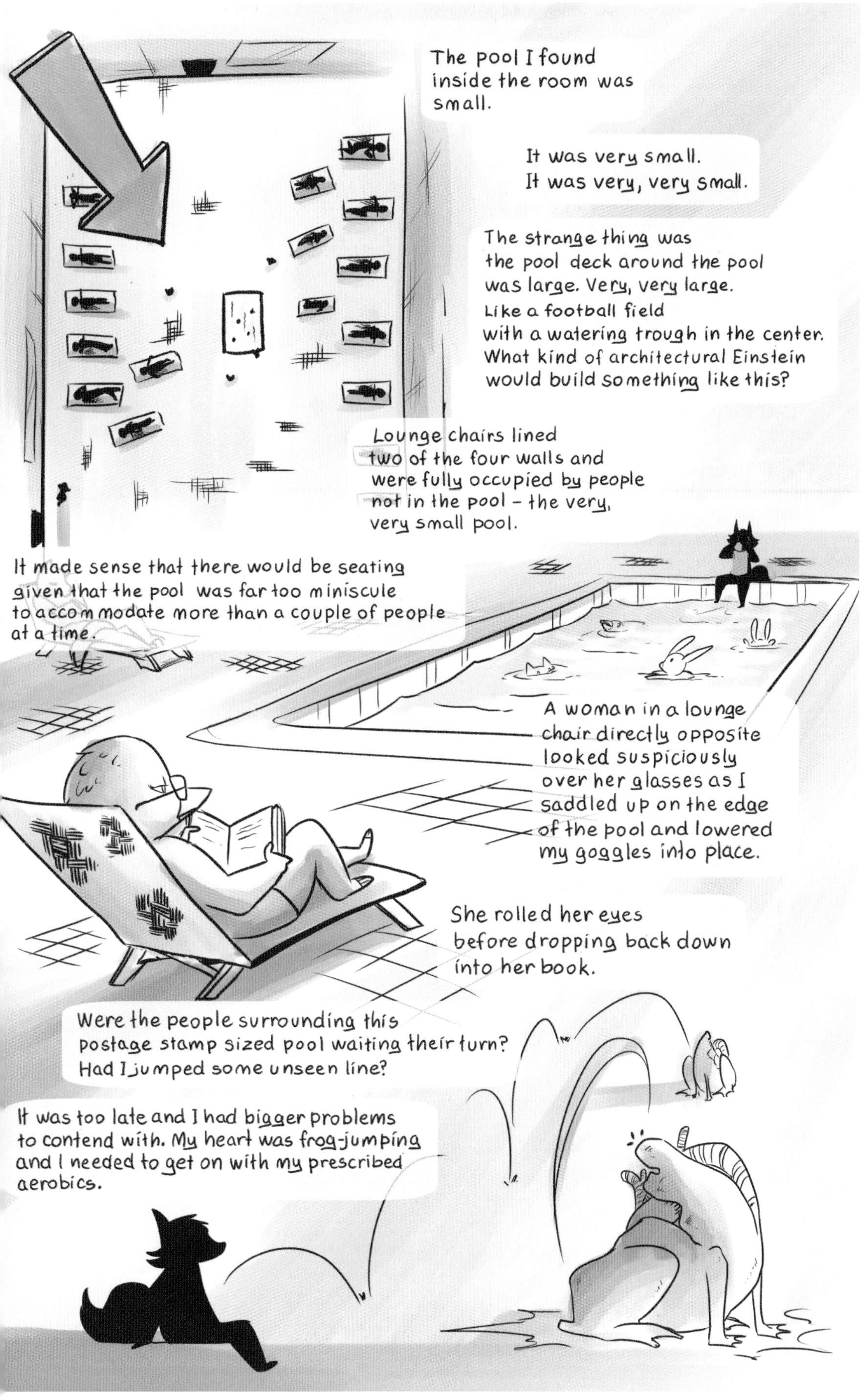

The pool I found inside the room was small.
It was very small.
It was very, very small.
The strange thing was the pool deck around the pool was large. Very, very large. Like a football field with a watering trough in the center. What kind of architectural Einstein would build something like this?
Lounge chairs lined two of the four walls and were fully occupied by people not in the pool - the very, very small pool.
It made sense that there would be seating given that the pool was far too miniscule to accommodate more than a couple of people at a time.
A woman in a lounge chair directly opposite looked suspiciously over her glasses as I saddled up on the edge of the pool and lowered my goggles into place.
She rolled her eyes before dropping back down into her book.
Were the people surrounding this postage stamp sized pool waiting their turn? Had I jumped some unseen line?
It was too late and I had bigger problems to contend with. My heart was frog-jumping and I needed to get on with my prescribed aerobics.

As a new swimmer, I wasn't fully comfortable with negotiating other swimmers in my lap lane, let alone a closet-sized, lane-less free-for-all. I watched as parents and kids zigged and zagged – some 80s video game daring me to try and make my way across it.

I picked my moment for the first length – left arm, right arm, left arm, right arm, breath, left arm – WALL. What? Impossible. Four and a half strokes and I was at the opposite side.

I turned back. Left, right, left, right, breath, left, WALL.

Not impossible. This pool was small as fuck.

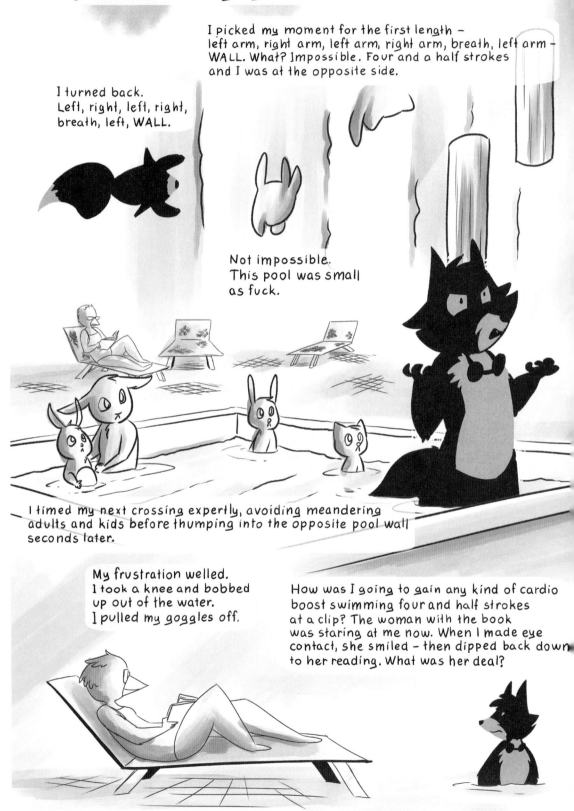

I timed my next crossing expertly, avoiding meandering adults and kids before thumping into the opposite pool wall seconds later.

My frustration welled. I took a knee and bobbed up out of the water. I pulled my goggles off.

How was I going to gain any kind of cardio boost swimming four and half strokes at a clip? The woman with the book was staring at me now. When I made eye contact, she smiled – then dipped back down to her reading. What was her deal?

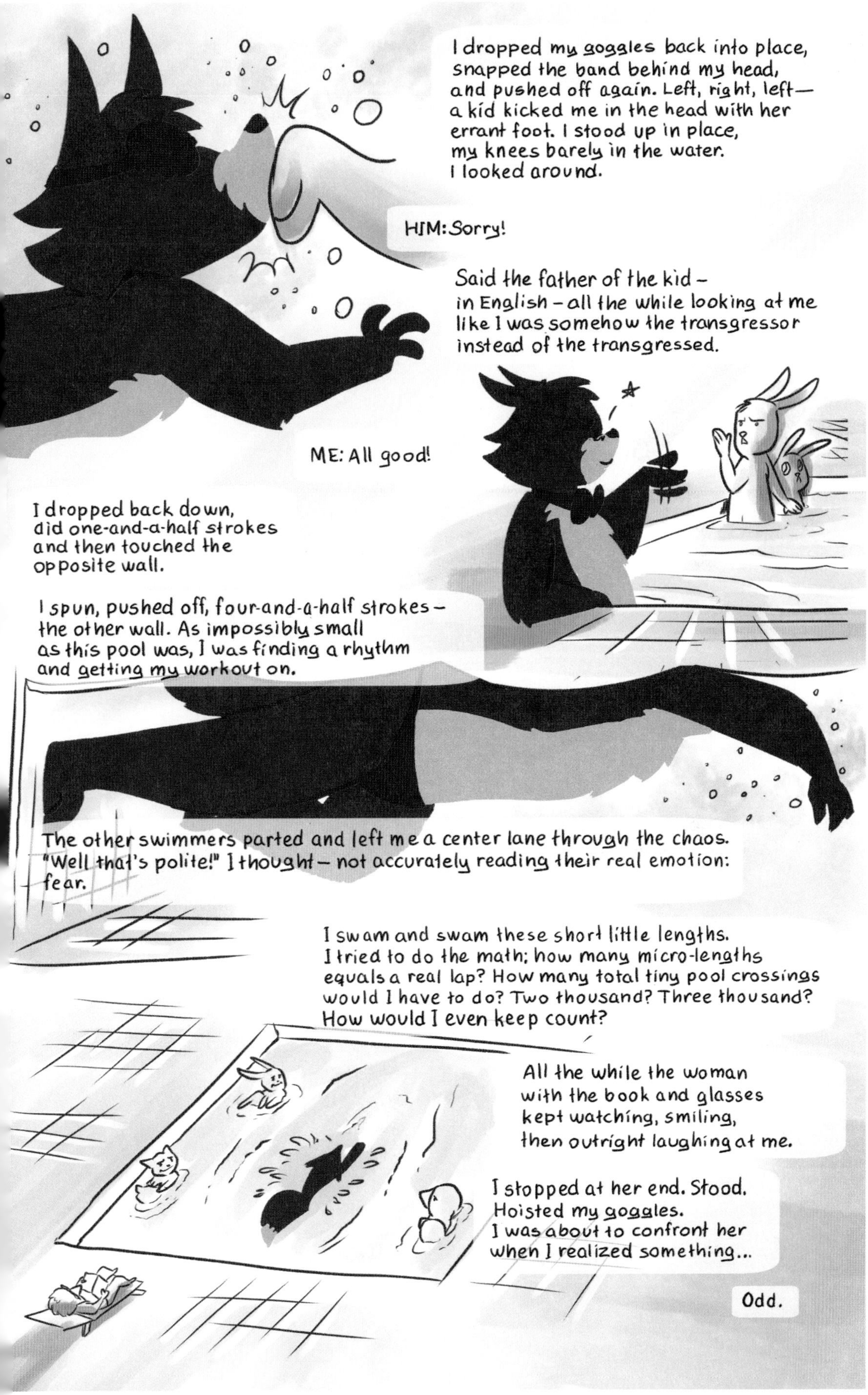
I dropped my goggles back into place, snapped the band behind my head, and pushed off again. Left, right, left— a kid kicked me in the head with her errant foot. I stood up in place, my knees barely in the water. I looked around.
HIM: Sorry!
Said the father of the kid – in English – all the while looking at me like I was somehow the transgressor instead of the transgressed.
ME: All good!
I dropped back down, did one-and-a-half strokes and then touched the opposite wall.
I spun, pushed off, four-and-a-half strokes – the other wall. As impossibly small as this pool was, I was finding a rhythm and getting my workout on.
The other swimmers parted and left me a center lane through the chaos. "Well that's polite!" I thought – not accurately reading their real emotion: fear.
I swam and swam these short little lengths. I tried to do the math: how many micro-lengths equals a real lap? How many total tiny pool crossings would I have to do? Two thousand? Three thousand? How would I even keep count?
All the while the woman with the book and glasses kept watching, smiling, then outright laughing at me.
I stopped at her end. Stood. Hoisted my goggles. I was about to confront her when I realized something...
Odd.

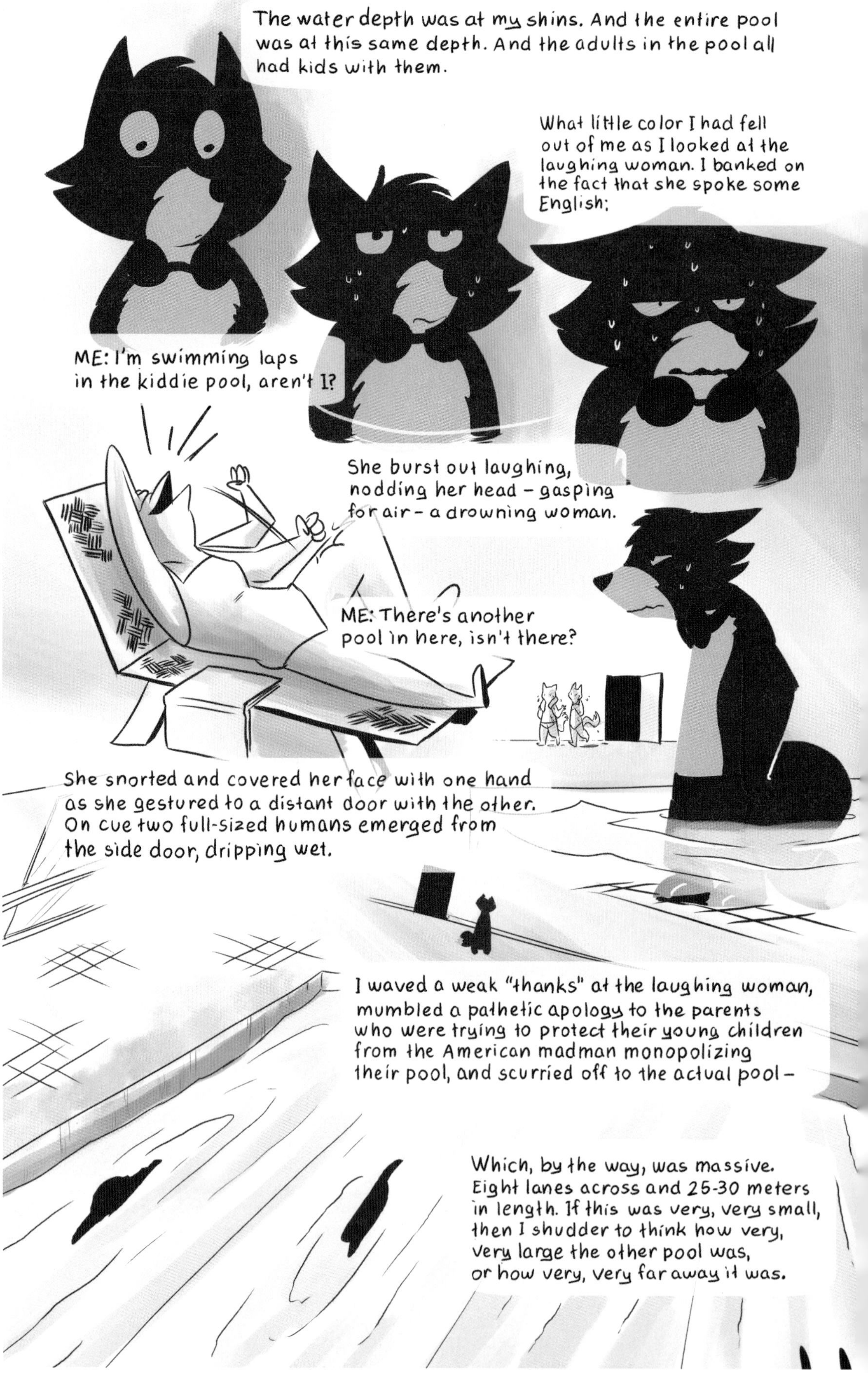
The water depth was at my shins. And the entire pool was at this same depth. And the adults in the pool all had kids with them.
What little color I had fell out of me as I looked at the laughing woman. I banked on the fact that she spoke some English:
ME: I'm swimming laps in the kiddie pool, aren't I?
She burst out laughing, nodding her head - gasping for air - a drowning woman.
ME: There's another pool in here, isn't there?
She snorted and covered her face with one hand as she gestured to a distant door with the other. On cue two full-sized humans emerged from the side door, dripping wet.
I waved a weak "thanks" at the laughing woman, mumbled a pathetic apology to the parents who were trying to protect their young children from the American madman monopolizing their pool, and scurried off to the actual pool -
Which, by the way, was massive. Eight lanes across and 25-30 meters in length. If this was very, very small, then I shudder to think how very, very large the other pool was, or how very, very far away it was.

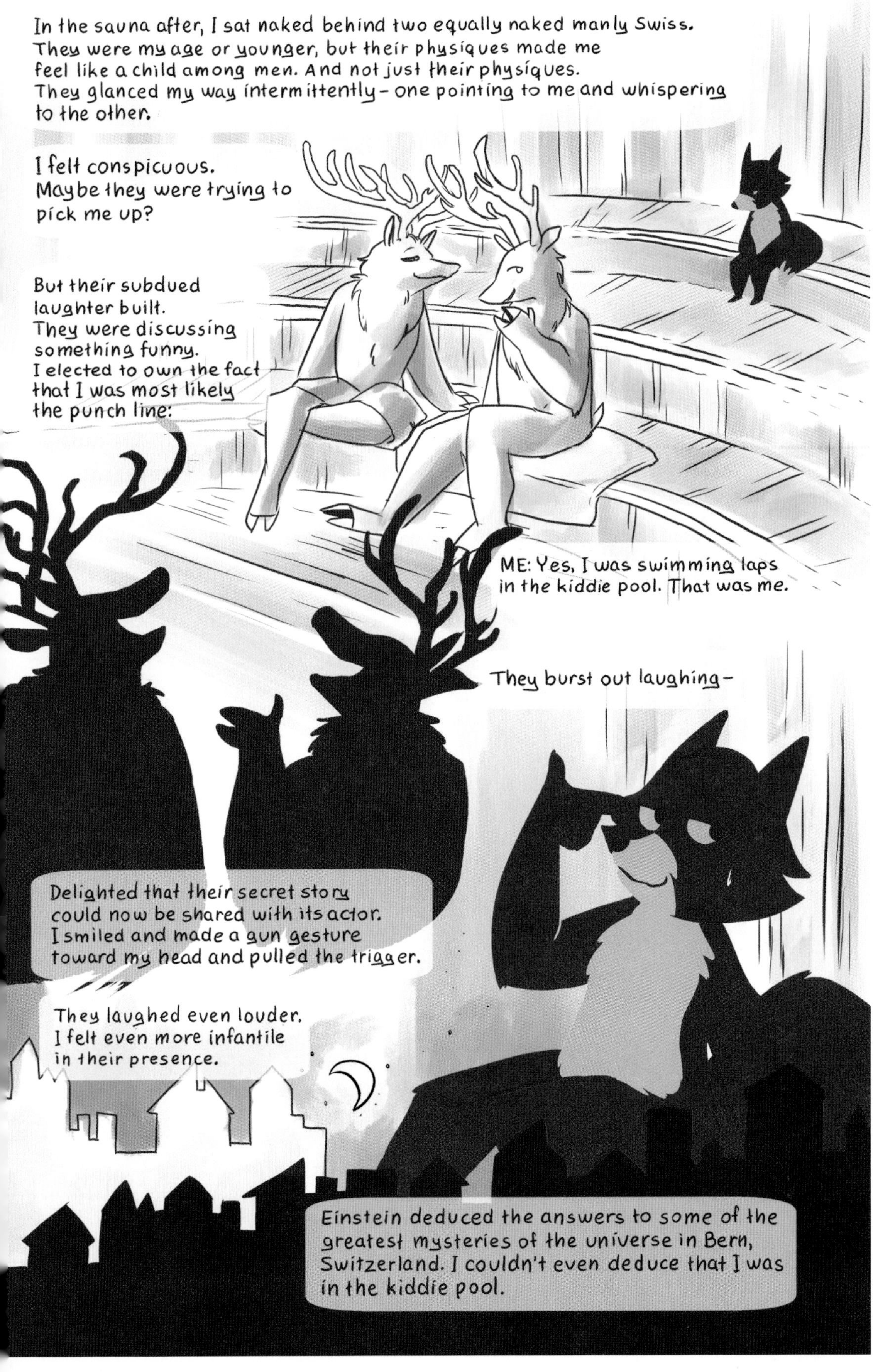
In the sauna after, I sat naked behind two equally naked manly Swiss. They were my age or younger, but their physiques made me feel like a child among men. And not just their physiques. They glanced my way intermittently – one pointing to me and whispering to the other.
I felt conspicuous. Maybe they were trying to pick me up?
But their subdued laughter built. They were discussing something funny. I elected to own the fact that I was most likely the punch line:
ME: Yes, I was swimming laps in the kiddie pool. That was me.
They burst out laughing–
Delighted that their secret story could now be shared with its actor. I smiled and made a gun gesture toward my head and pulled the trigger.
They laughed even louder. I felt even more infantile in their presence.
Einstein deduced the answers to some of the greatest mysteries of the universe in Bern, Switzerland. I couldn't even deduce that I was in the kiddie pool.

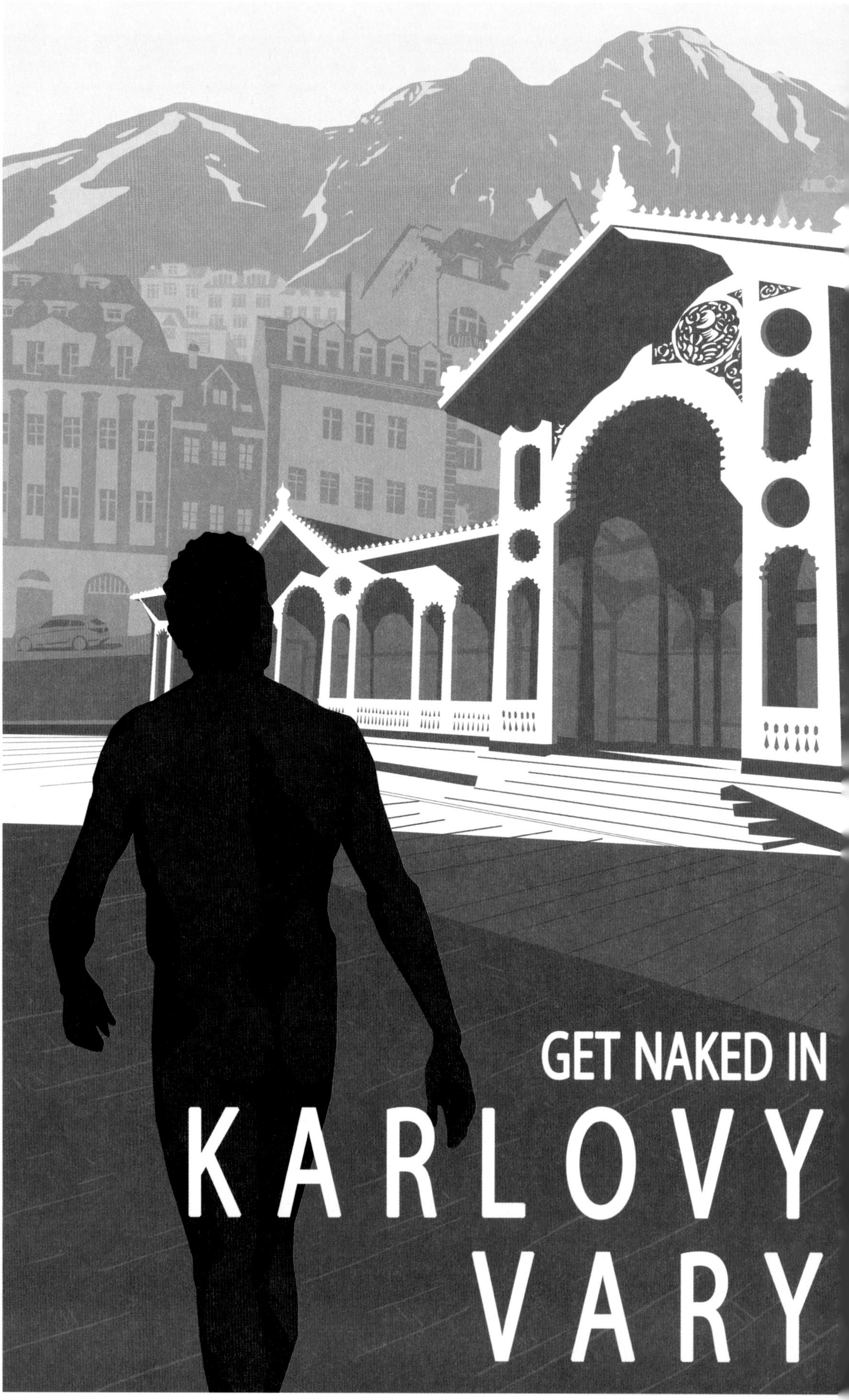
GET NAKED IN
KARLOVY
VARY

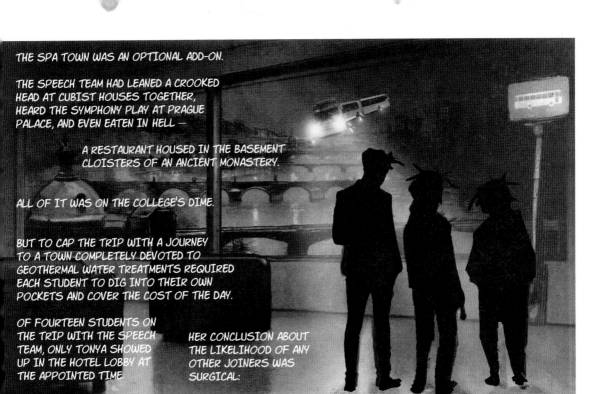

THE SPA TOWN WAS AN OPTIONAL ADD-ON.

THE SPEECH TEAM HAD LEANED A CROOKED HEAD AT CUBIST HOUSES TOGETHER, HEARD THE SYMPHONY PLAY AT PRAGUE PALACE, AND EVEN EATEN IN HELL —

A RESTAURANT HOUSED IN THE BASEMENT CLOISTERS OF AN ANCIENT MONASTERY.

ALL OF IT WAS ON THE COLLEGE'S DIME.

BUT TO CAP THE TRIP WITH A JOURNEY TO A TOWN COMPLETELY DEVOTED TO GEOTHERMAL WATER TREATMENTS REQUIRED EACH STUDENT TO DIG INTO THEIR OWN POCKETS AND COVER THE COST OF THE DAY.

OF FOURTEEN STUDENTS ON THE TRIP WITH THE SPEECH TEAM, ONLY TONYA SHOWED UP IN THE HOTEL LOBBY AT THE APPOINTED TIME.

HER CONCLUSION ABOUT THE LIKELIHOOD OF ANY OTHER JOINERS WAS SURGICAL:

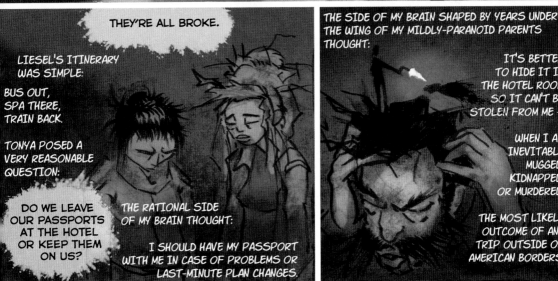

THEY'RE ALL BROKE.

LIESEL'S ITINERARY WAS SIMPLE:

BUS OUT, SPA THERE, TRAIN BACK.

TONYA POSED A VERY REASONABLE QUESTION:

DO WE LEAVE OUR PASSPORTS AT THE HOTEL OR KEEP THEM ON US?

THE RATIONAL SIDE OF MY BRAIN THOUGHT:

I SHOULD HAVE MY PASSPORT WITH ME IN CASE OF PROBLEMS OR LAST-MINUTE PLAN CHANGES.

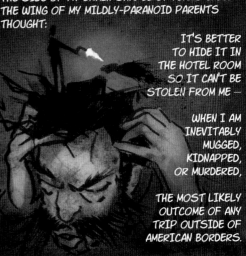

THE SIDE OF MY BRAIN SHAPED BY YEARS UNDER THE WING OF MY MILDLY-PARANOID PARENTS THOUGHT:

IT'S BETTER TO HIDE IT IN THE HOTEL ROOM SO IT CAN'T BE STOLEN FROM ME —

WHEN I AM INEVITABLY MUGGED, KIDNAPPED, OR MURDERED,

THE MOST LIKELY OUTCOME OF ANY TRIP OUTSIDE OF AMERICAN BORDERS.

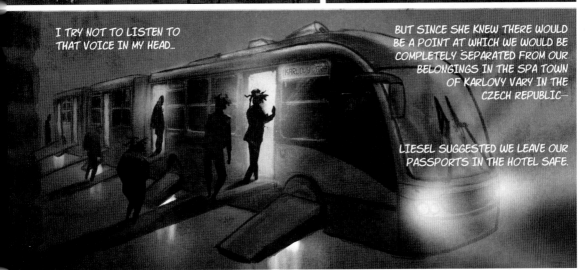

I TRY NOT TO LISTEN TO THAT VOICE IN MY HEAD...

BUT SINCE SHE KNEW THERE WOULD BE A POINT AT WHICH WE WOULD BE COMPLETELY SEPARATED FROM OUR BELONGINGS IN THE SPA TOWN OF KARLOVY VARY IN THE CZECH REPUBLIC—

LIESEL SUGGESTED WE LEAVE OUR PASSPORTS IN THE HOTEL SAFE.

AFTER 2 HOURS OF BUMPY
ROADS ON THE BUS —

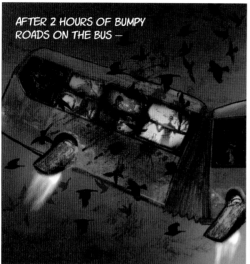

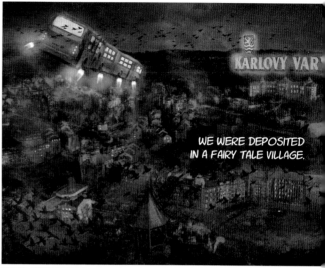

WE WERE DEPOSITED
IN A FAIRY TALE VILLAGE.

KARLOVY VARY

AFTER A WEEK OF THE INTERNATIONAL
SPEECH AND DEBATE CHAMPIONSHIPS...

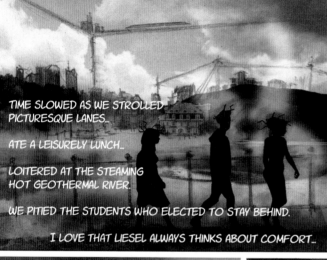

TIME SLOWED AS WE STROLLED
PICTURESQUE LANES...

ATE A LEISURELY LUNCH...

LOITERED AT THE STEAMING
HOT GEOTHERMAL RIVER.

WE PITIED THE STUDENTS WHO ELECTED TO STAY BEHIND.

I LOVE THAT LIESEL ALWAYS THINKS ABOUT COMFORT...

THERE COULD BE NO BETTER STRESS
BREAKER THAN THE MAGICAL SPA TOWN
OF KARLOVY VARY...

UNTIL LIESEL SPOTTED A CLOCK
IN THE TOWN SQUARE:

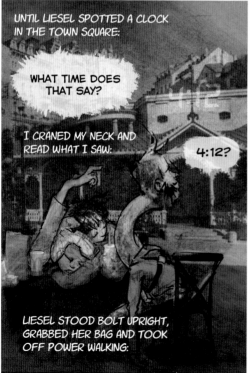

WHAT TIME DOES
THAT SAY?

I CRANED MY NECK AND
READ WHAT I SAW:

4:12?

LIESEL STOOD BOLT UPRIGHT,
GRABBED HER BAG AND TOOK
OFF POWER WALKING:

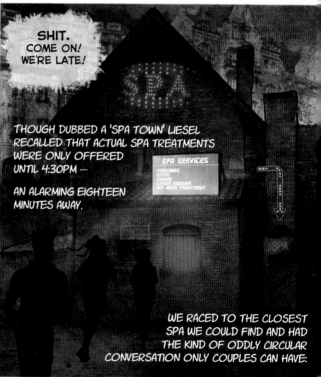

SHIT.
COME ON!
WE'RE LATE!

THOUGH DUBBED A 'SPA TOWN' LIESEL
RECALLED THAT ACTUAL SPA TREATMENTS
WERE ONLY OFFERED
UNTIL 4:30PM —

AN ALARMING EIGHTEEN
MINUTES AWAY.

SPA SERVICES
MASSAGES
BATHS
SAUNAS
STEAM SHOWER
HOT ROCK TREATMENT

WE RACED TO THE CLOSEST
SPA WE COULD FIND AND HAD
THE KIND OF ODDLY CIRCULAR
CONVERSATION ONLY COUPLES CAN HAVE:

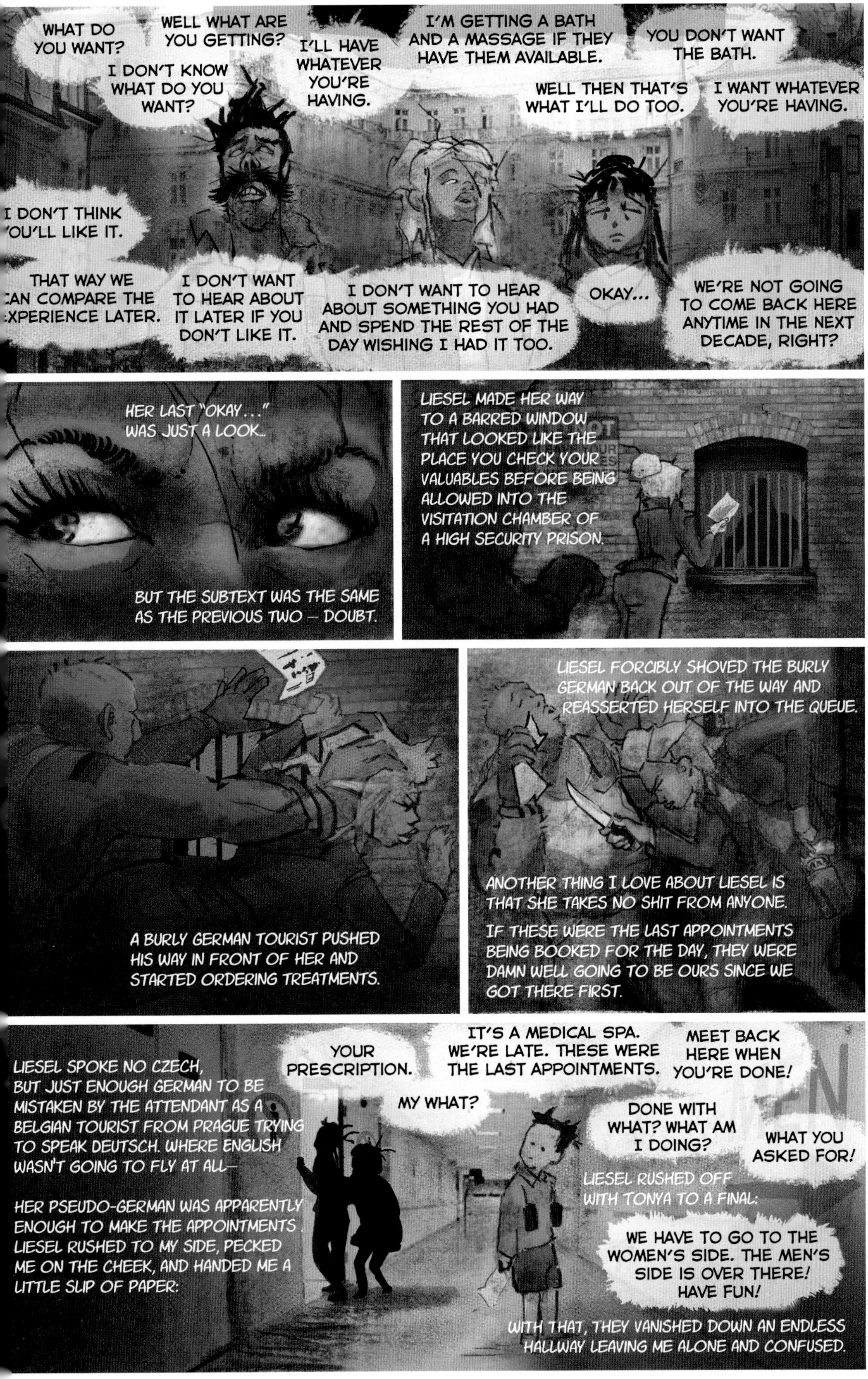
WHAT DO YOU WANT?
WELL WHAT ARE YOU GETTING?
I DON'T KNOW WHAT DO YOU WANT?
I'LL HAVE WHATEVER YOU'RE HAVING.
I'M GETTING A BATH AND A MASSAGE IF THEY HAVE THEM AVAILABLE.
YOU DON'T WANT THE BATH.
WELL THEN THAT'S WHAT I'LL DO TOO.
I WANT WHATEVER YOU'RE HAVING.
I DON'T THINK YOU'LL LIKE IT.
THAT WAY WE CAN COMPARE THE EXPERIENCE LATER.
I DON'T WANT TO HEAR ABOUT IT LATER IF YOU DON'T LIKE IT.
I DON'T WANT TO HEAR ABOUT SOMETHING YOU HAD AND SPEND THE REST OF THE DAY WISHING I HAD IT TOO.
OKAY...
WE'RE NOT GOING TO COME BACK HERE ANYTIME IN THE NEXT DECADE, RIGHT?
HER LAST "OKAY..." WAS JUST A LOOK..
BUT THE SUBTEXT WAS THE SAME AS THE PREVIOUS TWO – DOUBT.
LIESEL MADE HER WAY TO A BARRED WINDOW THAT LOOKED LIKE THE PLACE YOU CHECK YOUR VALUABLES BEFORE BEING ALLOWED INTO THE VISITATION CHAMBER OF A HIGH SECURITY PRISON.
A BURLY GERMAN TOURIST PUSHED HIS WAY IN FRONT OF HER AND STARTED ORDERING TREATMENTS.
LIESEL FORCIBLY SHOVED THE BURLY GERMAN BACK OUT OF THE WAY AND REASSERTED HERSELF INTO THE QUEUE.
ANOTHER THING I LOVE ABOUT LIESEL IS THAT SHE TAKES NO SHIT FROM ANYONE.
IF THESE WERE THE LAST APPOINTMENTS BEING BOOKED FOR THE DAY, THEY WERE DAMN WELL GOING TO BE OURS SINCE WE GOT THERE FIRST.
LIESEL SPOKE NO CZECH, BUT JUST ENOUGH GERMAN TO BE MISTAKEN BY THE ATTENDANT AS A BELGIAN TOURIST FROM PRAGUE TRYING TO SPEAK DEUTSCH. WHERE ENGLISH WASN'T GOING TO FLY AT ALL–
HER PSEUDO-GERMAN WAS APPARENTLY ENOUGH TO MAKE THE APPOINTMENTS. LIESEL RUSHED TO MY SIDE, PECKED ME ON THE CHEEK, AND HANDED ME A LITTLE SLIP OF PAPER:
YOUR PRESCRIPTION.
MY WHAT?
IT'S A MEDICAL SPA. WE'RE LATE. THESE WERE THE LAST APPOINTMENTS.
MEET BACK HERE WHEN YOU'RE DONE!
DONE WITH WHAT? WHAT AM I DOING?
WHAT YOU ASKED FOR!
LIESEL RUSHED OFF WITH TONYA TO A FINAL:
WE HAVE TO GO TO THE WOMEN'S SIDE. THE MEN'S SIDE IS OVER THERE! HAVE FUN!
WITH THAT, THEY VANISHED DOWN AN ENDLESS HALLWAY LEAVING ME ALONE AND CONFUSED.

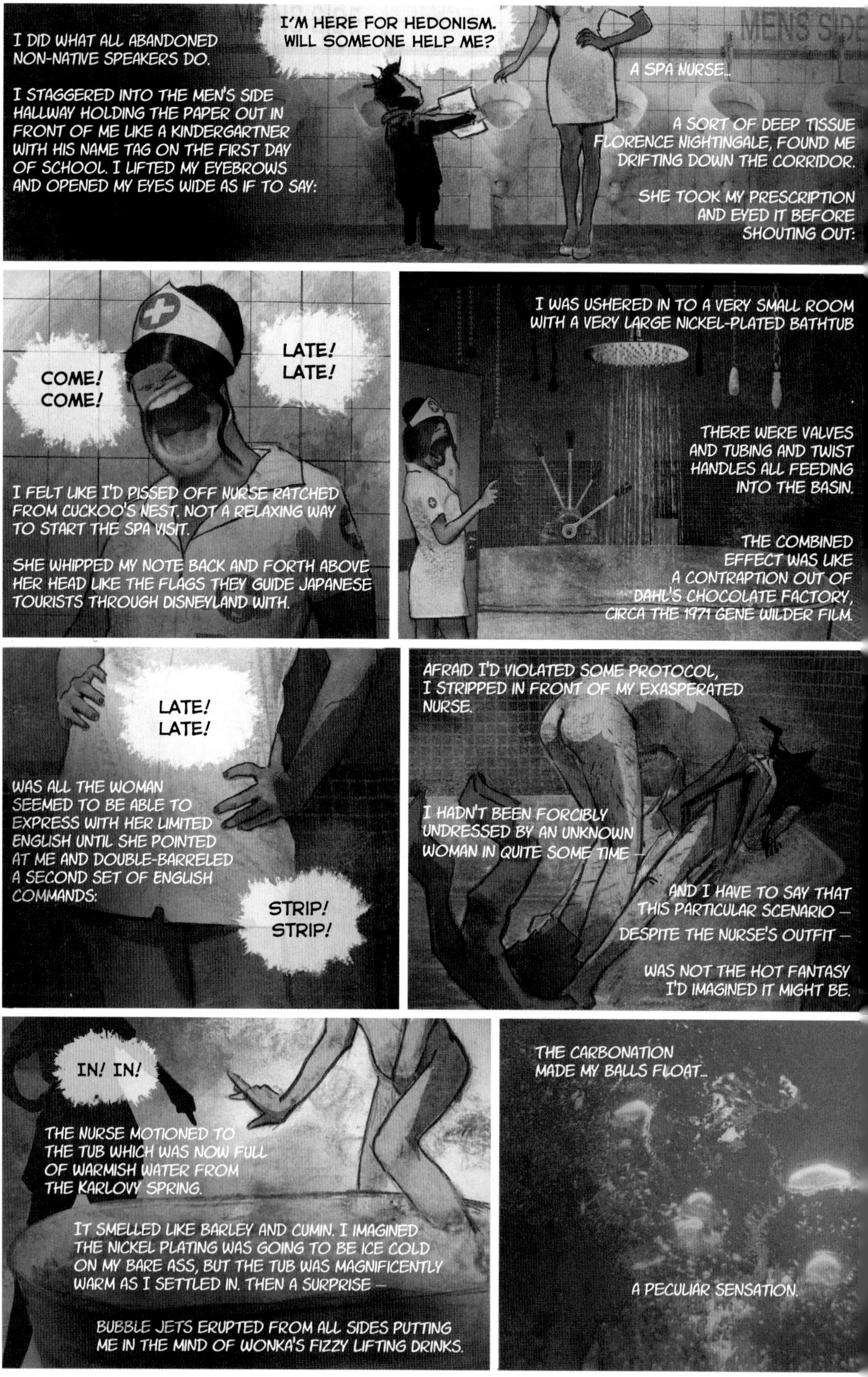

I DID WHAT ALL ABANDONED NON-NATIVE SPEAKERS DO.
I STAGGERED INTO THE MEN'S SIDE HALLWAY HOLDING THE PAPER OUT IN FRONT OF ME LIKE A KINDERGARTNER WITH HIS NAME TAG ON THE FIRST DAY OF SCHOOL. I LIFTED MY EYEBROWS AND OPENED MY EYES WIDE AS IF TO SAY:
I'M HERE FOR HEDONISM. WILL SOMEONE HELP ME?
MEN'S SIDE
A SPA NURSE...
A SORT OF DEEP TISSUE FLORENCE NIGHTINGALE, FOUND ME DRIFTING DOWN THE CORRIDOR.
SHE TOOK MY PRESCRIPTION AND EYED IT BEFORE SHOUTING OUT:
COME! COME!
LATE! LATE!
I FELT LIKE I'D PISSED OFF NURSE RATCHED FROM CUCKOO'S NEST. NOT A RELAXING WAY TO START THE SPA VISIT.
SHE WHIPPED MY NOTE BACK AND FORTH ABOVE HER HEAD LIKE THE FLAGS THEY GUIDE JAPANESE TOURISTS THROUGH DISNEYLAND WITH.
I WAS USHERED IN TO A VERY SMALL ROOM WITH A VERY LARGE NICKEL-PLATED BATHTUB
THERE WERE VALVES AND TUBING AND TWIST HANDLES ALL FEEDING INTO THE BASIN.
THE COMBINED EFFECT WAS LIKE A CONTRAPTION OUT OF DAHL'S CHOCOLATE FACTORY, CIRCA THE 1971 GENE WILDER FILM.
LATE! LATE!
WAS ALL THE WOMAN SEEMED TO BE ABLE TO EXPRESS WITH HER LIMITED ENGLISH UNTIL SHE POINTED AT ME AND DOUBLE-BARRELED A SECOND SET OF ENGLISH COMMANDS:
STRIP! STRIP!
AFRAID I'D VIOLATED SOME PROTOCOL, I STRIPPED IN FRONT OF MY EXASPERATED NURSE.
I HADN'T BEEN FORCIBLY UNDRESSED BY AN UNKNOWN WOMAN IN QUITE SOME TIME –
AND I HAVE TO SAY THAT THIS PARTICULAR SCENARIO –
DESPITE THE NURSE'S OUTFIT –
WAS NOT THE HOT FANTASY I'D IMAGINED IT MIGHT BE.
IN! IN!
THE NURSE MOTIONED TO THE TUB WHICH WAS NOW FULL OF WARMISH WATER FROM THE KARLOVY SPRING.
IT SMELLED LIKE BARLEY AND CUMIN. I IMAGINED THE NICKEL PLATING WAS GOING TO BE ICE COLD ON MY BARE ASS, BUT THE TUB WAS MAGNIFICENTLY WARM AS I SETTLED IN. THEN A SURPRISE –
BUBBLE JETS ERUPTED FROM ALL SIDES PUTTING ME IN THE MIND OF WONKA'S FIZZY LIFTING DRINKS.
THE CARBONATION MADE MY BALLS FLOAT...
A PECULIAR SENSATION.

PULL. PULL.
PULL NOW?
NO! NO!
SHE CAUTIONED WITH GESTICULATIONS.
PULL. PULL. PULL THE ROPE?
YES. YES.
NOW?
NO! NO!
AGAIN WITH THE FLAILING ARMS AND UNRELENTINGLY DISAPPROVING EYEBROWS.
AFTER. AFTER!
AND WITH THAT SHE HIT A BUTTON, HURRIED OUT, AND CLOSED THE DOOR.
I HAD NO IDEA WHAT WAS HAPPENING. WHAT WAS THE ROPE FOR? WHEN DO I PULL IT?
WHAT WOULD HAPPEN WHEN I DID?
I DECIDED MY BEST COURSE WAS TO SIMPLY WAIT UNTIL THE WOMAN RETURNED AND YELLED TWO MORE THINGS AT ME. SO I DID JUST THAT AND NODDED OFF IN THE TUB.
IT WAS BLISS UNTIL...
I WAS AWAKENED BY
LATE! LATE! PULL! PULL!
THE NURSE WAS BACK AND SHE WAS NOT PLEASED. RED-CHEEKED, SHE WAS A WHIRLWIND OF ANXIETY AND HARSH FACIAL EXPRESSIONS ALL DIRECTED AT ME.
I STOOD UP IN THE TUB, PULLED THE CHAIN, AND A RUBE GOLDBERG SYSTEM OF PULLEYS AND CHAINS LIFTED THE TUB FLAPPER...
WATER RUSHED OUT WITH THE FORCE OF MATTER BEING SUCKED INTO A BLACK HOLE. MY FEET WENT OUT AND I SPLASHED BACK DOWN INTO THE TUB LANDING HARD ON MY TAIL BONE.
NO! NO! OUT! OUT!
THE WOMAN SAID, MISTAKING MY FALL FOR ADDITIONAL WATER FROLICKING.
I WRENCHED MYSELF UP OUT OF THE TUB.
COME! COME!
THE WOMAN MOTIONED THE DOOR WITH SWEEPING GESTURES. I FOLLOWED —
BUT WAIT — I WAS NAKED — DO I DRESS OR...?
FROM OUTSIDE, AN ANSWER:
LATE! LATE! HURRY! HURRY!
CLEARLY TEMPORAL TENSION WAS ON THE MAIN MENU FOR CZECH SPAS.
SINCE I WAS ON THE MEN'S SIDE, I SIMPLY GRABBED MY CLOTHES, JUMBLED THEM UP IN A BALL, AND RACED OUT INTO THE HALLWAY WHERE—

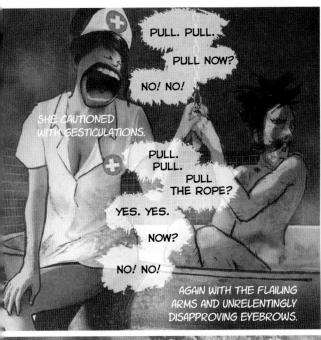

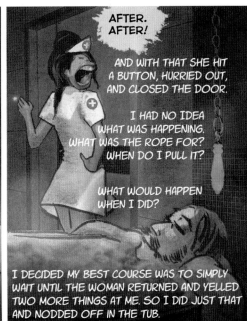

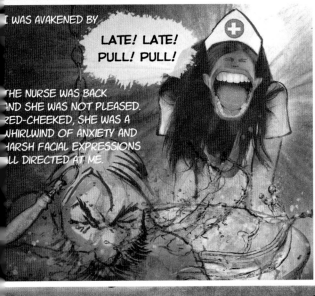

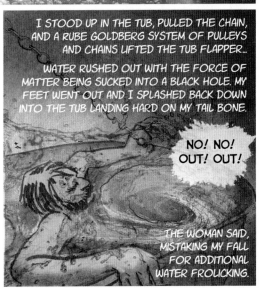

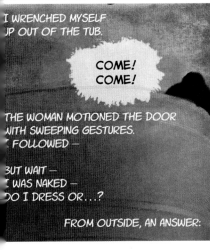

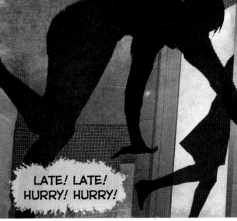

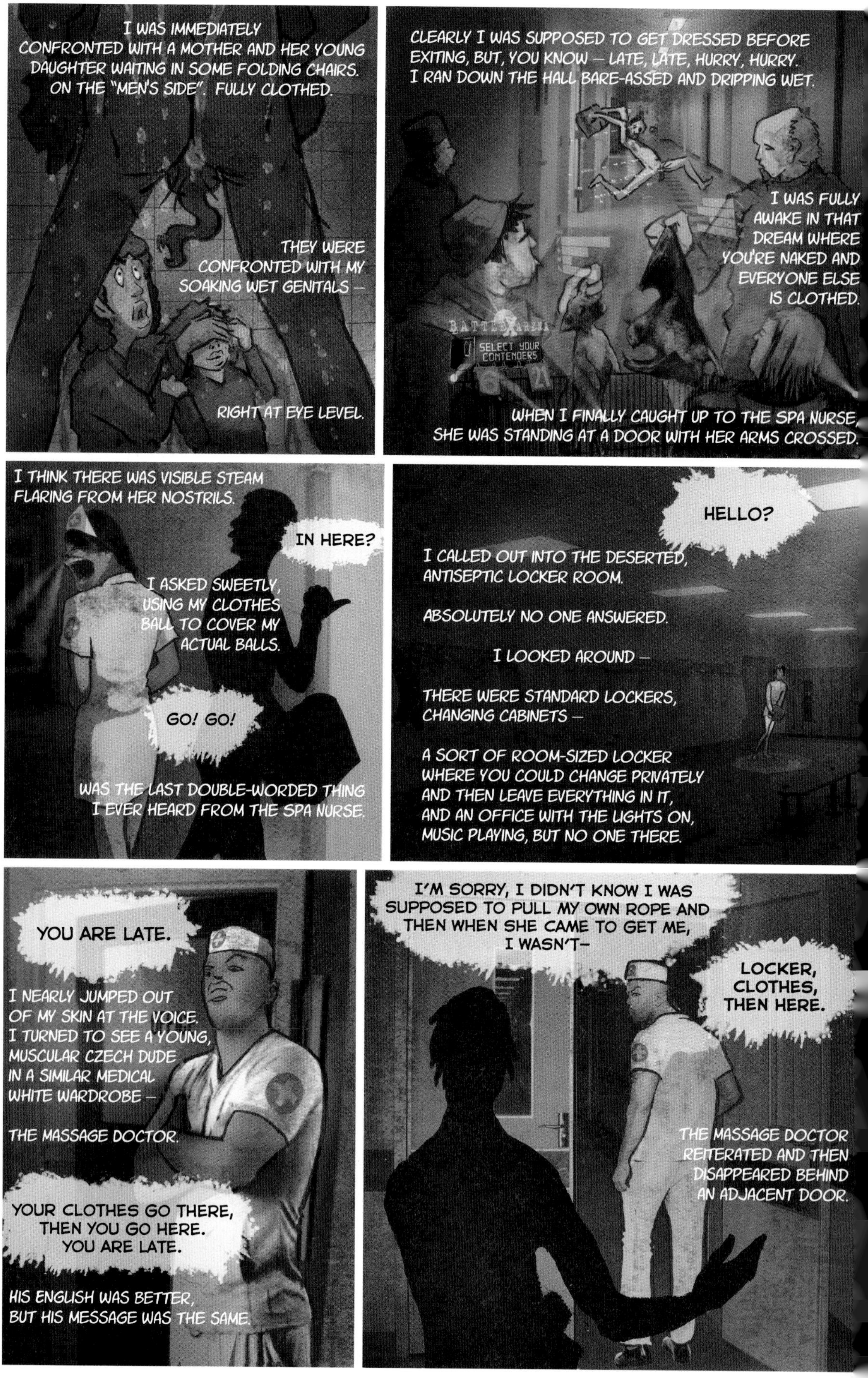
I WAS IMMEDIATELY CONFRONTED WITH A MOTHER AND HER YOUNG DAUGHTER WAITING IN SOME FOLDING CHAIRS. ON THE "MEN'S SIDE". FULLY CLOTHED.
THEY WERE CONFRONTED WITH MY SOAKING WET GENITALS –
RIGHT AT EYE LEVEL.
CLEARLY I WAS SUPPOSED TO GET DRESSED BEFORE EXITING, BUT, YOU KNOW – LATE, LATE, HURRY, HURRY. I RAN DOWN THE HALL BARE-ASSED AND DRIPPING WET.
I WAS FULLY AWAKE IN THAT DREAM WHERE YOU'RE NAKED AND EVERYONE ELSE IS CLOTHED.
SELECT YOUR CONTENDERS
WHEN I FINALLY CAUGHT UP TO THE SPA NURSE, SHE WAS STANDING AT A DOOR WITH HER ARMS CROSSED.
I THINK THERE WAS VISIBLE STEAM FLARING FROM HER NOSTRILS.
IN HERE?
I ASKED SWEETLY, USING MY CLOTHES BALL TO COVER MY ACTUAL BALLS.
GO! GO!
WAS THE LAST DOUBLE-WORDED THING I EVER HEARD FROM THE SPA NURSE.
HELLO?
I CALLED OUT INTO THE DESERTED, ANTISEPTIC LOCKER ROOM.
ABSOLUTELY NO ONE ANSWERED.
I LOOKED AROUND –
THERE WERE STANDARD LOCKERS, CHANGING CABINETS –
A SORT OF ROOM-SIZED LOCKER WHERE YOU COULD CHANGE PRIVATELY AND THEN LEAVE EVERYTHING IN IT, AND AN OFFICE WITH THE LIGHTS ON, MUSIC PLAYING, BUT NO ONE THERE.
YOU ARE LATE.
I NEARLY JUMPED OUT OF MY SKIN AT THE VOICE. I TURNED TO SEE A YOUNG, MUSCULAR CZECH DUDE IN A SIMILAR MEDICAL WHITE WARDROBE –
THE MASSAGE DOCTOR.
YOUR CLOTHES GO THERE, THEN YOU GO HERE. YOU ARE LATE.
HIS ENGLISH WAS BETTER, BUT HIS MESSAGE WAS THE SAME.
I'M SORRY, I DIDN'T KNOW I WAS SUPPOSED TO PULL MY OWN ROPE AND THEN WHEN SHE CAME TO GET ME, I WASN'T–
LOCKER, CLOTHES, THEN HERE.
THE MASSAGE DOCTOR REITERATED AND THEN DISAPPEARED BEHIND AN ADJACENT DOOR.

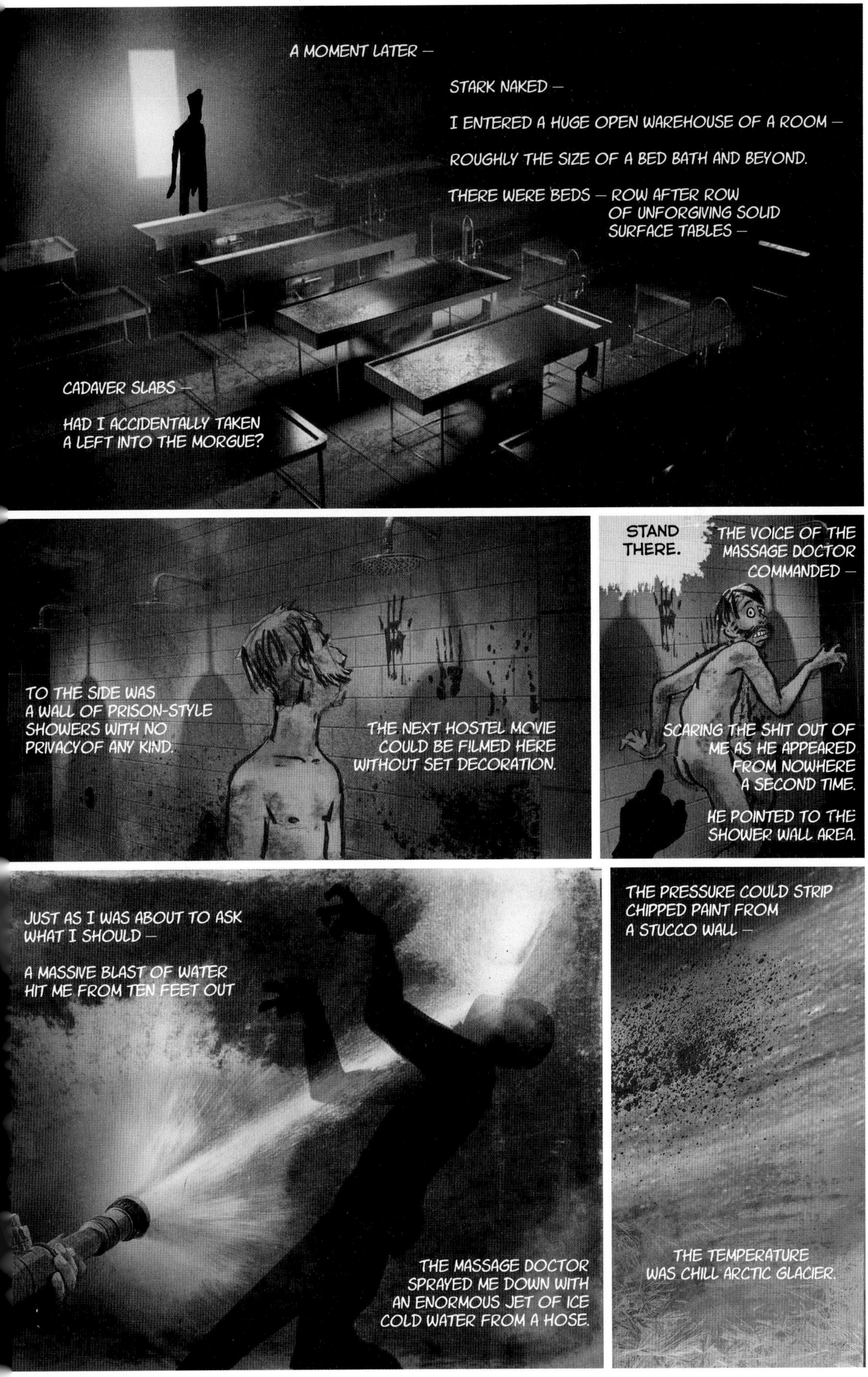
A MOMENT LATER –
STARK NAKED –
I ENTERED A HUGE OPEN WAREHOUSE OF A ROOM –
ROUGHLY THE SIZE OF A BED BATH AND BEYOND.
THERE WERE BEDS – ROW AFTER ROW OF UNFORGIVING SOLID SURFACE TABLES –
CADAVER SLABS –
HAD I ACCIDENTALLY TAKEN A LEFT INTO THE MORGUE?
TO THE SIDE WAS A WALL OF PRISON-STYLE SHOWERS WITH NO PRIVACYOF ANY KIND.
THE NEXT HOSTEL MOVIE COULD BE FILMED HERE WITHOUT SET DECORATION.
STAND THERE.
THE VOICE OF THE MASSAGE DOCTOR COMMANDED –
SCARING THE SHIT OUT OF ME AS HE APPEARED FROM NOWHERE A SECOND TIME.
HE POINTED TO THE SHOWER WALL AREA.
JUST AS I WAS ABOUT TO ASK WHAT I SHOULD –
A MASSIVE BLAST OF WATER HIT ME FROM TEN FEET OUT
THE MASSAGE DOCTOR SPRAYED ME DOWN WITH AN ENORMOUS JET OF ICE COLD WATER FROM A HOSE.
THE PRESSURE COULD STRIP CHIPPED PAINT FROM A STUCCO WALL –
THE TEMPERATURE WAS CHILL ARCTIC GLACIER.

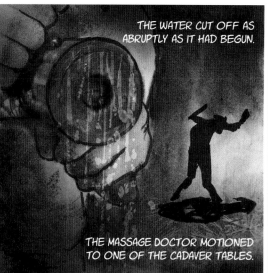

THE WATER CUT OFF AS ABRUPTLY AS IT HAD BEGUN.

THE MASSAGE DOCTOR MOTIONED TO ONE OF THE CADAVER TABLES.

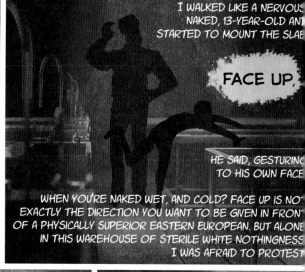

I WALKED LIKE A NERVOUS NAKED, 13-YEAR-OLD AND STARTED TO MOUNT THE SLAB.

FACE UP,

HE SAID, GESTURING TO HIS OWN FACE.

WHEN YOU'RE NAKED WET, AND COLD? FACE UP IS NOT EXACTLY THE DIRECTION YOU WANT TO BE GIVEN IN FRONT OF A PHYSICALLY SUPERIOR EASTERN EUROPEAN. BUT ALONE IN THIS WAREHOUSE OF STERILE WHITE NOTHINGNESS I WAS AFRAID TO PROTEST.

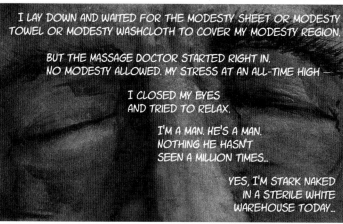

I LAY DOWN AND WAITED FOR THE MODESTY SHEET OR MODESTY TOWEL OR MODESTY WASHCLOTH TO COVER MY MODESTY REGION.

BUT THE MASSAGE DOCTOR STARTED RIGHT IN. NO MODESTY ALLOWED. MY STRESS AT AN ALL-TIME HIGH —

I CLOSED MY EYES AND TRIED TO RELAX.

I'M A MAN. HE'S A MAN. NOTHING HE HASN'T SEEN A MILLION TIMES...

YES, I'M STARK NAKED IN A STERILE WHITE WAREHOUSE TODAY...

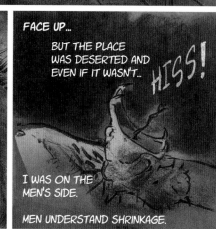

FACE UP...

BUT THE PLACE WAS DESERTED AND EVEN IF IT WASN'T...

HISS!

I WAS ON THE MEN'S SIDE.

MEN UNDERSTAND SHRINKAGE.

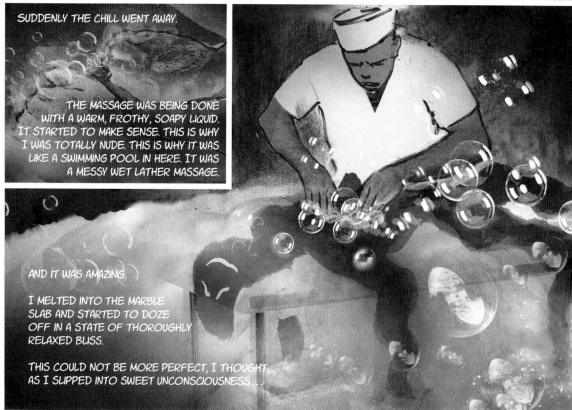

SUDDENLY THE CHILL WENT AWAY.

THE MASSAGE WAS BEING DONE WITH A WARM, FROTHY, SOAPY LIQUID. IT STARTED TO MAKE SENSE. THIS IS WHY I WAS TOTALLY NUDE. THIS IS WHY IT WAS LIKE A SWIMMING POOL IN HERE. IT WAS A MESSY WET LATHER MASSAGE.

AND IT WAS AMAZING.

I MELTED INTO THE MARBLE SLAB AND STARTED TO DOZE OFF IN A STATE OF THOROUGHLY RELAXED BLISS.

THIS COULD NOT BE MORE PERFECT, I THOUGHT, AS I SLIPPED INTO SWEET UNCONSCIOUSNESS...

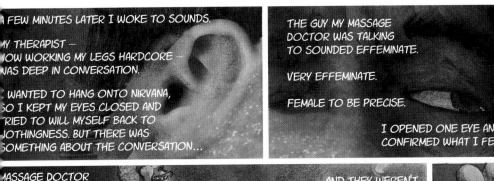

A FEW MINUTES LATER I WOKE TO SOUNDS.
MY THERAPIST — NOW WORKING MY LEGS HARDCORE — WAS DEEP IN CONVERSATION.
I WANTED TO HANG ONTO NIRVANA, SO I KEPT MY EYES CLOSED AND TRIED TO WILL MYSELF BACK TO NOTHINGNESS. BUT THERE WAS SOMETHING ABOUT THE CONVERSATION...
THE GUY MY MASSAGE DOCTOR WAS TALKING TO SOUNDED EFFEMINATE.
VERY EFFEMINATE.
FEMALE TO BE PRECISE.
I OPENED ONE EYE AND CONFIRMED WHAT I FEARED.
MASSAGE DOCTOR WAS TALKING TO A TALL BLONDE WOMAN —
NOT IN A NURSE OUTFIT — MORE LIKE A VISITING FRIEND —
INCHES FROM MY EXTREMELY EXPOSED GROIN.
AND THEY WEREN'T JUST TALKING...
THEY WERE LAUGHING...
AND HE WAS RUBBING...
AND SHE WAS POINTING...
AND THEY WERE TALKING AND LAUGHING AND I WAS SPRAWLED OUT FACE UP...
I HAD A DECISION TO MAKE.
MODESTY? OR ECSTASY?
I CHOSE ECSTASY.
I DECIDED THEN AND THERE THAT THIS WAS AS NAKED I'D EVER BEEN —
AS NAKED AS I COULD EVER BE.
I WONDERED IF IT WAS POSSIBLE TO BE MORE NAKED THAN THIS.
NEVER ASK FATE QUESTIONS THAT MIGHT GET ANSWERED THAT NIGHT.
I MET BACK UP WITH LIESEL AND TONYA IN THE CENTER HALL AFTER.
MENS SIDE
THEY WERE BRIGHT-EYED AND LAUGHING.
HAVING A SPA BUDDY AND A LITTLE GERMAN AT THEIR DISPOSAL MADE FOR A VERY DIFFERENT EXPERIENCE ON THE WOMEN'S SIDE.
BUT AS WE LEFT THE SPA IN SEARCH OF OUR TRAIN —
WE FOUND THAT THE LANGUAGE BARRIER THAT WAS SLIGHTLY PRESENT WHILE THE SUN WAS UP BECAME ABSURDLY PRONOUNCED WHEN TWILIGHT SET IN.
Praha
Ohře
Teplá
ENTER
OPEN
Skalná
Ostrov
Františkovy Lázně
Karlovarský
THERE WERE NO OTHER TOURISTS AROUND AND DIRECTIONS WERE HARD TO COME BY.
KARLOVY VARY
WITH ONLY MINUTES TO SPARE WE RACED TO WHAT WE HOPED WAS OUR TRAIN STATION.

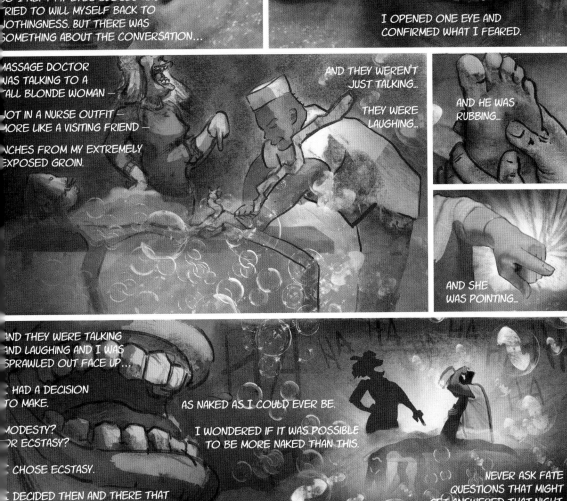

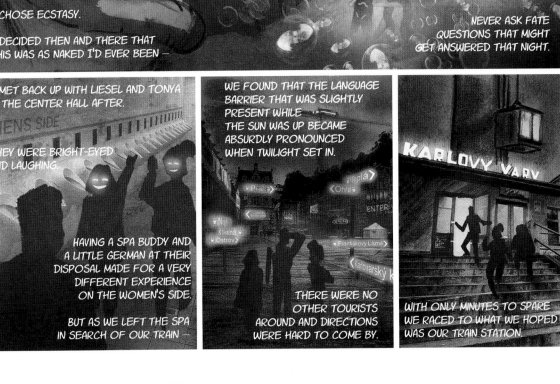

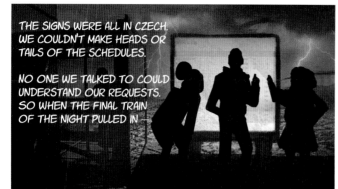

THE SIGNS WERE ALL IN CZECH. WE COULDN'T MAKE HEADS OR TAILS OF THE SCHEDULES.

NO ONE WE TALKED TO COULD UNDERSTAND OUR REQUESTS. SO WHEN THE FINAL TRAIN OF THE NIGHT PULLED IN —

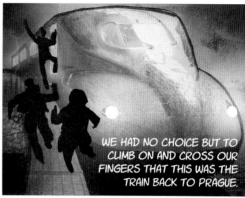

WE HAD NO CHOICE BUT TO CLIMB ON AND CROSS OUR FINGERS THAT THIS WAS THE TRAIN BACK TO PRAGUE.

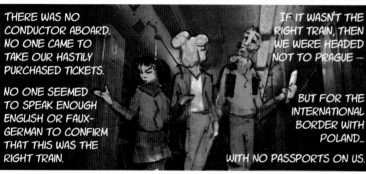

THERE WAS NO CONDUCTOR ABOARD. NO ONE CAME TO TAKE OUR HASTILY PURCHASED TICKETS.

NO ONE SEEMED TO SPEAK ENOUGH ENGLISH OR FAUX-GERMAN TO CONFIRM THAT THIS WAS THE RIGHT TRAIN.

IF IT WASN'T THE RIGHT TRAIN, THEN WE WERE HEADED NOT TO PRAGUE —

BUT FOR THE INTERNATIONAL BORDER WITH POLAND...

WITH NO PASSPORTS ON US.

WE HAD A LITTLE CARD GAME WITH US THAT WE USED TO KILL TIME WITH TONYA.

IT ALSO KEPT ME FROM YELLING OUT:

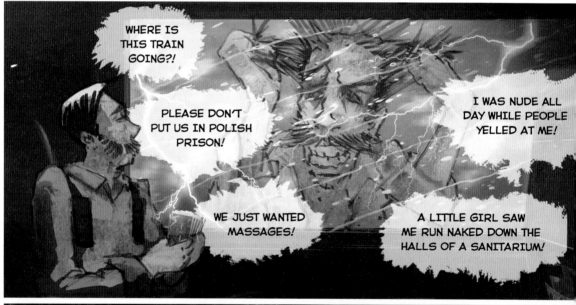

WHERE IS THIS TRAIN GOING?!

PLEASE DON'T PUT US IN POLISH PRISON!

WE JUST WANTED MASSAGES!

I WAS NUDE ALL DAY WHILE PEOPLE YELLED AT ME!

A LITTLE GIRL SAW ME RUN NAKED DOWN THE HALLS OF A SANITARIUM!

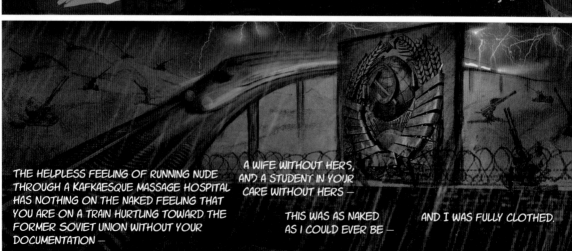

THE HELPLESS FEELING OF RUNNING NUDE THROUGH A KAFKAESQUE MASSAGE HOSPITAL HAS NOTHING ON THE NAKED FEELING THAT YOU ARE ON A TRAIN HURTLING TOWARD THE FORMER SOVIET UNION WITHOUT YOUR DOCUMENTATION —

A WIFE WITHOUT HERS, AND A STUDENT IN YOUR CARE WITHOUT HERS —

THIS WAS AS NAKED AS I COULD EVER BE —

AND I WAS FULLY CLOTHED.

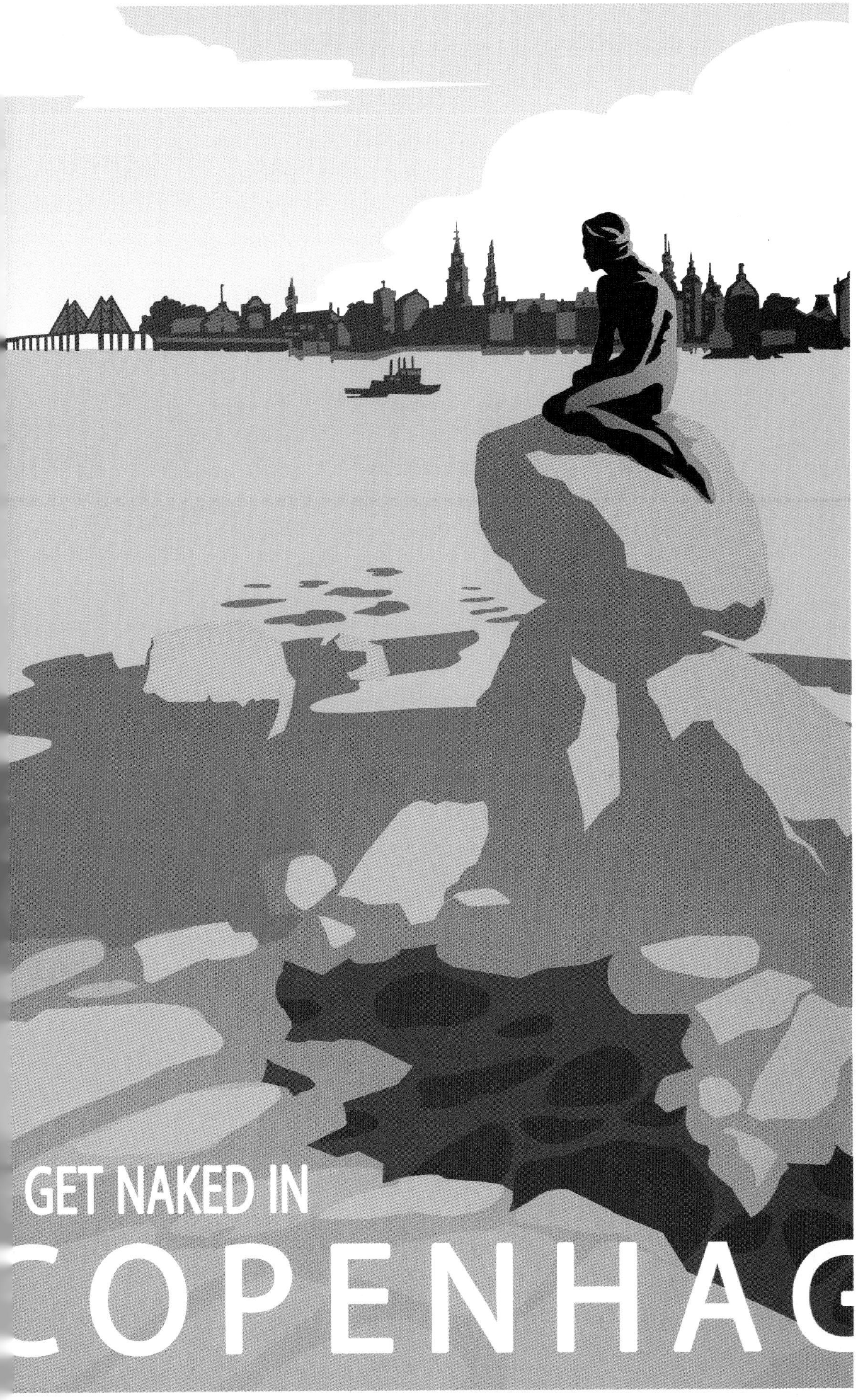
GET NAKED IN
COPENHAG

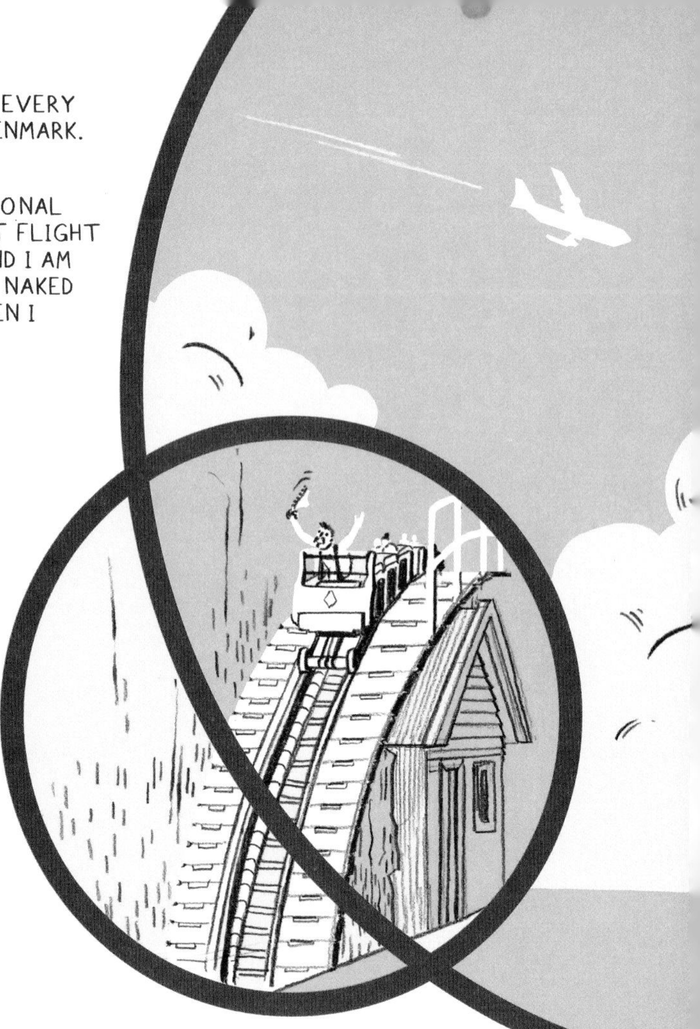

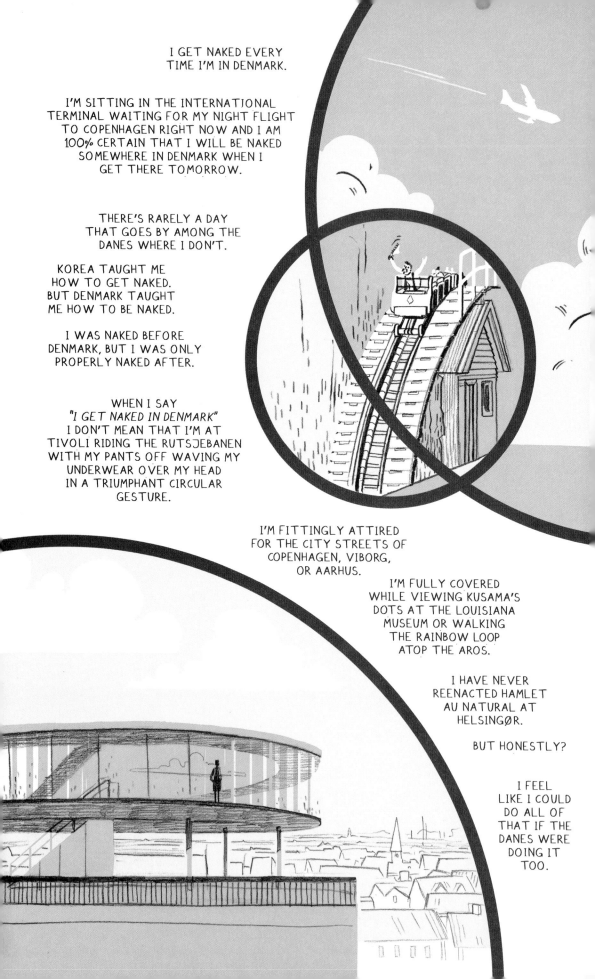

I GET NAKED EVERY TIME I'M IN DENMARK.

I'M SITTING IN THE INTERNATIONAL TERMINAL WAITING FOR MY NIGHT FLIGHT TO COPENHAGEN RIGHT NOW AND I AM 100% CERTAIN THAT I WILL BE NAKED SOMEWHERE IN DENMARK WHEN I GET THERE TOMORROW.

THERE'S RARELY A DAY THAT GOES BY AMONG THE DANES WHERE I DON'T.

KOREA TAUGHT ME HOW TO GET NAKED. BUT DENMARK TAUGHT ME HOW TO BE NAKED.

I WAS NAKED BEFORE DENMARK, BUT I WAS ONLY PROPERLY NAKED AFTER.

WHEN I SAY *"I GET NAKED IN DENMARK"* I DON'T MEAN THAT I'M AT TIVOLI RIDING THE RUTSJEBANEN WITH MY PANTS OFF WAVING MY UNDERWEAR OVER MY HEAD IN A TRIUMPHANT CIRCULAR GESTURE.

I'M FITTINGLY ATTIRED FOR THE CITY STREETS OF COPENHAGEN, VIBORG, OR AARHUS.

I'M FULLY COVERED WHILE VIEWING KUSAMA'S DOTS AT THE LOUISIANA MUSEUM OR WALKING THE RAINBOW LOOP ATOP THE AROS.

I HAVE NEVER REENACTED HAMLET AU NATURAL AT HELSINGØR.

BUT HONESTLY?

I FEEL LIKE I COULD DO ALL OF THAT IF THE DANES WERE DOING IT TOO.

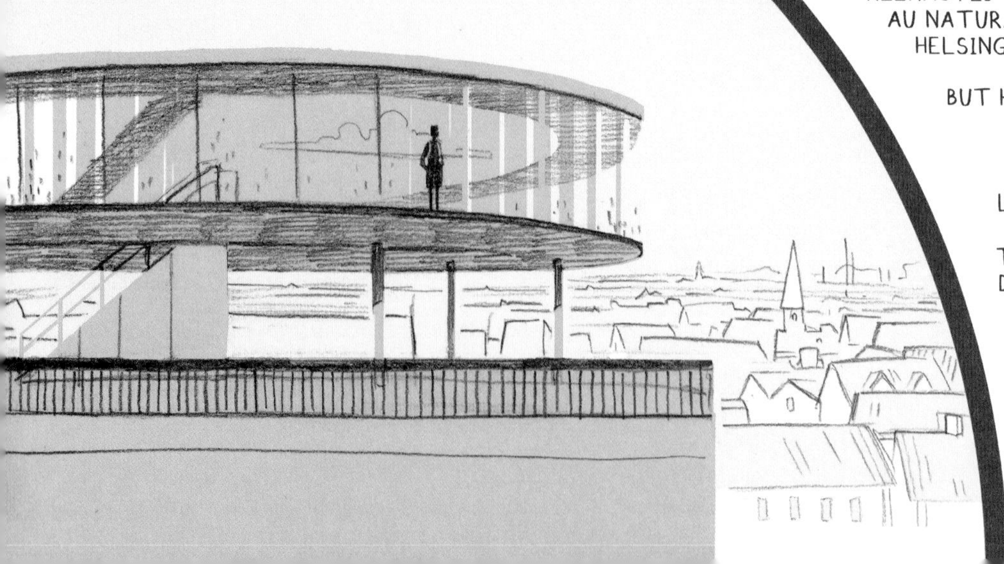

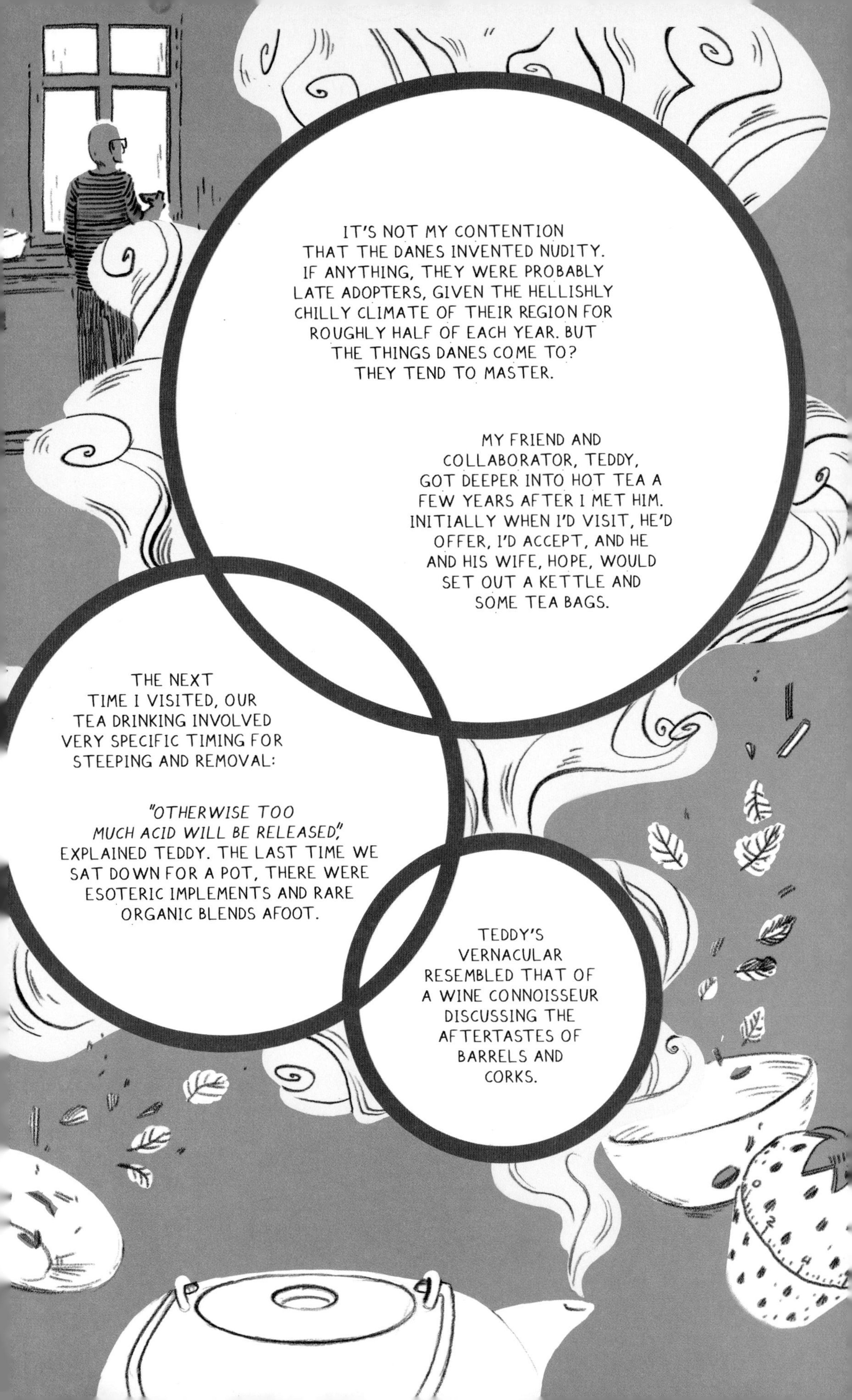
IT'S NOT MY CONTENTION THAT THE DANES INVENTED NUDITY. IF ANYTHING, THEY WERE PROBABLY LATE ADOPTERS, GIVEN THE HELLISHLY CHILLY CLIMATE OF THEIR REGION FOR ROUGHLY HALF OF EACH YEAR. BUT THE THINGS DANES COME TO? THEY TEND TO MASTER.
MY FRIEND AND COLLABORATOR, TEDDY, GOT DEEPER INTO HOT TEA A FEW YEARS AFTER I MET HIM. INITIALLY WHEN I'D VISIT, HE'D OFFER, I'D ACCEPT, AND HE AND HIS WIFE, HOPE, WOULD SET OUT A KETTLE AND SOME TEA BAGS.
THE NEXT TIME I VISITED, OUR TEA DRINKING INVOLVED VERY SPECIFIC TIMING FOR STEEPING AND REMOVAL:
"OTHERWISE TOO MUCH ACID WILL BE RELEASED," EXPLAINED TEDDY. THE LAST TIME WE SAT DOWN FOR A POT, THERE WERE ESOTERIC IMPLEMENTS AND RARE ORGANIC BLENDS AFOOT.
TEDDY'S VERNACULAR RESEMBLED THAT OF A WINE CONNOISSEUR DISCUSSING THE AFTERTASTES OF BARRELS AND CORKS.

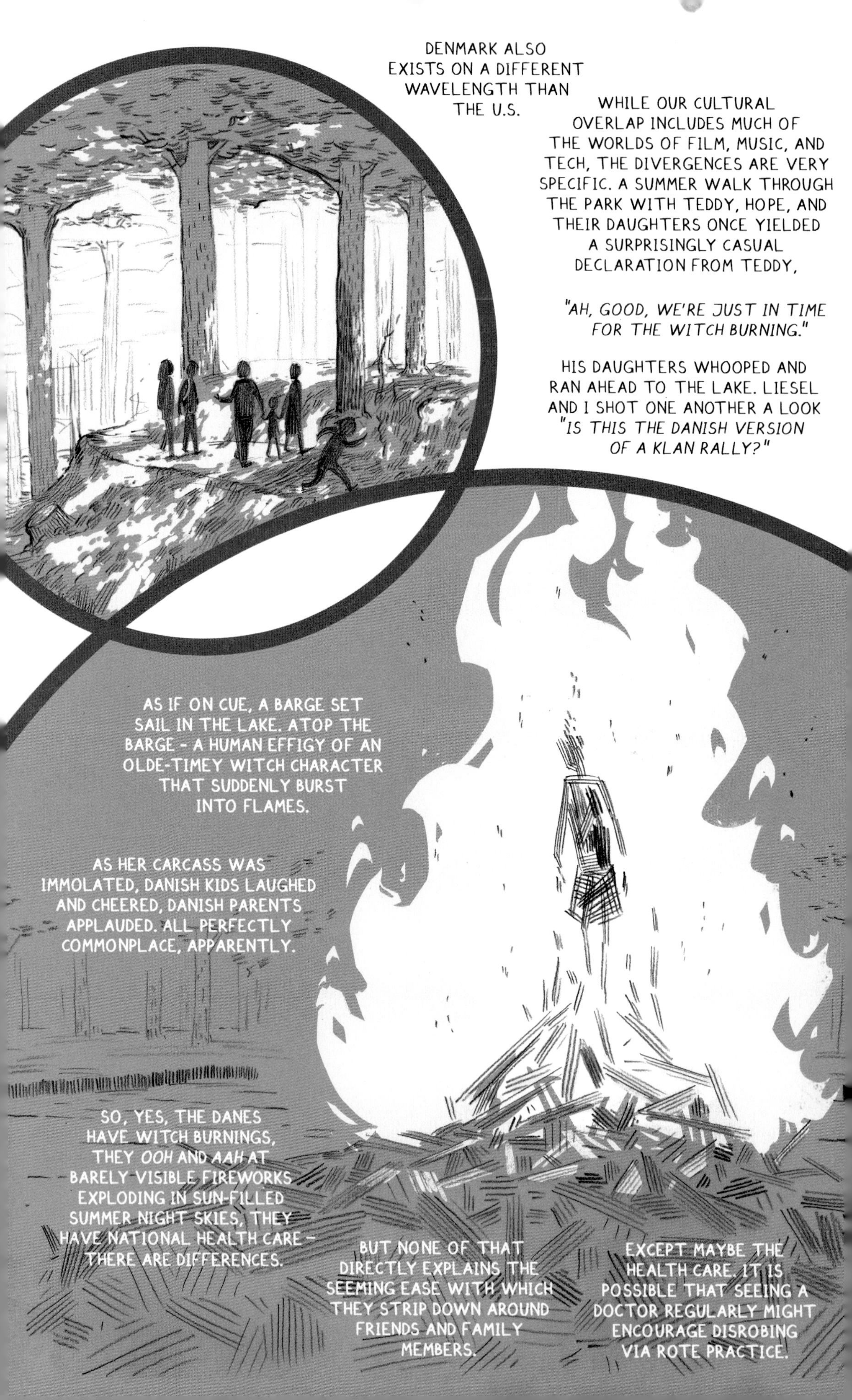
DENMARK ALSO EXISTS ON A DIFFERENT WAVELENGTH THAN THE U.S.
WHILE OUR CULTURAL OVERLAP INCLUDES MUCH OF THE WORLDS OF FILM, MUSIC, AND TECH, THE DIVERGENCES ARE VERY SPECIFIC. A SUMMER WALK THROUGH THE PARK WITH TEDDY, HOPE, AND THEIR DAUGHTERS ONCE YIELDED A SURPRISINGLY CASUAL DECLARATION FROM TEDDY,
"AH, GOOD, WE'RE JUST IN TIME FOR THE WITCH BURNING."
HIS DAUGHTERS WHOOPED AND RAN AHEAD TO THE LAKE. LIESEL AND I SHOT ONE ANOTHER A LOOK *"IS THIS THE DANISH VERSION OF A KLAN RALLY?"*
AS IF ON CUE, A BARGE SET SAIL IN THE LAKE. ATOP THE BARGE - A HUMAN EFFIGY OF AN OLDE-TIMEY WITCH CHARACTER THAT SUDDENLY BURST INTO FLAMES.
AS HER CARCASS WAS IMMOLATED, DANISH KIDS LAUGHED AND CHEERED, DANISH PARENTS APPLAUDED. ALL PERFECTLY COMMONPLACE, APPARENTLY.
SO, YES, THE DANES HAVE WITCH BURNINGS, THEY *OOH* AND *AAH* AT BARELY VISIBLE FIREWORKS EXPLODING IN SUN-FILLED SUMMER NIGHT SKIES, THEY HAVE NATIONAL HEALTH CARE - THERE ARE DIFFERENCES.
BUT NONE OF THAT DIRECTLY EXPLAINS THE SEEMING EASE WITH WHICH THEY STRIP DOWN AROUND FRIENDS AND FAMILY MEMBERS.
EXCEPT MAYBE THE HEALTH CARE. IT IS POSSIBLE THAT SEEING A DOCTOR REGULARLY MIGHT ENCOURAGE DISROBING VIA ROTE PRACTICE.

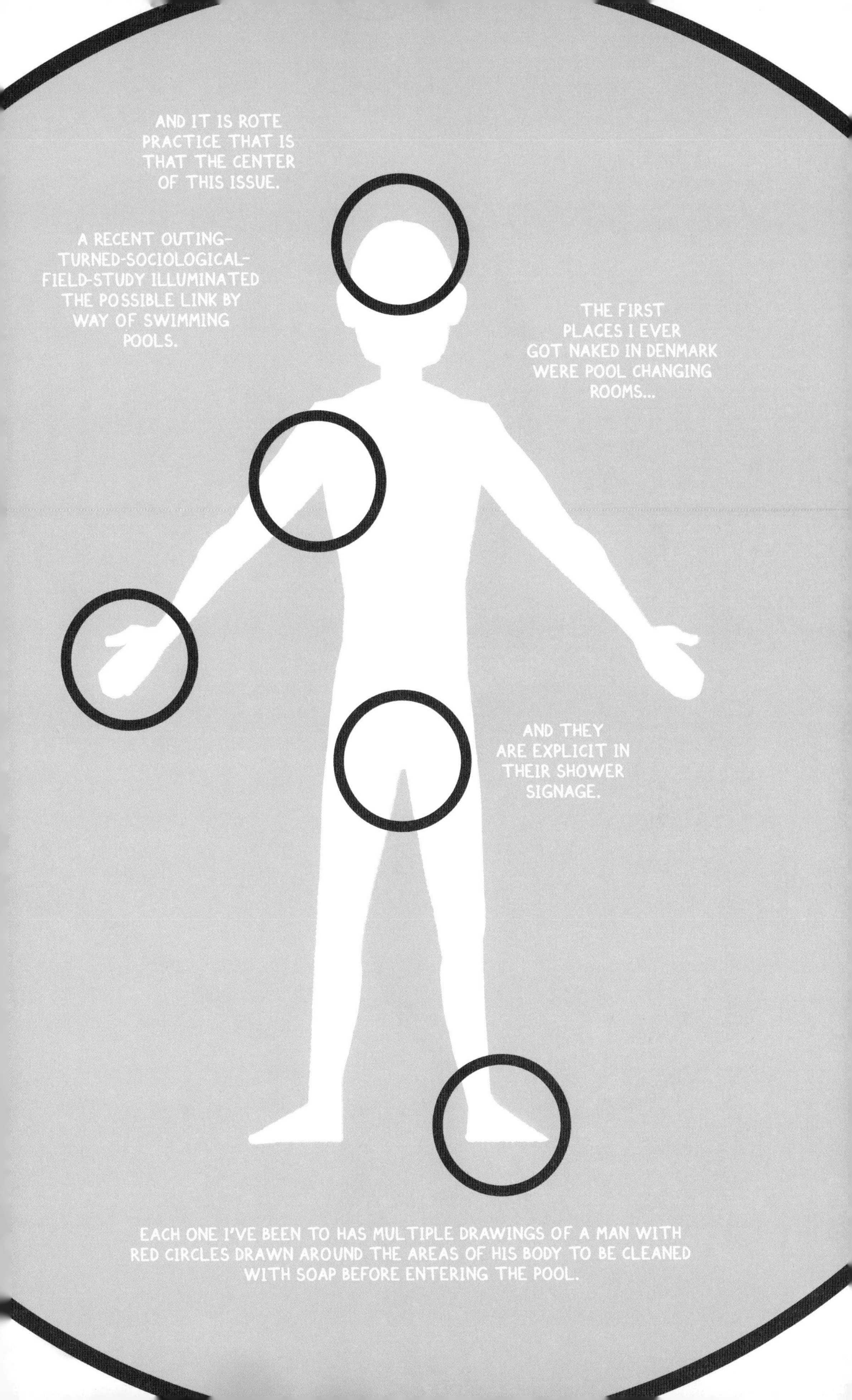

AND IT IS ROTE
PRACTICE THAT IS
THAT THE CENTER
OF THIS ISSUE.

A RECENT OUTING-
TURNED-SOCIOLOGICAL-
FIELD-STUDY ILLUMINATED
THE POSSIBLE LINK BY
WAY OF SWIMMING
POOLS.

THE FIRST
PLACES I EVER
GOT NAKED IN DENMARK
WERE POOL CHANGING
ROOMS...

AND THEY
ARE EXPLICIT IN
THEIR SHOWER
SIGNAGE.

EACH ONE I'VE BEEN TO HAS MULTIPLE DRAWINGS OF A MAN WITH
RED CIRCLES DRAWN AROUND THE AREAS OF HIS BODY TO BE CLEANED
WITH SOAP BEFORE ENTERING THE POOL.

THE MAN IN THE DRAWING IS NUDE, WHICH MAY SEEM OBVIOUS TO NON-AMERICANS, BUT I CAN ASSURE YOU THAT IN THE U.S.A., MOST POOL-GOERS SHOWER IN THEIR SWIMMING SUITS SO AS NOT TO HAVE TO GET NAKED.

MANY ALSO CHANGE INTO SAID SUITS BY WRAPPING A TOWEL AROUND THEIR WAIST AND SHIMMYING OUT OF THEIR UNDERWEAR AND INTO THEIR BOARD SHORTS – ALL WITHOUT EVER REMOVING THE TOWEL.

IF THERE WAS STILL A VAUDEVILLE CIRCUIT, THIS QUICK CHANGE ACT WOULD BE ON IT.

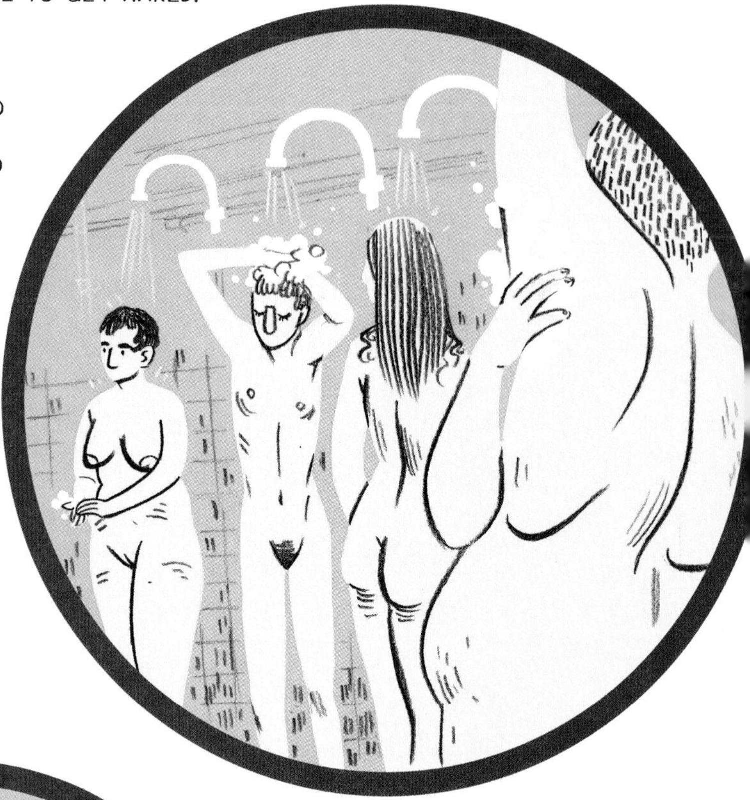

IN DENMARK, THERE'S AN EXACT INVERSE. PEOPLE WILL STRIP DOWN AT THEIR LOCKERS, CHANGE INTO SWIMSUITS, WALK TO THE SHOWERS, STRIP OFF THE SWIMSUITS AGAIN, BATHE, AND THEN REPLACE THEIR SUITS ONCE MORE.

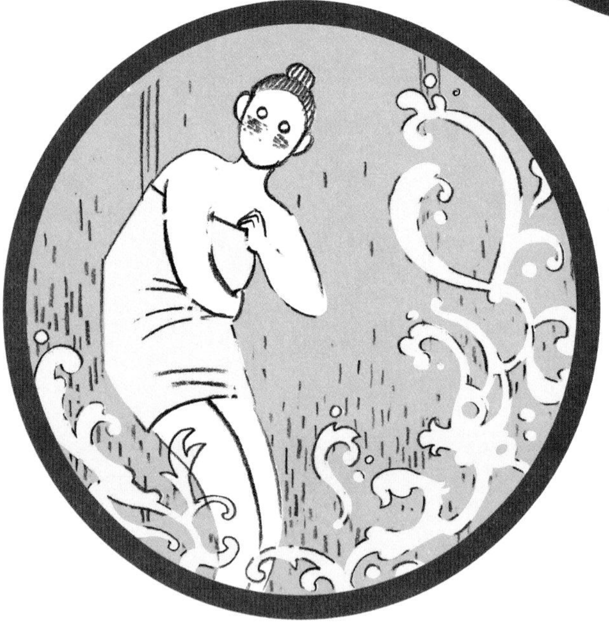

DENMARK'S DOUBLE-NAKED IN THIS PROCESS IS A SORT OF PER CAPITA "*CARBON BALANCING*" FOR AMERICA'S ZERO-NAKED AT SWIMMING POOLS STATUS QUO.

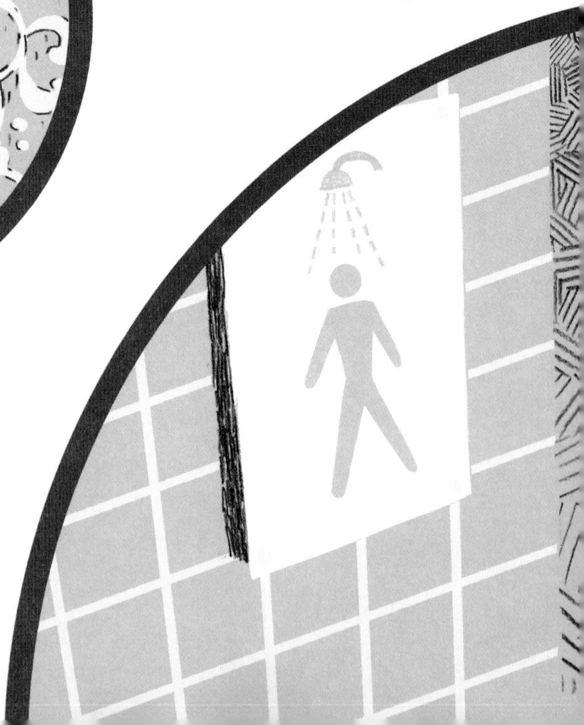

BUT HOW IS IT THAT EACH AND EVERY DANE ASCRIBES TO THIS FULL-ON, FULL MONTY SHOWERING RITUAL? IN AMERICA, RULES LIKE THIS ARE POSTED TO BE BROKEN.

A RECENT SWIM AT COPENHAGEN'S OBRO HALLEN POOL PROVIDED SOME ANSWERS...

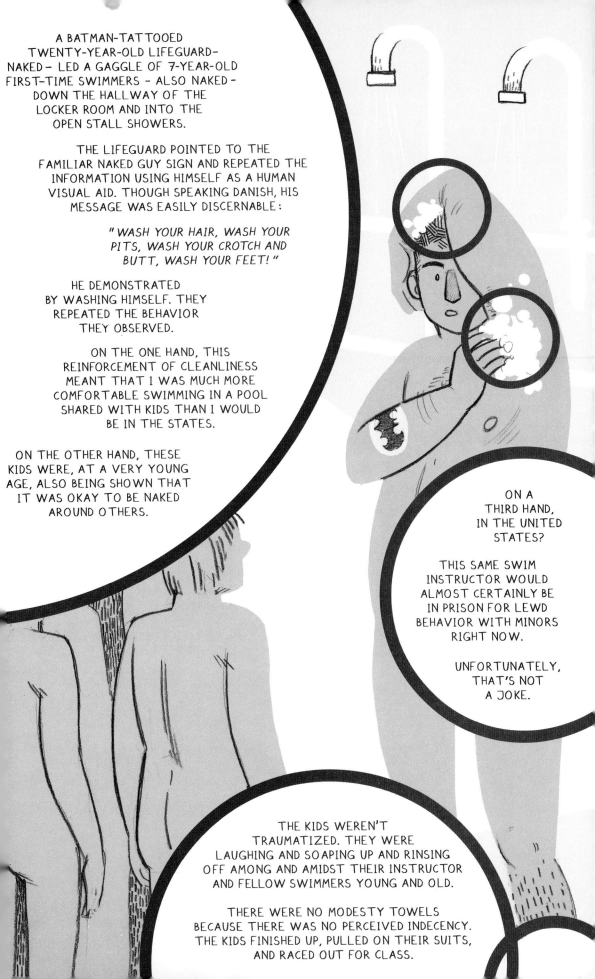

A BATMAN-TATTOOED TWENTY-YEAR-OLD LIFEGUARD- NAKED – LED A GAGGLE OF 7-YEAR-OLD FIRST-TIME SWIMMERS - ALSO NAKED - DOWN THE HALLWAY OF THE LOCKER ROOM AND INTO THE OPEN STALL SHOWERS.

THE LIFEGUARD POINTED TO THE FAMILIAR NAKED GUY SIGN AND REPEATED THE INFORMATION USING HIMSELF AS A HUMAN VISUAL AID. THOUGH SPEAKING DANISH, HIS MESSAGE WAS EASILY DISCERNABLE:

"WASH YOUR HAIR, WASH YOUR PITS, WASH YOUR CROTCH AND BUTT, WASH YOUR FEET!"

HE DEMONSTRATED BY WASHING HIMSELF. THEY REPEATED THE BEHAVIOR THEY OBSERVED.

ON THE ONE HAND, THIS REINFORCEMENT OF CLEANLINESS MEANT THAT I WAS MUCH MORE COMFORTABLE SWIMMING IN A POOL SHARED WITH KIDS THAN I WOULD BE IN THE STATES.

ON THE OTHER HAND, THESE KIDS WERE, AT A VERY YOUNG AGE, ALSO BEING SHOWN THAT IT WAS OKAY TO BE NAKED AROUND OTHERS.

ON A THIRD HAND, IN THE UNITED STATES?

THIS SAME SWIM INSTRUCTOR WOULD ALMOST CERTAINLY BE IN PRISON FOR LEWD BEHAVIOR WITH MINORS RIGHT NOW.

UNFORTUNATELY, THAT'S NOT A JOKE.

THE KIDS WEREN'T TRAUMATIZED. THEY WERE LAUGHING AND SOAPING UP AND RINSING OFF AMONG AND AMIDST THEIR INSTRUCTOR AND FELLOW SWIMMERS YOUNG AND OLD.

THERE WERE NO MODESTY TOWELS BECAUSE THERE WAS NO PERCEIVED INDECENCY. THE KIDS FINISHED UP, PULLED ON THEIR SUITS, AND RACED OUT FOR CLASS.

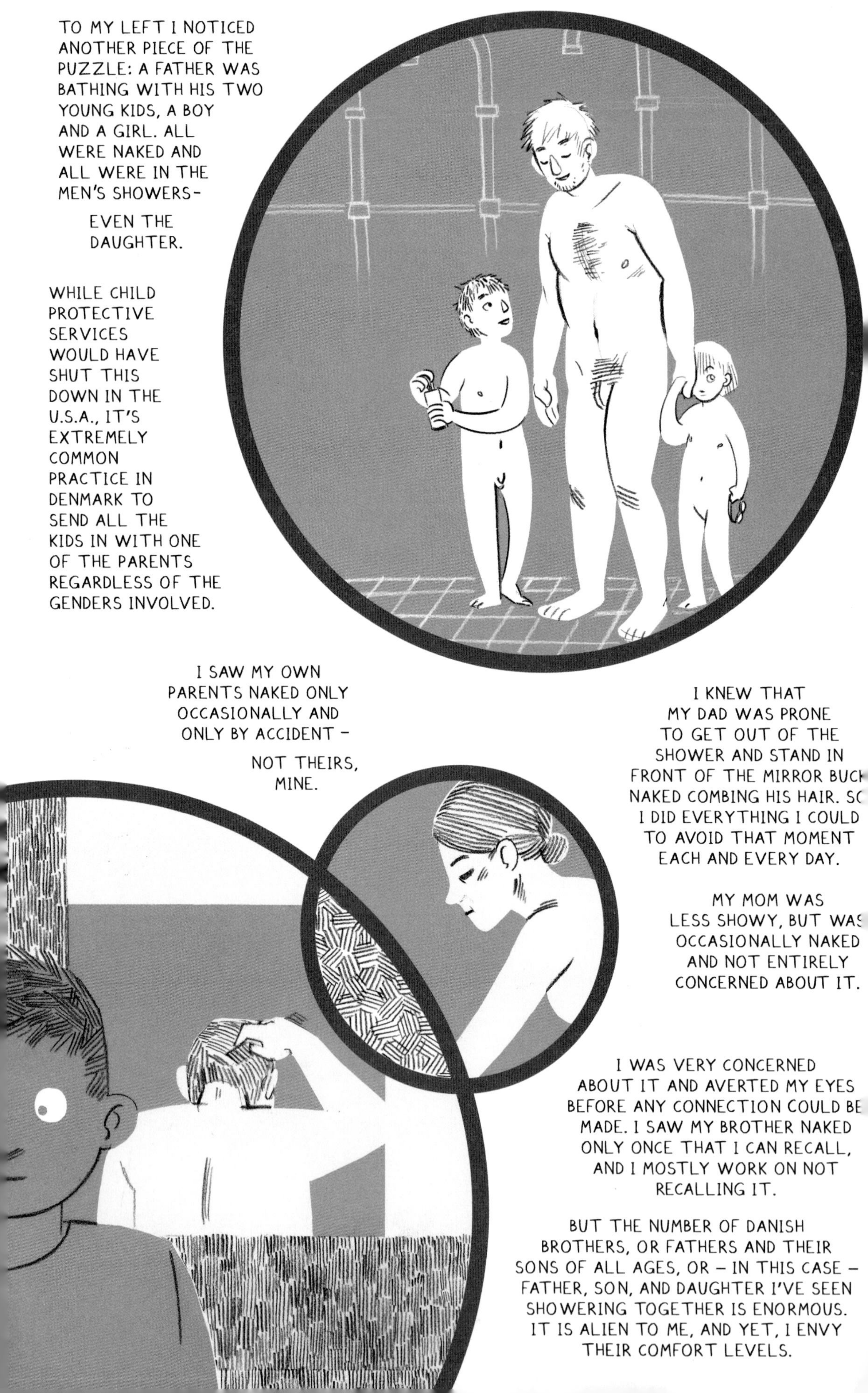

TO MY LEFT I NOTICED ANOTHER PIECE OF THE PUZZLE: A FATHER WAS BATHING WITH HIS TWO YOUNG KIDS, A BOY AND A GIRL. ALL WERE NAKED AND ALL WERE IN THE MEN'S SHOWERS—

EVEN THE DAUGHTER.

WHILE CHILD PROTECTIVE SERVICES WOULD HAVE SHUT THIS DOWN IN THE U.S.A., IT'S EXTREMELY COMMON PRACTICE IN DENMARK TO SEND ALL THE KIDS IN WITH ONE OF THE PARENTS REGARDLESS OF THE GENDERS INVOLVED.

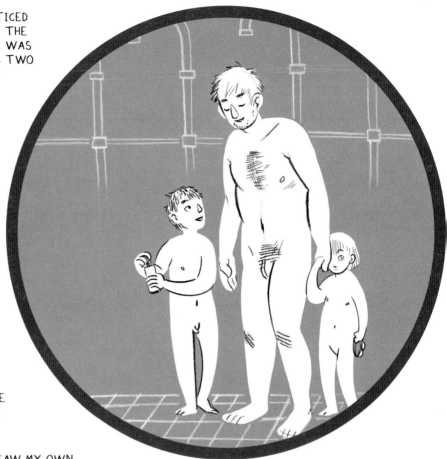

I SAW MY OWN PARENTS NAKED ONLY OCCASIONALLY AND ONLY BY ACCIDENT –

NOT THEIRS, MINE.

I KNEW THAT MY DAD WAS PRONE TO GET OUT OF THE SHOWER AND STAND IN FRONT OF THE MIRROR BUCK NAKED COMBING HIS HAIR. SO I DID EVERYTHING I COULD TO AVOID THAT MOMENT EACH AND EVERY DAY.

MY MOM WAS LESS SHOWY, BUT WAS OCCASIONALLY NAKED AND NOT ENTIRELY CONCERNED ABOUT IT.

I WAS VERY CONCERNED ABOUT IT AND AVERTED MY EYES BEFORE ANY CONNECTION COULD BE MADE. I SAW MY BROTHER NAKED ONLY ONCE THAT I CAN RECALL, AND I MOSTLY WORK ON NOT RECALLING IT.

BUT THE NUMBER OF DANISH BROTHERS, OR FATHERS AND THEIR SONS OF ALL AGES, OR – IN THIS CASE – FATHER, SON, AND DAUGHTER I'VE SEEN SHOWERING TOGETHER IS ENORMOUS. IT IS ALIEN TO ME, AND YET, I ENVY THEIR COMFORT LEVELS.

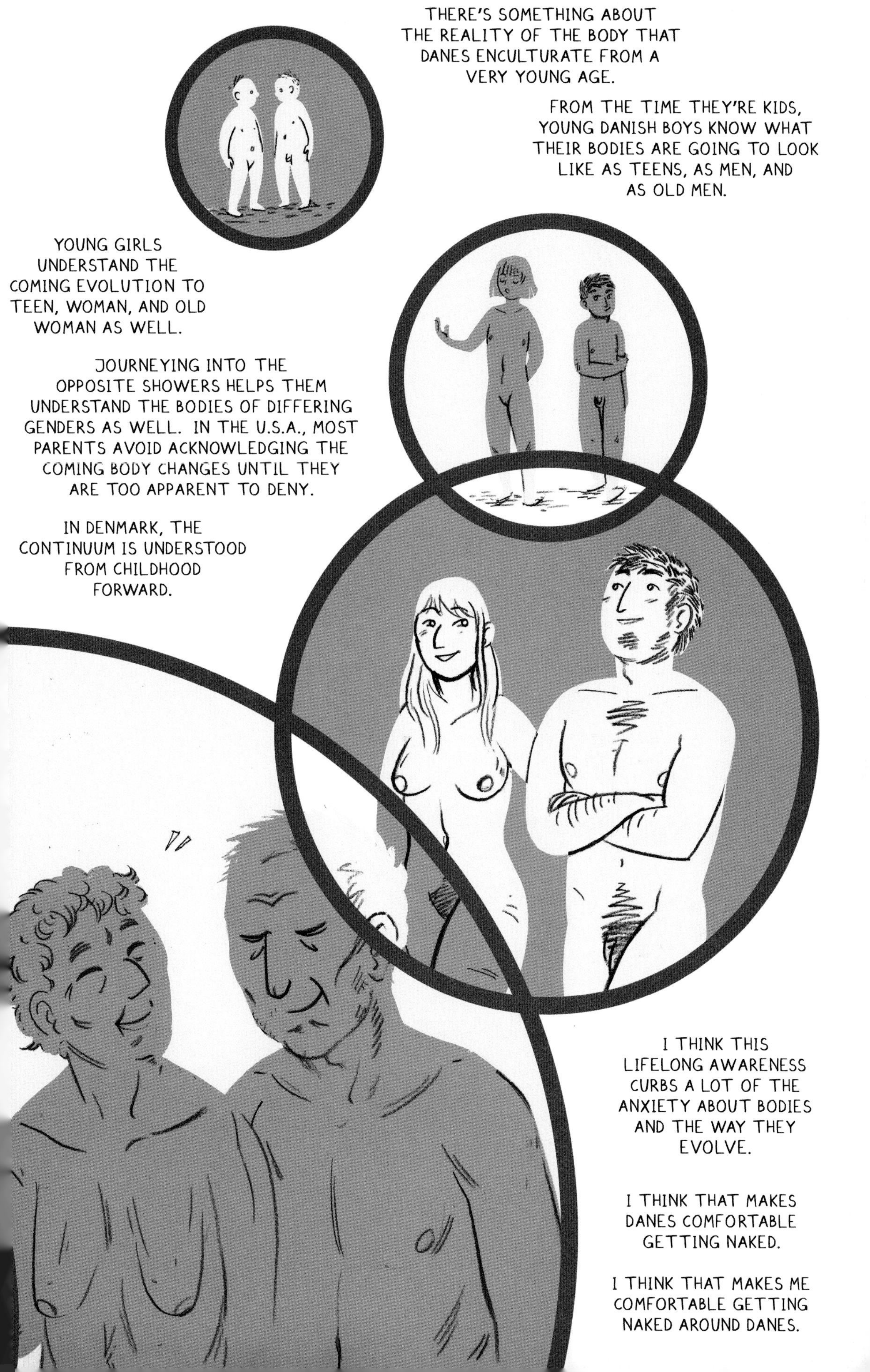
THERE'S SOMETHING ABOUT THE REALITY OF THE BODY THAT DANES ENCULTURATE FROM A VERY YOUNG AGE.
FROM THE TIME THEY'RE KIDS, YOUNG DANISH BOYS KNOW WHAT THEIR BODIES ARE GOING TO LOOK LIKE AS TEENS, AS MEN, AND AS OLD MEN.
YOUNG GIRLS UNDERSTAND THE COMING EVOLUTION TO TEEN, WOMAN, AND OLD WOMAN AS WELL.
JOURNEYING INTO THE OPPOSITE SHOWERS HELPS THEM UNDERSTAND THE BODIES OF DIFFERING GENDERS AS WELL. IN THE U.S.A., MOST PARENTS AVOID ACKNOWLEDGING THE COMING BODY CHANGES UNTIL THEY ARE TOO APPARENT TO DENY.
IN DENMARK, THE CONTINUUM IS UNDERSTOOD FROM CHILDHOOD FORWARD.
I THINK THIS LIFELONG AWARENESS CURBS A LOT OF THE ANXIETY ABOUT BODIES AND THE WAY THEY EVOLVE.
I THINK THAT MAKES DANES COMFORTABLE GETTING NAKED.
I THINK THAT MAKES ME COMFORTABLE GETTING NAKED AROUND DANES.

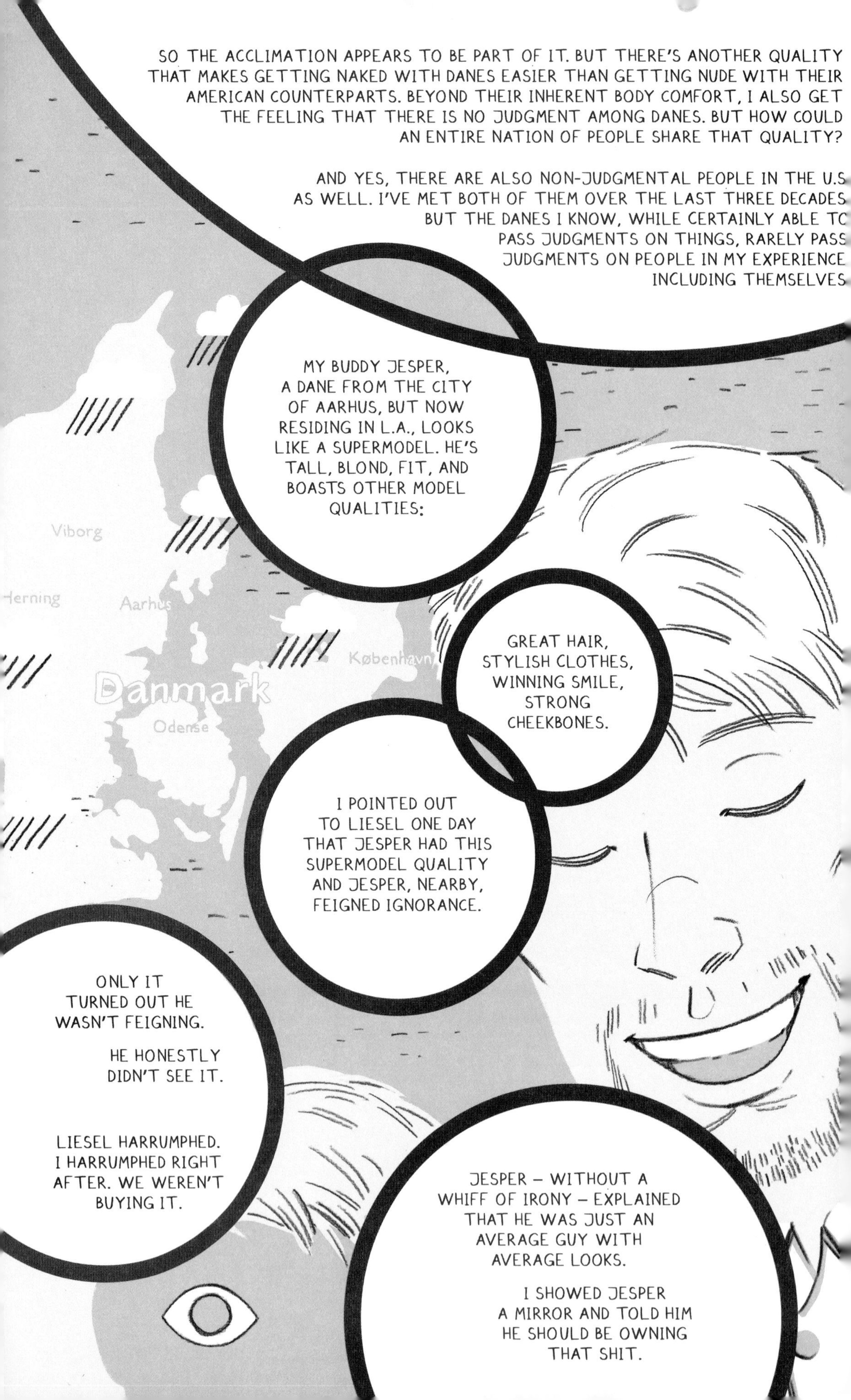
SO THE ACCLIMATION APPEARS TO BE PART OF IT. BUT THERE'S ANOTHER QUALITY THAT MAKES GETTING NAKED WITH DANES EASIER THAN GETTING NUDE WITH THEIR AMERICAN COUNTERPARTS. BEYOND THEIR INHERENT BODY COMFORT, I ALSO GET THE FEELING THAT THERE IS NO JUDGMENT AMONG DANES. BUT HOW COULD AN ENTIRE NATION OF PEOPLE SHARE THAT QUALITY?
AND YES, THERE ARE ALSO NON-JUDGMENTAL PEOPLE IN THE U.S AS WELL. I'VE MET BOTH OF THEM OVER THE LAST THREE DECADES BUT THE DANES I KNOW, WHILE CERTAINLY ABLE TO PASS JUDGMENTS ON THINGS, RARELY PASS JUDGMENTS ON PEOPLE IN MY EXPERIENCE INCLUDING THEMSELVES
MY BUDDY JESPER, A DANE FROM THE CITY OF AARHUS, BUT NOW RESIDING IN L.A., LOOKS LIKE A SUPERMODEL. HE'S TALL, BLOND, FIT, AND BOASTS OTHER MODEL QUALITIES:
Viborg
Herning
Aarhus
København
Danmark
Odense
GREAT HAIR, STYLISH CLOTHES, WINNING SMILE, STRONG CHEEKBONES.
I POINTED OUT TO LIESEL ONE DAY THAT JESPER HAD THIS SUPERMODEL QUALITY AND JESPER, NEARBY, FEIGNED IGNORANCE.
ONLY IT TURNED OUT HE WASN'T FEIGNING.
HE HONESTLY DIDN'T SEE IT.
LIESEL HARRUMPHED. I HARRUMPHED RIGHT AFTER. WE WEREN'T BUYING IT.
JESPER – WITHOUT A WHIFF OF IRONY – EXPLAINED THAT HE WAS JUST AN AVERAGE GUY WITH AVERAGE LOOKS.
I SHOWED JESPER A MIRROR AND TOLD HIM HE SHOULD BE OWNING THAT SHIT.

"DANES,"

JESPER SAID,

"ARE RAISED
TO NOT BE
BOASTFUL."

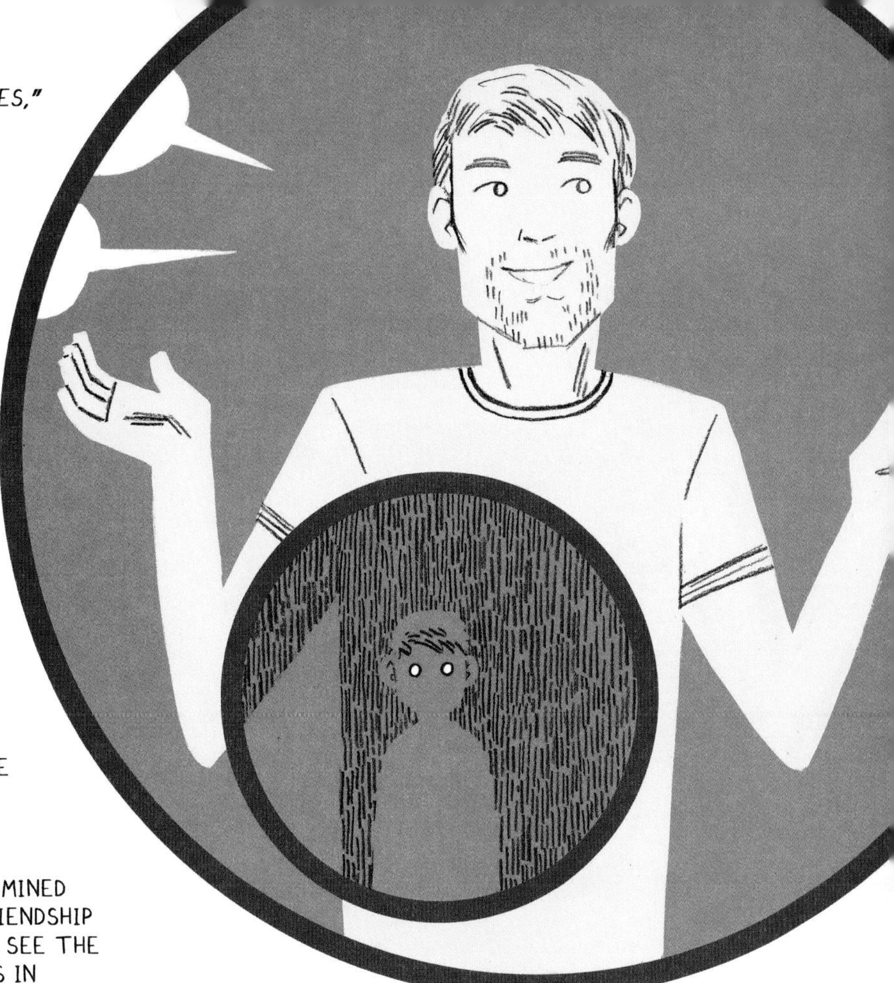

HE EXPLAINED THAT AS A KID, HE WAS CONDITIONED NOT TO EXTOLL HIS OWN VIRTUES; NOT EVEN TO ACKNOWLEDGE THEM WHEN THEY WERE CALLED OUT BY OTHERS.

IT SEEMED A BIT MUCH TO BUY INTO – AN ENTIRE CULTURE DEVOID OF COMPETITIVE ONE-UPMANSHIP?

BUT WHEN I REEXAMINED MY DECADES-LONG FRIENDSHIP WITH TEDDY, I COULD SEE THE SAME QUALITIES IN HIM AS WELL.

ONE OF THE MOST TALENTED COMIC ARTISTS IN THE WORLD, TEDDY IS 99% UNABLE TO ACCEPT A COMPLIMENT.

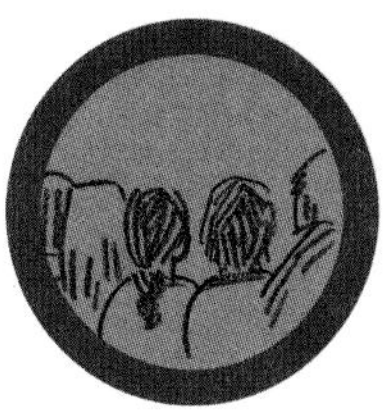

THE SAME QUALITY WAS PRESENT IN OTHER DANES I'D INTERACTED WITH OVER THE YEARS AS WELL ...

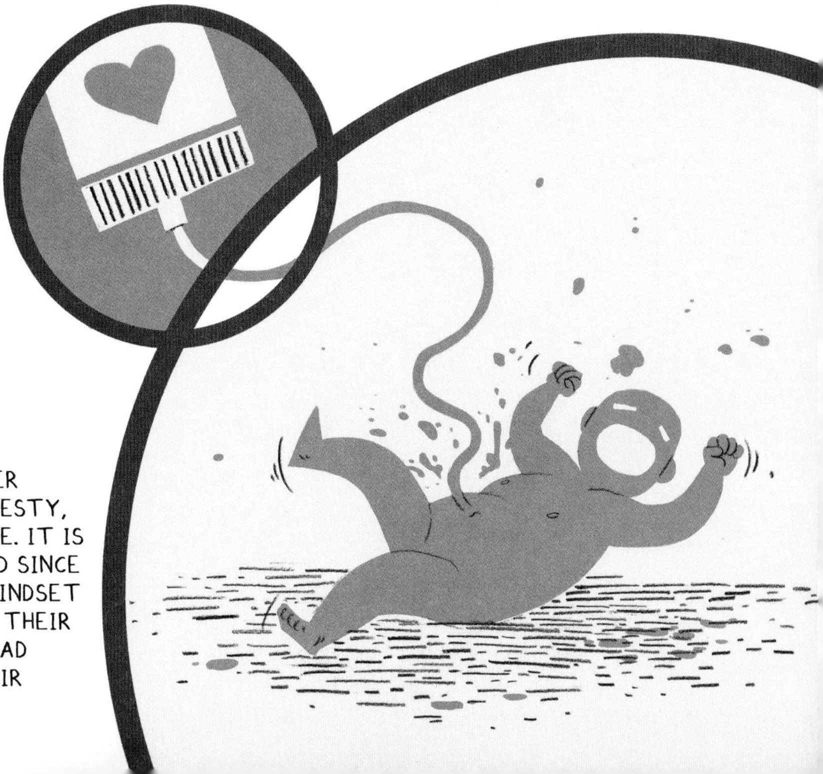

ARTISTS, ANIMATORS, STUDENTS – THEY ALL SHARED THIS REFRESHING LACK OF SELF-AGGRANDIZEMENT THAT IS PRACTICALLY FED VIA INTRAVENOUS DRIP INTO AMERICANS FROM THE MOMENT THEY'RE BORN.

WHILE IT MIGHT SEEM TO AN OUTSIDER THAT THIS IS FALSE MODESTY, IT IS THE EXACT OPPOSITE. IT IS TRUE MODESTY. INSTILLED SINCE BIRTH, IT IS AN ACTUAL MINDSET THAT GROUNDS DANES IN THEIR COMMONALITY INSTEAD OF UNDERLINING THEIR SEPARATIONS.

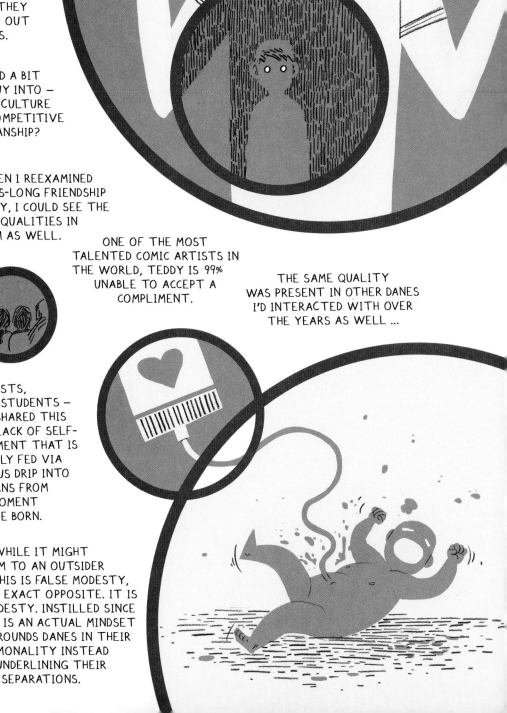

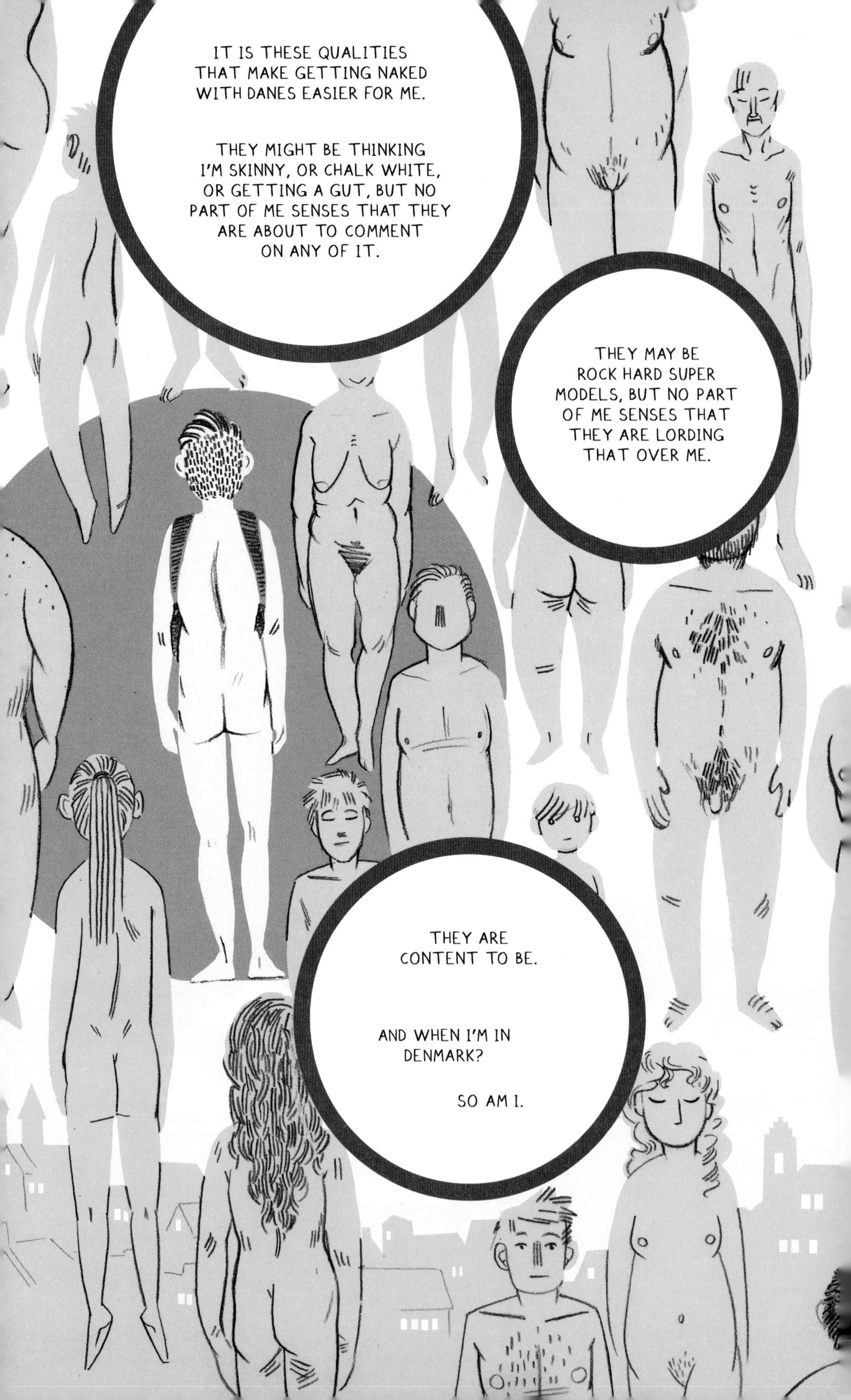
IT IS THESE QUALITIES THAT MAKE GETTING NAKED WITH DANES EASIER FOR ME.
THEY MIGHT BE THINKING I'M SKINNY, OR CHALK WHITE, OR GETTING A GUT, BUT NO PART OF ME SENSES THAT THEY ARE ABOUT TO COMMENT ON ANY OF IT.
THEY MAY BE ROCK HARD SUPER MODELS, BUT NO PART OF ME SENSES THAT THEY ARE LORDING THAT OVER ME.
THEY ARE CONTENT TO BE.
AND WHEN I'M IN DENMARK?
SO AM I.

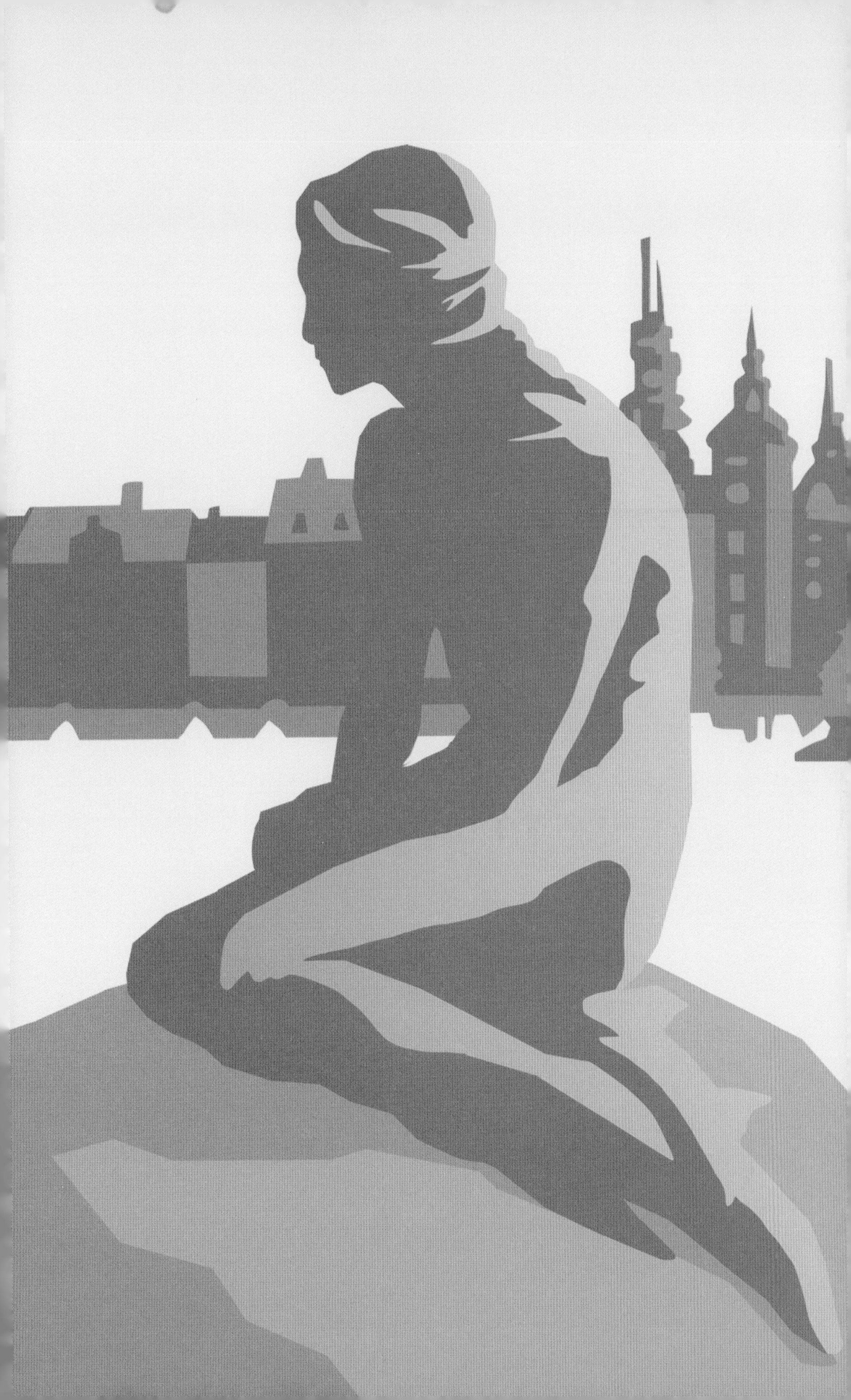

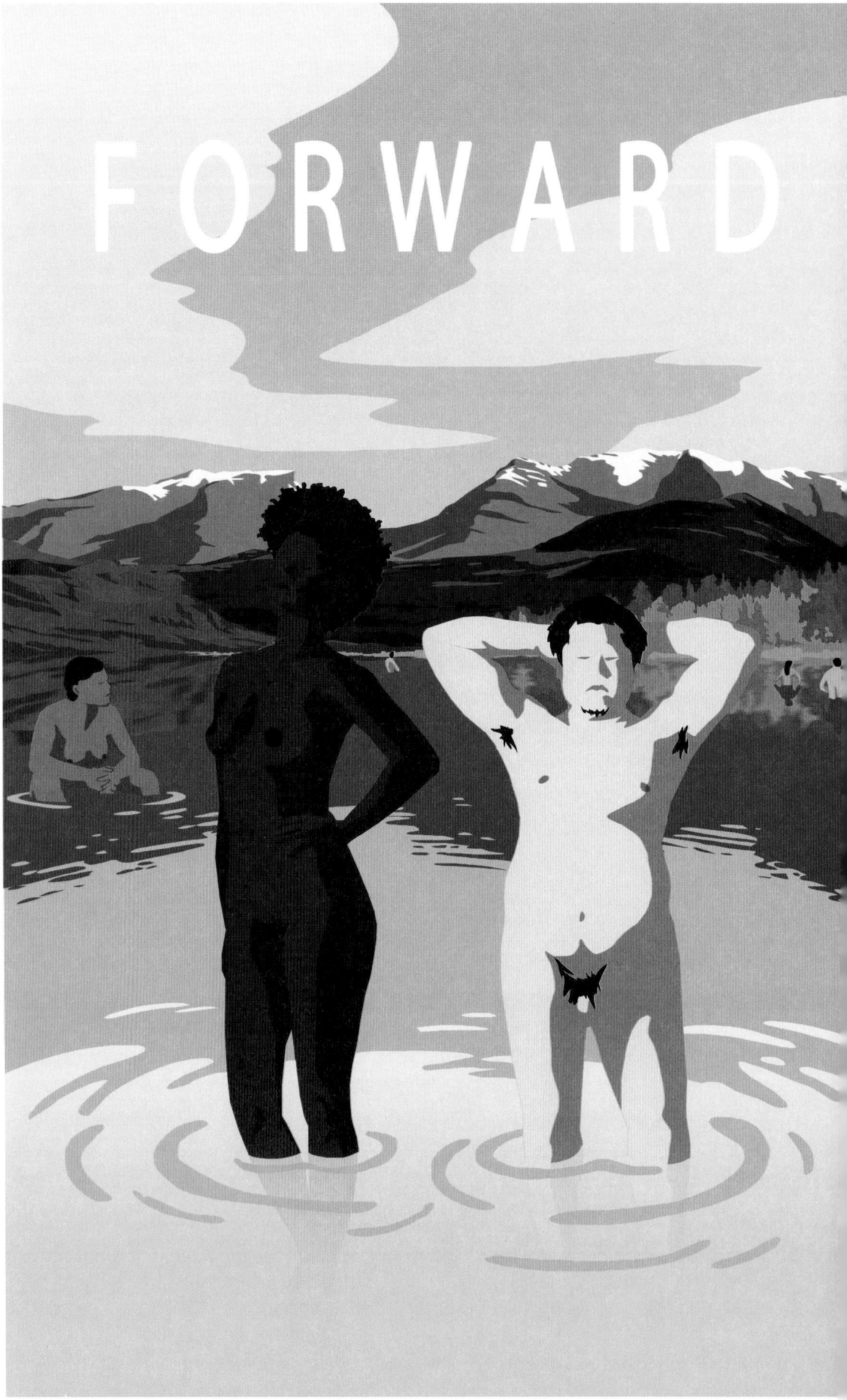
FORWARD

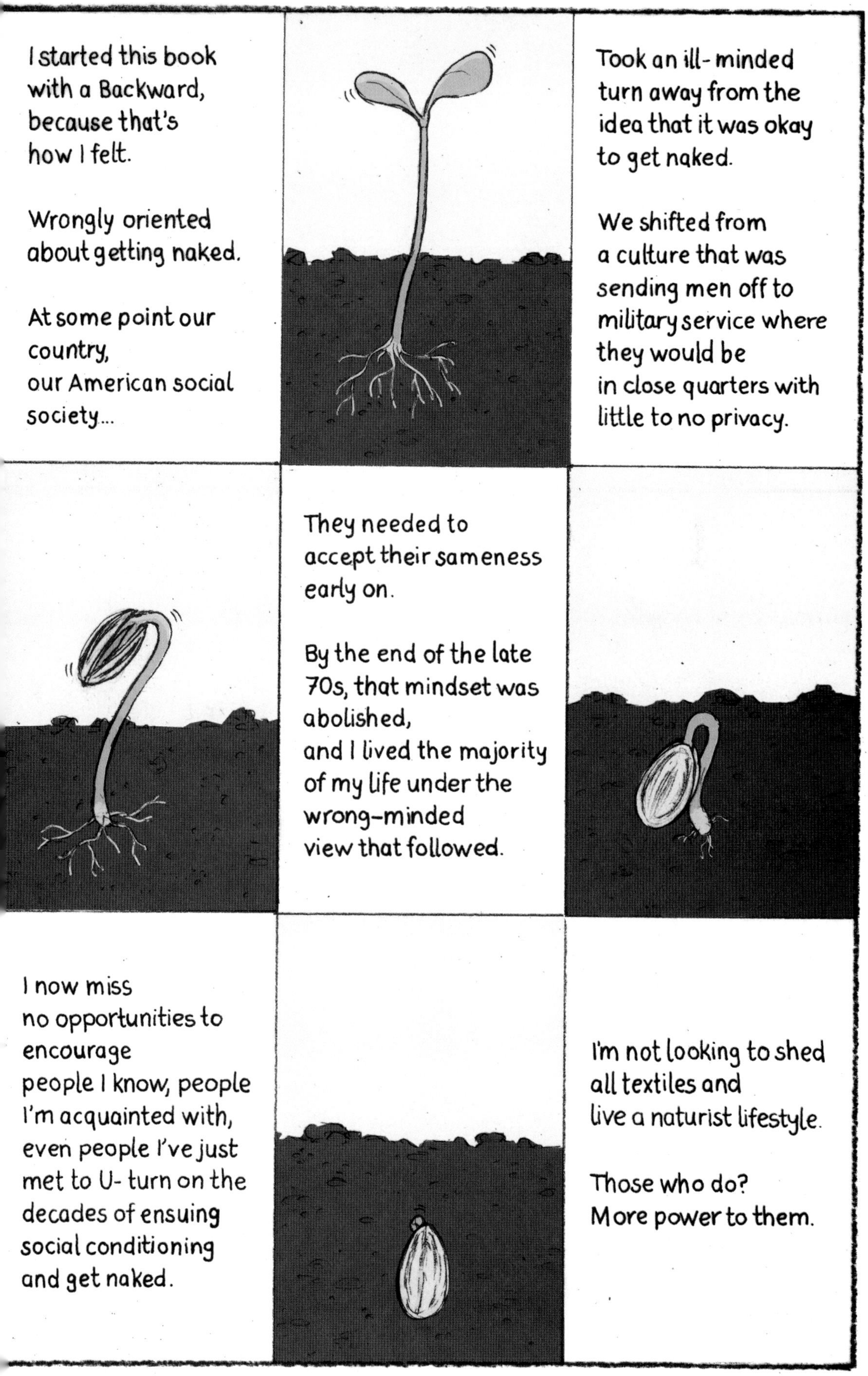

I started this book with a Backward, because that's how I felt.

Wrongly oriented about getting naked.

At some point our country, our American social society...

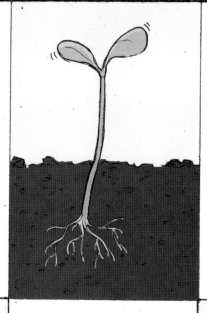

Took an ill-minded turn away from the idea that it was okay to get naked.

We shifted from a culture that was sending men off to military service where they would be in close quarters with little to no privacy.

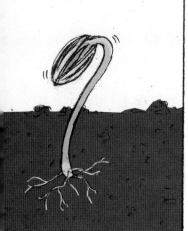

They needed to accept their sameness early on.

By the end of the late 70s, that mindset was abolished, and I lived the majority of my life under the wrong-minded view that followed.

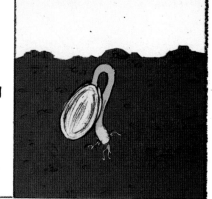

I now miss no opportunities to encourage people I know, people I'm acquainted with, even people I've just met to U-turn on the decades of ensuing social conditioning and get naked.

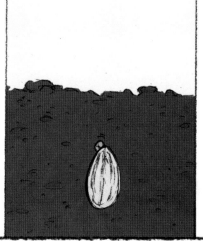

I'm not looking to shed all textiles and live a naturist lifestyle.

Those who do? More power to them.

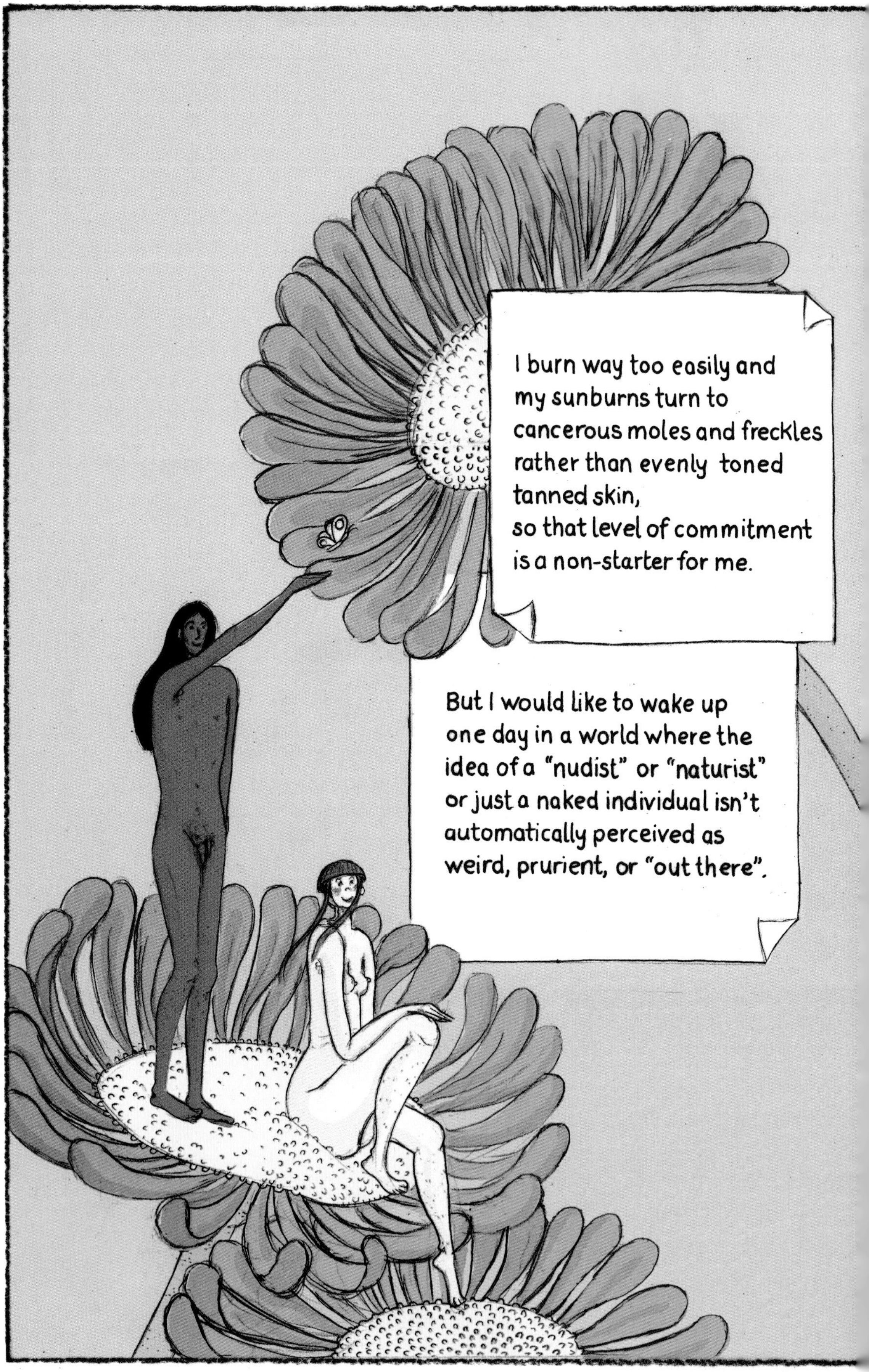
I burn way too easily and my sunburns turn to cancerous moles and freckles rather than evenly toned tanned skin, so that level of commitment is a non-starter for me.
But I would like to wake up one day in a world where the idea of a "nudist" or "naturist" or just a naked individual isn't automatically perceived as weird, prurient, or "out there".

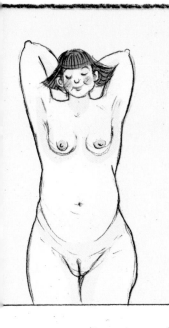

I've invited literally hundreds of people to Korean Spas in LA.

The "first time getting naked" demo tends to shake out into three distinct groups:

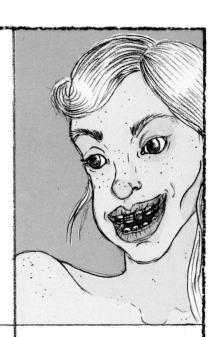

A very small portion of people think nothing about the fact that they will get naked arround others.

They're in the door, out of their clothes, and down the hall having barely registered that anything changed about their person.

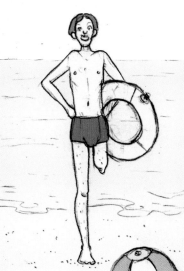

Then there are those in the "mildly uneasy crew." They tend to make a passing joke or a "Well, here we go," or a "Never thought I'd be doing this." They hesitate a moment then commit.

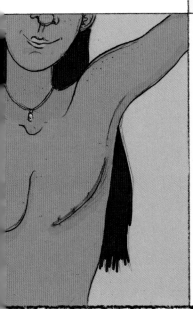

They're not instantaneously at ease, but by the end of a cycle through the wet pools and saunas, they tend to express a "I don't know what I was worried about" kind of sentiment.

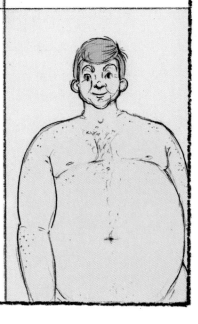

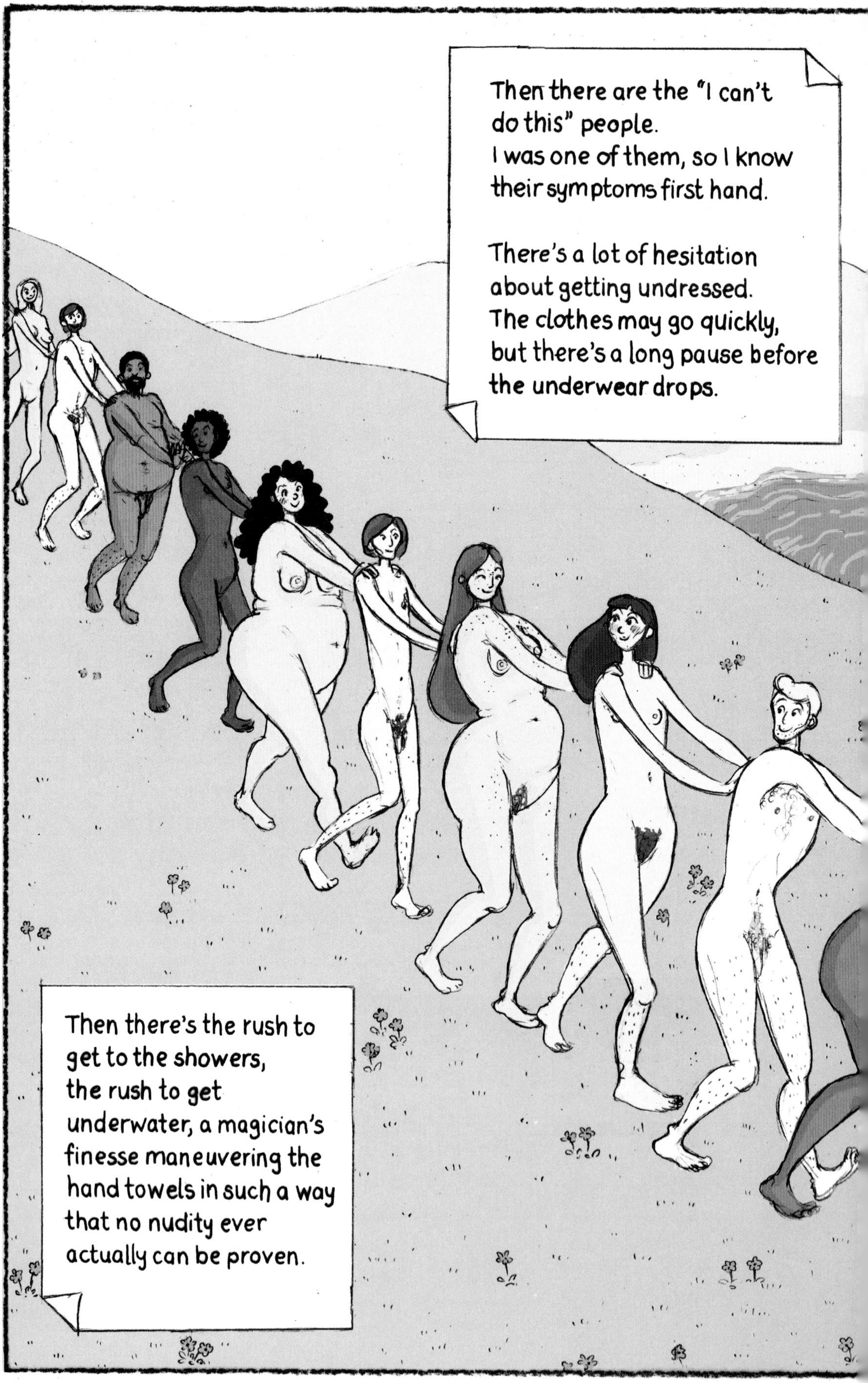
Then there are the "I can't do this" people.
I was one of them, so I know their symptoms first hand.
There's a lot of hesitation about getting undressed.
The clothes may go quickly, but there's a long pause before the underwear drops.
Then there's the rush to get to the showers, the rush to get underwater, a magician's finesse maneuvering the hand towels in such a way that no nudity ever actually can be proven.

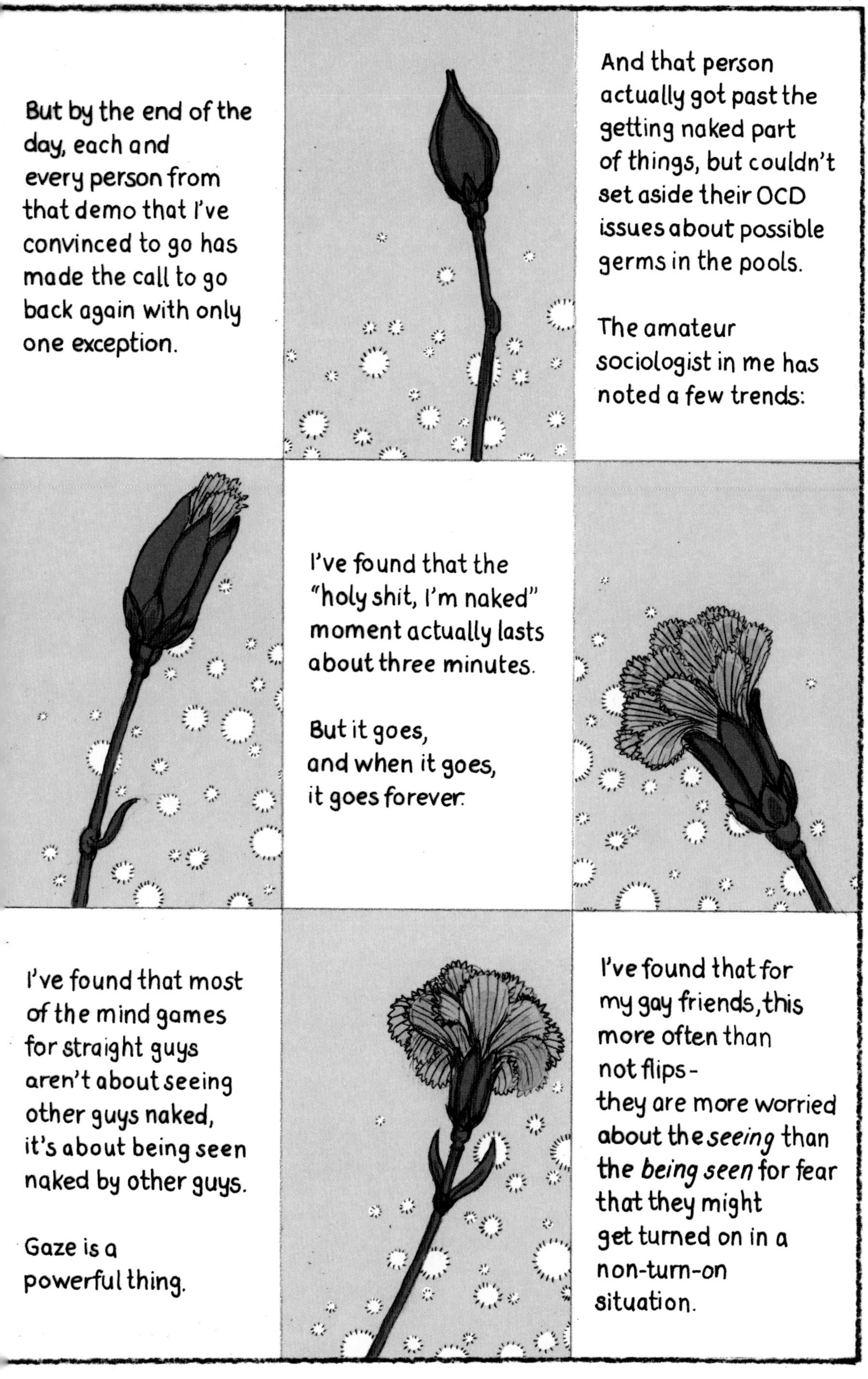

But by the end of the day, each and every person from that demo that I've convinced to go has made the call to go back again with only one exception.

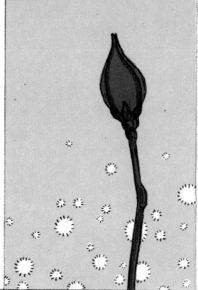

And that person actually got past the getting naked part of things, but couldn't set aside their OCD issues about possible germs in the pools.

The amateur sociologist in me has noted a few trends:

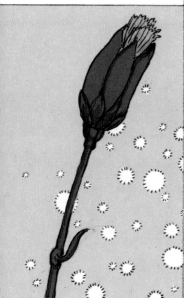

I've found that the "holy shit, I'm naked" moment actually lasts about three minutes.

But it goes, and when it goes, it goes forever.

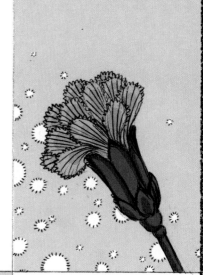

I've found that most of the mind games for straight guys aren't about seeing other guys naked, it's about being seen naked by other guys.

Gaze is a powerful thing.

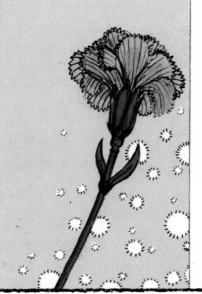

I've found that for my gay friends, this more often than not flips - they are more worried about the *seeing* than the *being seen* for fear that they might get turned on in a non-turn-on situation.

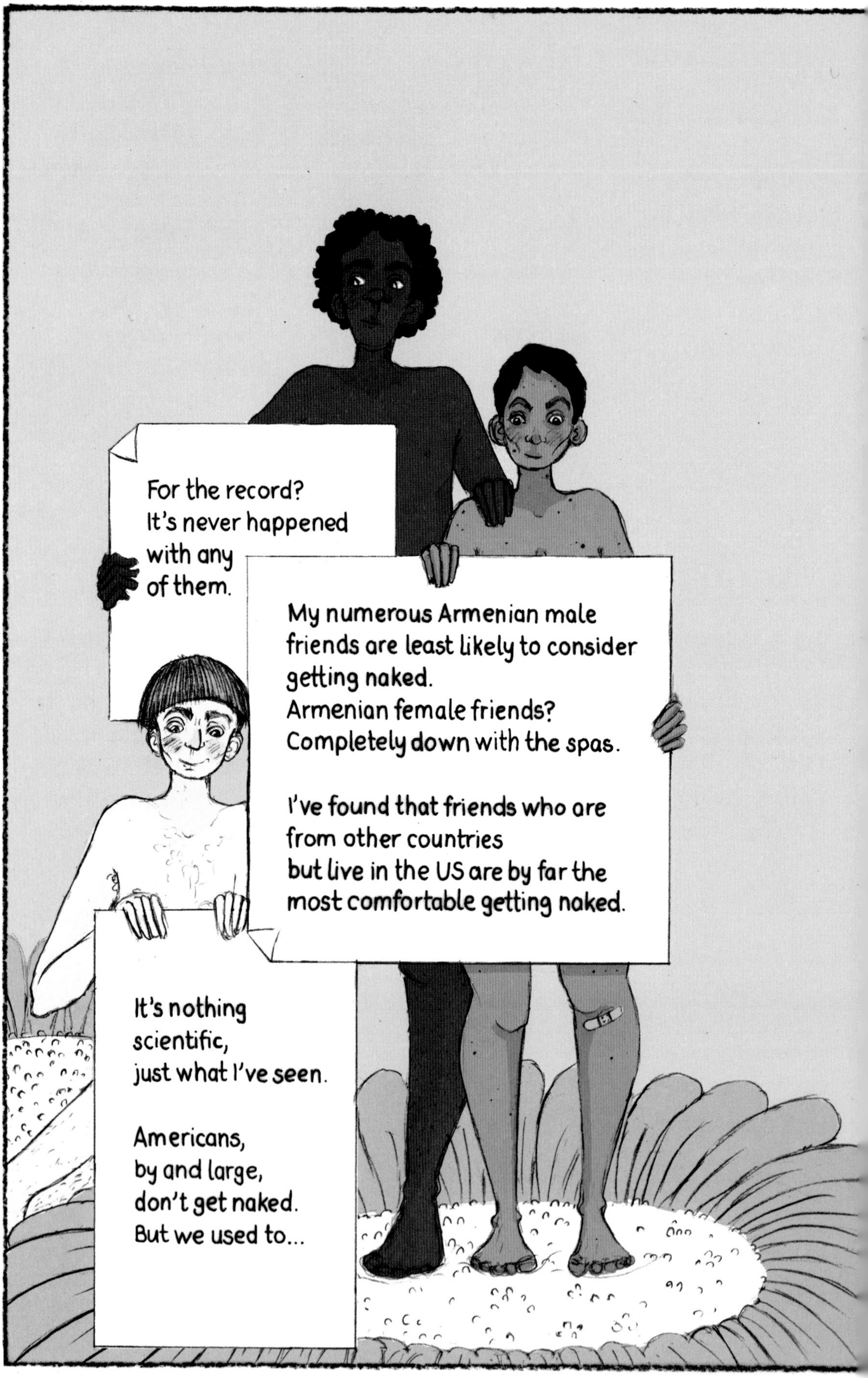
For the record? It's never happened with any of them.
My numerous Armenian male friends are least likely to consider getting naked.
Armenian female friends? Completely down with the spas.
I've found that friends who are from other countries but live in the US are by far the most comfortable getting naked.
It's nothing scientific, just what I've seen.
Americans, by and large, don't get naked. But we used to...

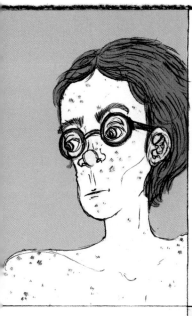

And the shift away from a willingness to bare ourselves was a giant step backward for our individual and collective wellbeing.

I'm taking a step forward.

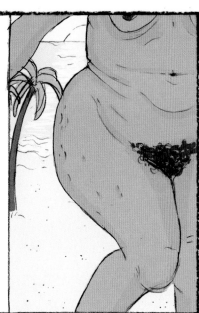

This shouldn't be confused with the notion that I will always be nude. I like clothes and I will most often be wearing some.

What I'm getting at is more general.

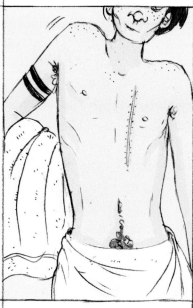

Going forward, I won't shy away from situations where I have to get naked.

This doesn't mean I'll be seeking out as many off-the-wall naked adventures as possible.

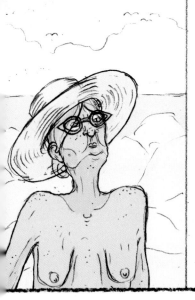

I definitely will not naked bungee jump.

But it has nothing to do with the naked part. It has everything to do with the bungee part.

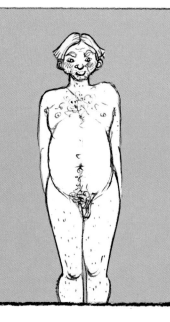

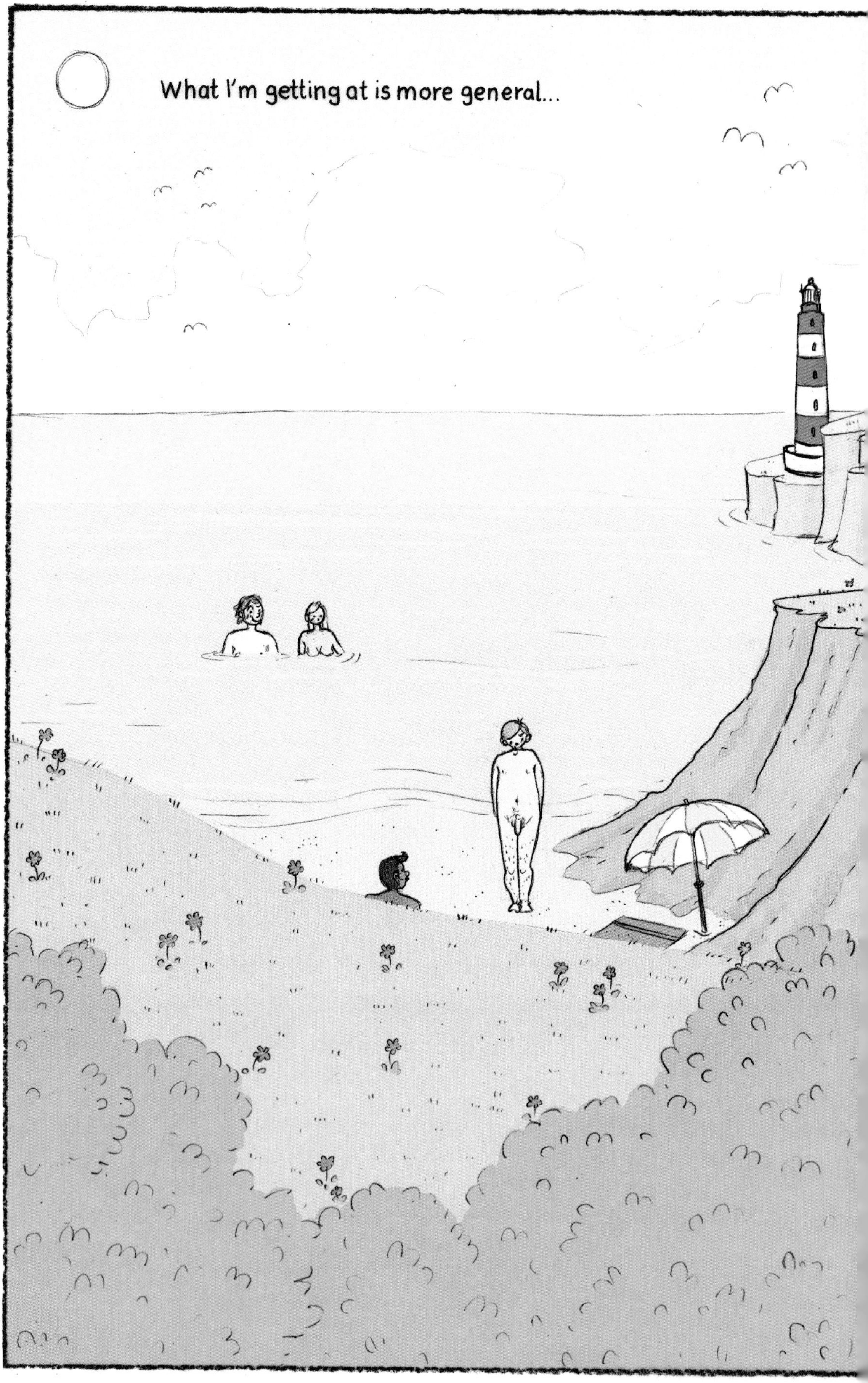
What I'm getting at is more general...

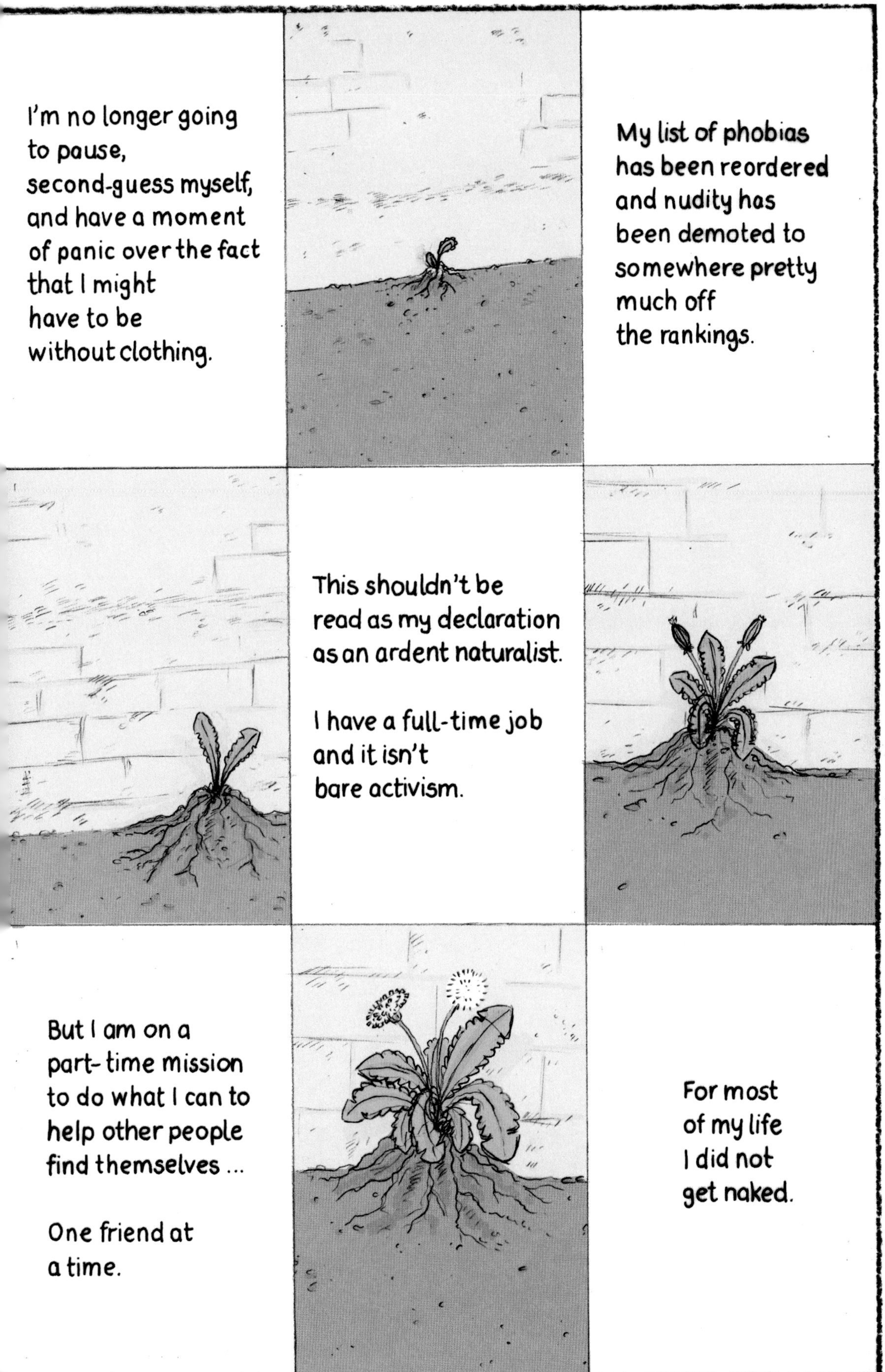
I'm no longer going to pause, second-guess myself, and have a moment of panic over the fact that I might have to be without clothing.
My list of phobias has been reordered and nudity has been demoted to somewhere pretty much off the rankings.
This shouldn't be read as my declaration as an ardent naturalist.
I have a full-time job and it isn't bare activism.
But I am on a part-time mission to do what I can to help other people find themselves ...
One friend at a time.
For most of my life I did not get naked.

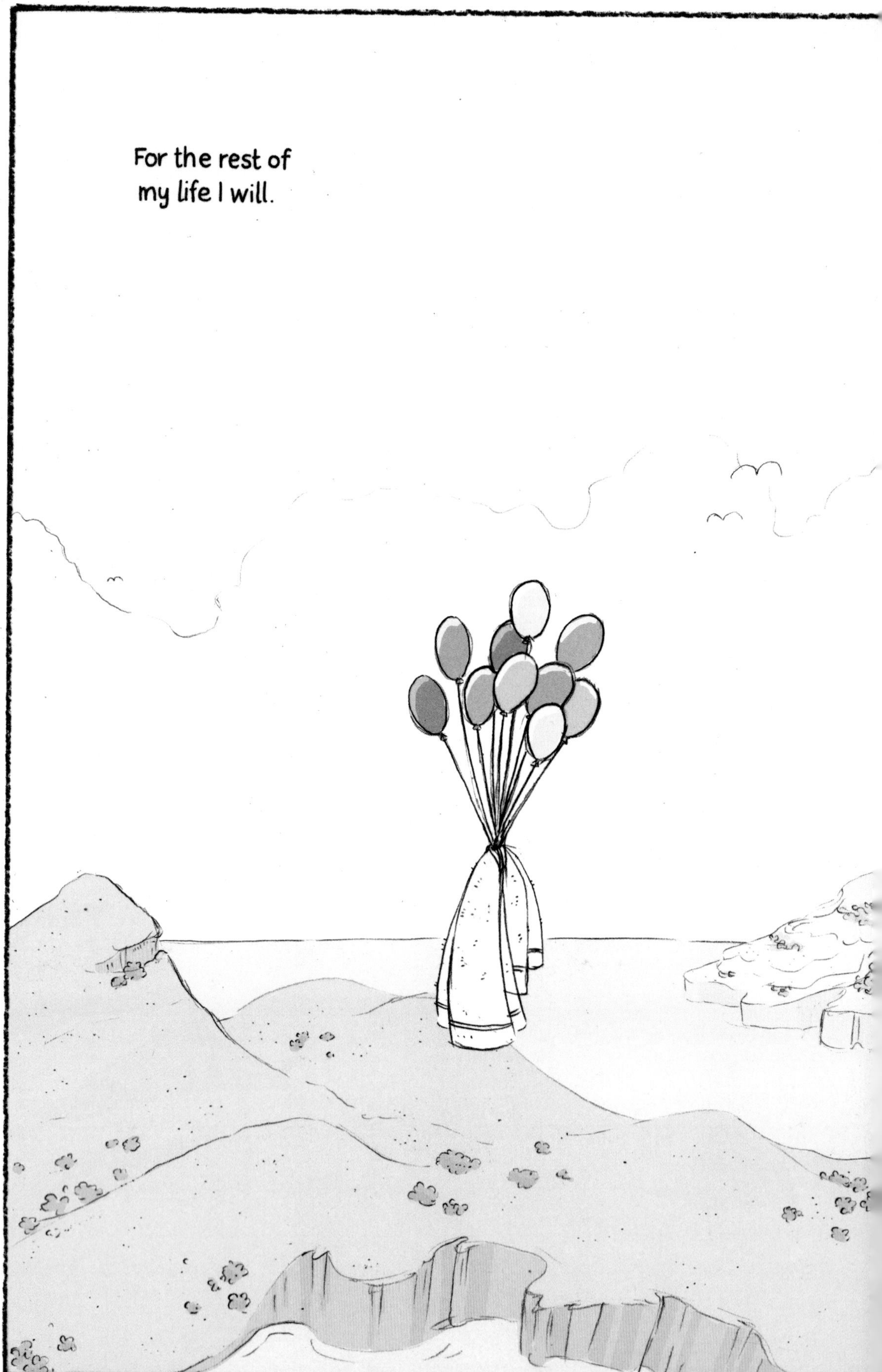
For the rest of my life I will.

creator biographies

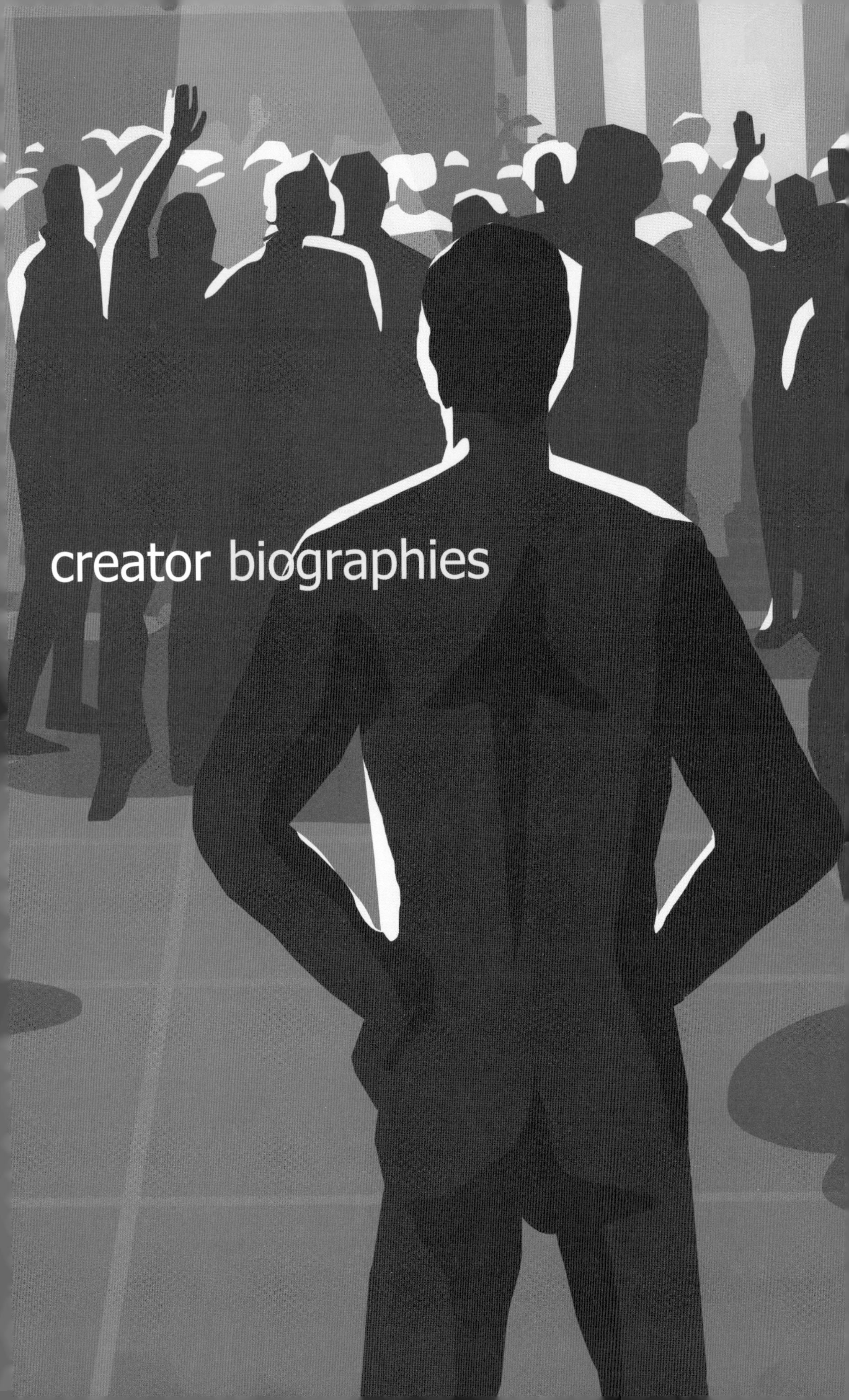

ESSAYS

Steven Terence Seagle was born in Mississippi,
grew up in Colorado, and lives in California.

Steven loves drum corps, ice water, and Liesel.

Steven would like to thank his friends mentioned in the
essays for their role in these adventures,
his parents, and all the fine people at
The Animation Workshop, Viborg.

The last place Steven got naked was in a sensory
deprivation float tank... which is an essay for later.

Steven's other books for grown-ups include *KAFKA*, *Genius*,
it's a bird..., *Solstice*, *The Crusades*, *House of Secrets*,
American Virgin, and *The Red Diary/The RE[a]D Diary*.

For younger folk he co-created
Camp Midnight, *Batula*,
Ben 10, and *Big Hero 6*.

twitter: @ManOfActionEnt
facebook: ManOfActionEnt

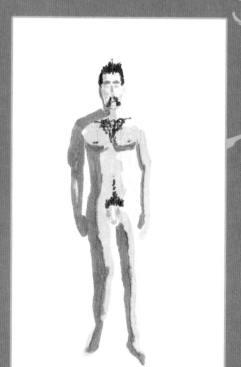

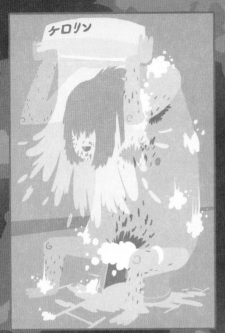

Mads Skovbakke is from the windy west of Denmark -
Nørre Nissum to be specific.

Mads enjoys Japanese bathhouses, dancing, and baking.

Mads would like to thank his family - the whole bunch -
his study-buddies at The Animation Workshop, along with
Peter Dyring-Olsen, Morten Thorning, and Erik Barkman.

The last place Mads got naked was earlier this morning.
This is true whenever you read this text, as Mads likes to enjoy his
freedom to sleep 'au naturale' - as they say in France.

You will find his work in a bunch of teaching
and informational material around Denmark,
as well as in the school zine 'Cyclops',
where he runs the production alongside Erlend and Silja -
both contributors to this comic.
His work will also be found in the fierce and fiery souls
of the next generation of comics artists
as he teaches across all of Denmark.

madsskovbakke.strikingly.com
twitter: @madsskovbakke
instagram: @madsellegårdskovbakke
Facebook: madsscribbles

BACKWARD

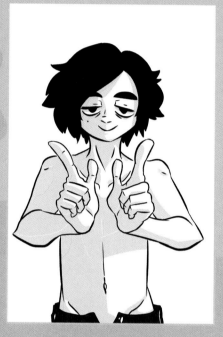

Fred Tornager is from Falster, Denmark.

Fred enjoys making cool comics, eating delicious food, and taking long walks while listening to music.

Fred would like to thank Fred for creating something great and also their dog for being a big supporter and constant source of love and loyalty.

The last place Fred got **naked** was in the shower, of course.

Tornager.com
twitter: @Freddietornager
instagram: @fred_tornager
tumblr: Freddie-tornager.tumblr.com

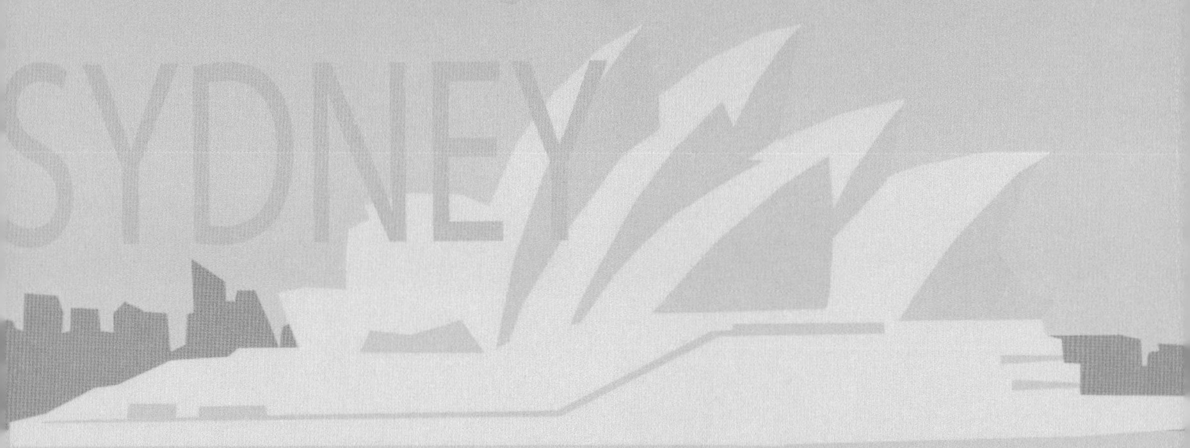

Thorbjørn (Thor) Petersen is from the Danish town of Viborg.

Thor enjoys drawing dynamic cartoon-action, doing martial arts, and spending time with his girlfriend.

Thor would like to thank all of his classmates, family, and friends for their support and encouragement in his pursuit to become a professional cartoonist and illustrator.

The last time Thor was naked was in the shower of his residence - a place where nobody is watching (he thinks, anyway!).

Thor has done E-book cover illustrations for Danish publishing house Lindhardt og Ringhof and has contributed to the professional comics anthology *Fiesta Magasinet*. He also does freelance logo and tattoo design.

artofthebear.carbonmade.com
tumblr: teebear-comix.tumblr.com

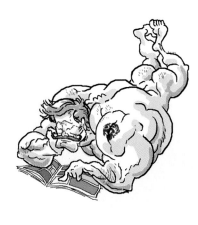

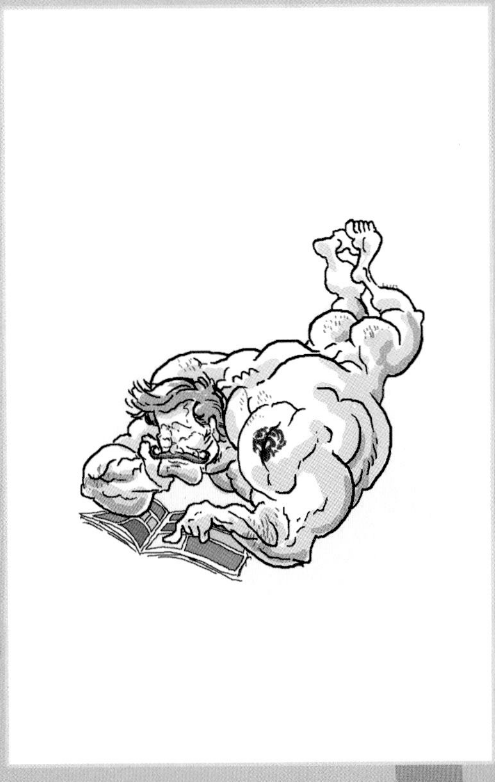

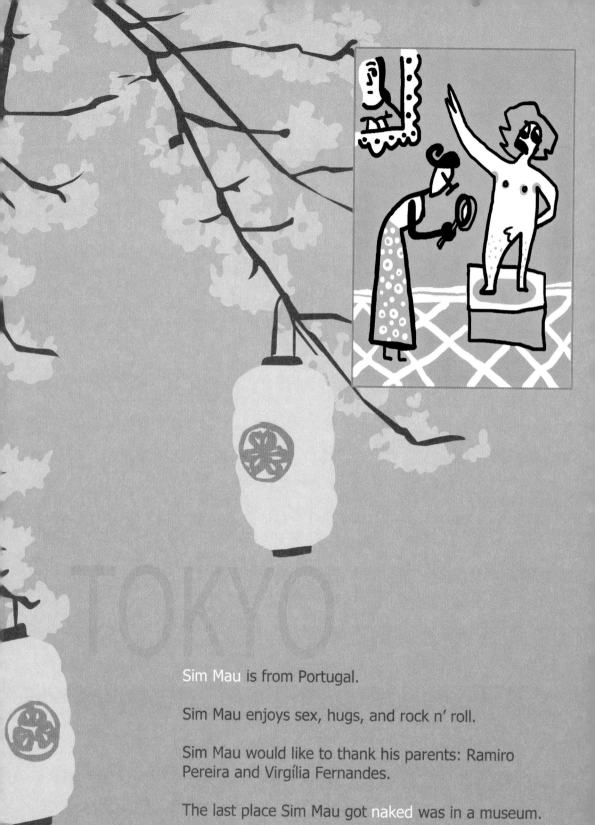

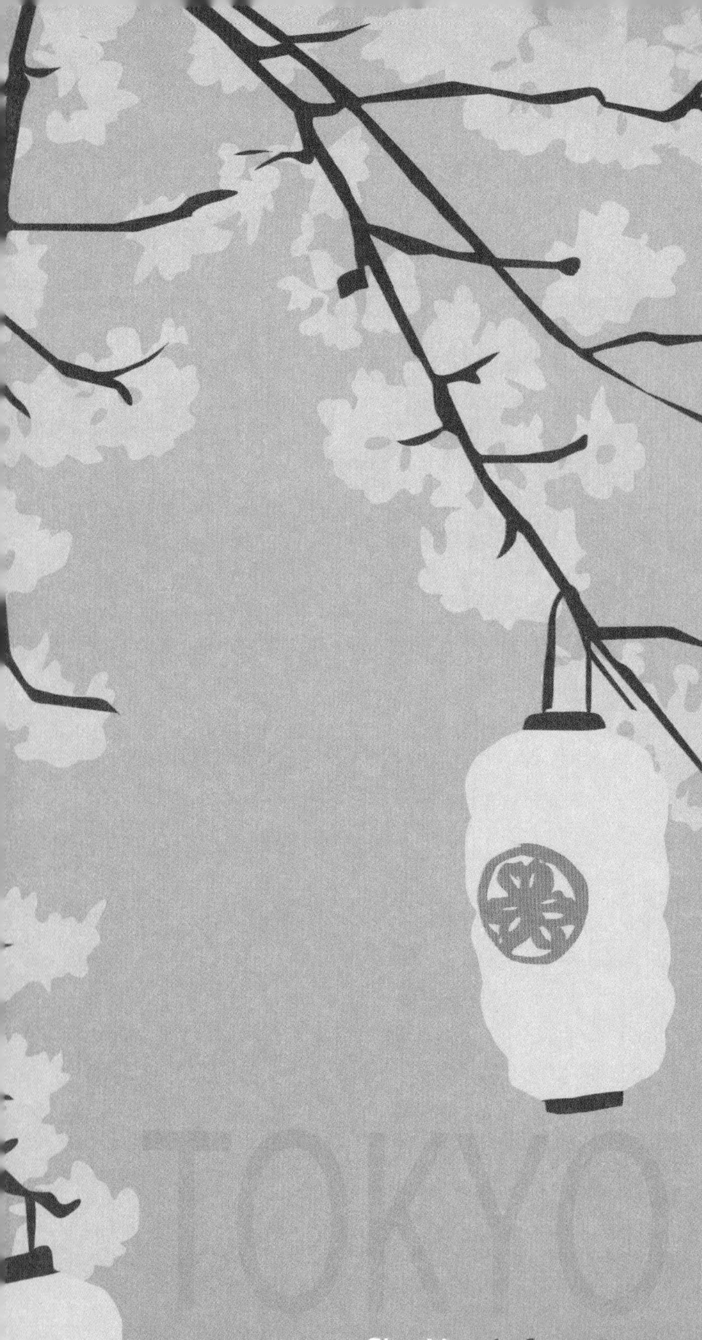
TOKYO

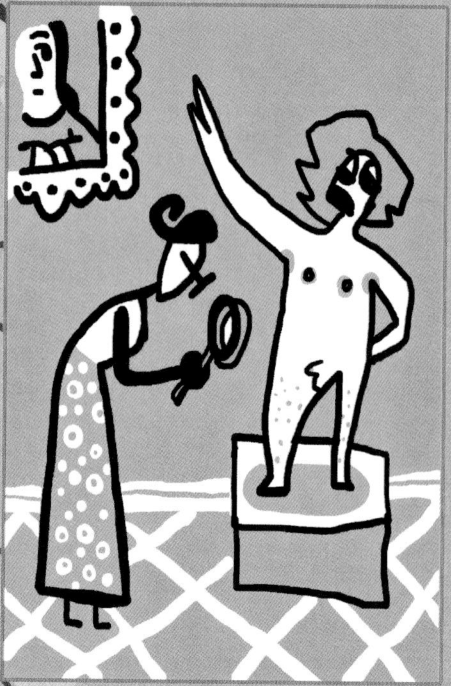

Sim Mau is from Portugal.

Sim Mau enjoys sex, hugs, and rock n' roll.

Sim Mau would like to thank his parents: Ramiro Pereira and Virgília Fernandes.

The last place Sim Mau got naked was in a museum.

Sim Mau's work has been presented in *Revista Gerador* #15 (Portugal)

twitter: @Sim_Mau_333
tumblr: sim-mau.tumblr.com
instagram: @sim_mau

ALICANTE

Rebekka Davidsen Hestbæk is from Nordskov, Denmark.

Rebekka enjoys ice cream, 80s music, and sleeping in.

Rebekka would like to thank her family for always supporting her.

The last place Rebekka got naked was just her ankles, but in that cold, she's never felt more nude.

Rebekka has previously worked on covers for children's books.

tumblr: rebekkadraws.tumblr.com

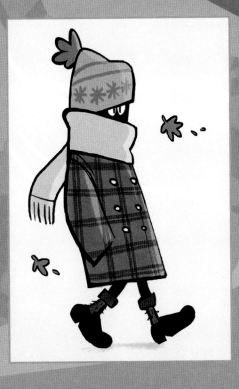

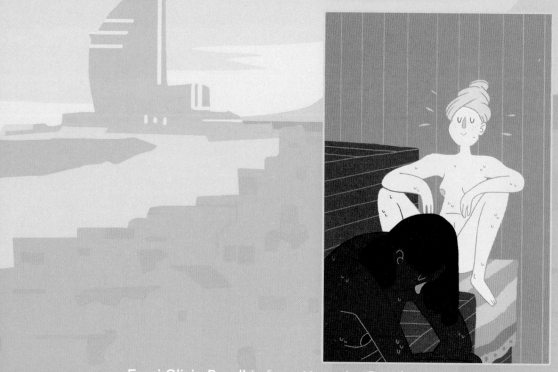

Emei Olivia Burell is from Uppsala, Sweden.

Emei enjoys Lindy Hop, pomelos, and bike rides.

Emei would like to thank her family, her friends at The Animation Workshop, and Erik Barkman.

The last place Emei got naked was in a Sauna, where she realized she had never been so comfortable getting naked as she is now.

Emei debuted her first graphic novel *Berättelser om Yunnan* in 2017. Her work has also appeared in *Adventure Time Comics*, *Hip Hop Family Tree*, *Studygroupcomics*, and a number of publications in Sweden, Denmark, the UK, and Chile.

emeiburell.strikingly.com
twitter: @emeiburell
instagram: @emeiburell
tumblr: @emeiburell
medium: @emeiburell
facebook: emeiart

BARCELONA

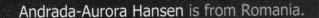

Andrada-Aurora Hansen is from Romania.

Aurora enjoys painting, hot tea, and eerie folk tales.

Aurora would like to thank her husband, Mark Hansen,
as well as her family and friends.

Aurora's work has previously appeared in *Roomies*
written by Karen vad Bruun.

The last place Aurora got naked was in preparation
for a shower in her bathroom
where she - incidentally - slipped and fell.

instagram: @ahansenart
tumbler: @ahansenart
twitter: @AuroraSketches

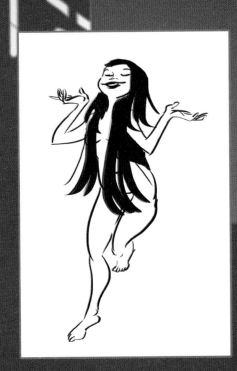

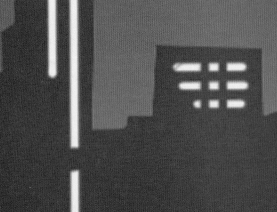

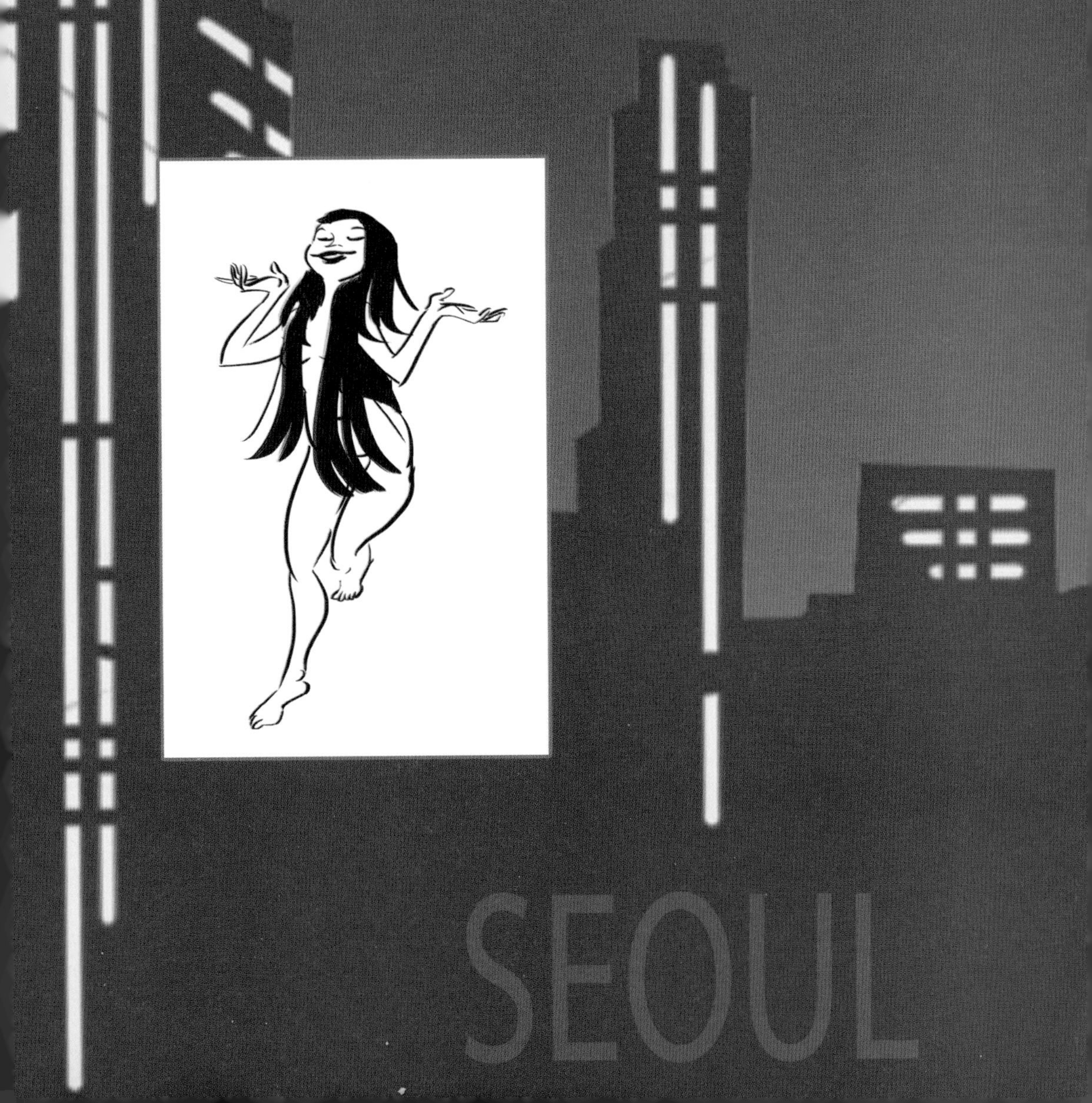

SEOUL

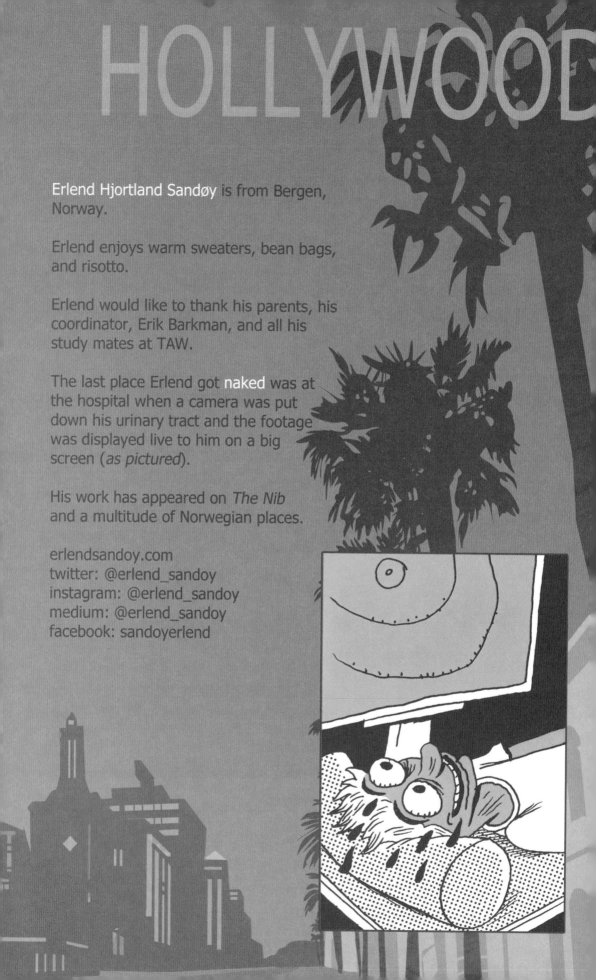

Erlend Hjortland Sandøy is from Bergen, Norway.

Erlend enjoys warm sweaters, bean bags, and risotto.

Erlend would like to thank his parents, his coordinator, Erik Barkman, and all his study mates at TAW.

The last place Erlend got naked was at the hospital when a camera was put down his urinary tract and the footage was displayed live to him on a big screen (*as pictured*).

His work has appeared on *The Nib* and a multitude of Norwegian places.

erlendsandoy.com
twitter: @erlend_sandoy
instagram: @erlend_sandoy
medium: @erlend_sandoy
facebook: sandoyerlend

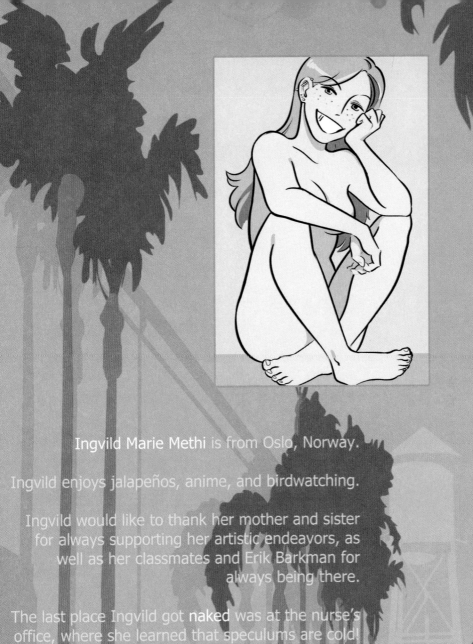

Ingvild Marie Methi is from Oslo, Norway.

Ingvild enjoys jalapeños, anime, and birdwatching.

Ingvild would like to thank her mother and sister for always supporting her artistic endeavors, as well as her classmates and Erik Barkman for always being there.

The last place Ingvild got naked was at the nurse's office, where she learned that speculums are cold!

Her work has appeared in various Norwegian comic magazines.

Immethi.strikingly.com
tumblr: immethi.tumblr.com

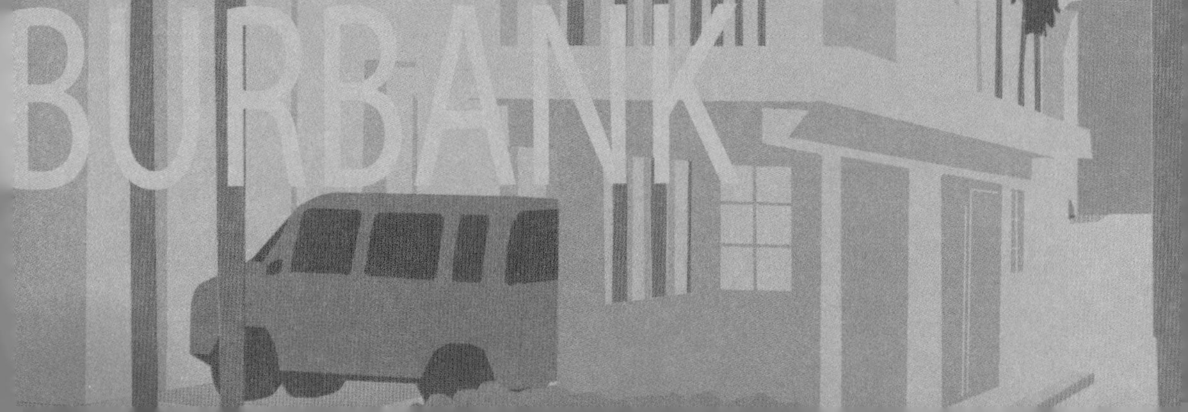

BURBANK

Thomas Vium is from Denmark.

Thomas enjoys nature, exploration, and paying attention to details around us.

Thomas would like to thank Naja.

The last place Thomas got "naked" was a few minutes ago when his daughter asked him yet another question about life he couldn't answer.

www.thomasvium.com

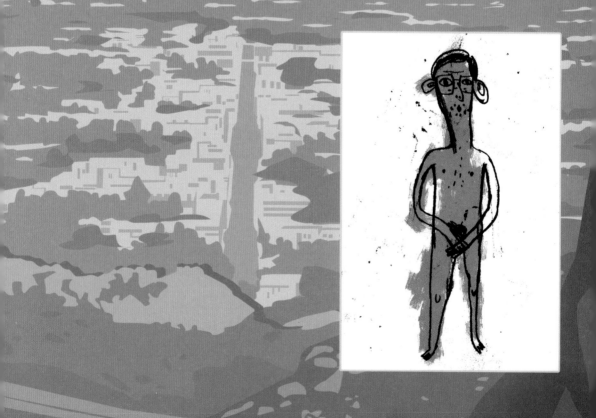

Christoffer Hammer is from Aalborg, Denmark.

Christoffer enjoys western cartoons, homemade food, and videogames.

Christoffer would like to thank his parents, his coorodinator Erik Barkman, and all his study mates at TAW.

The last place Christoffer was naked was in the men's shower at the local swimming hall in Viborg where he - by his own doing and without any help - got himself naked along with a bunch of other men he did not know.

More of his work can be found at:

christofferhammer.strikingly.com
mickeymonster.Deviantart
twitter: Christoffrrr

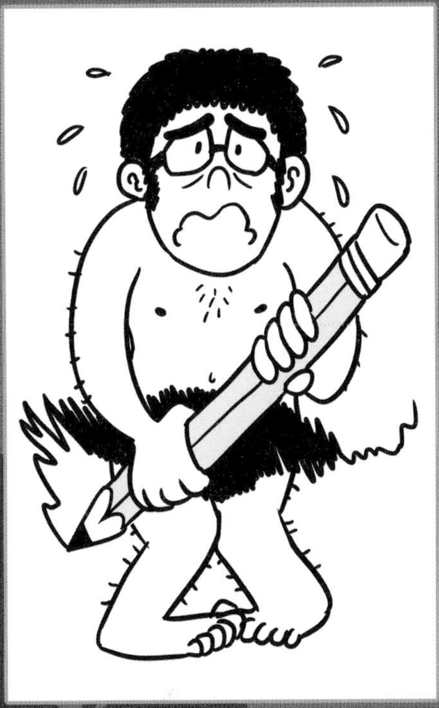

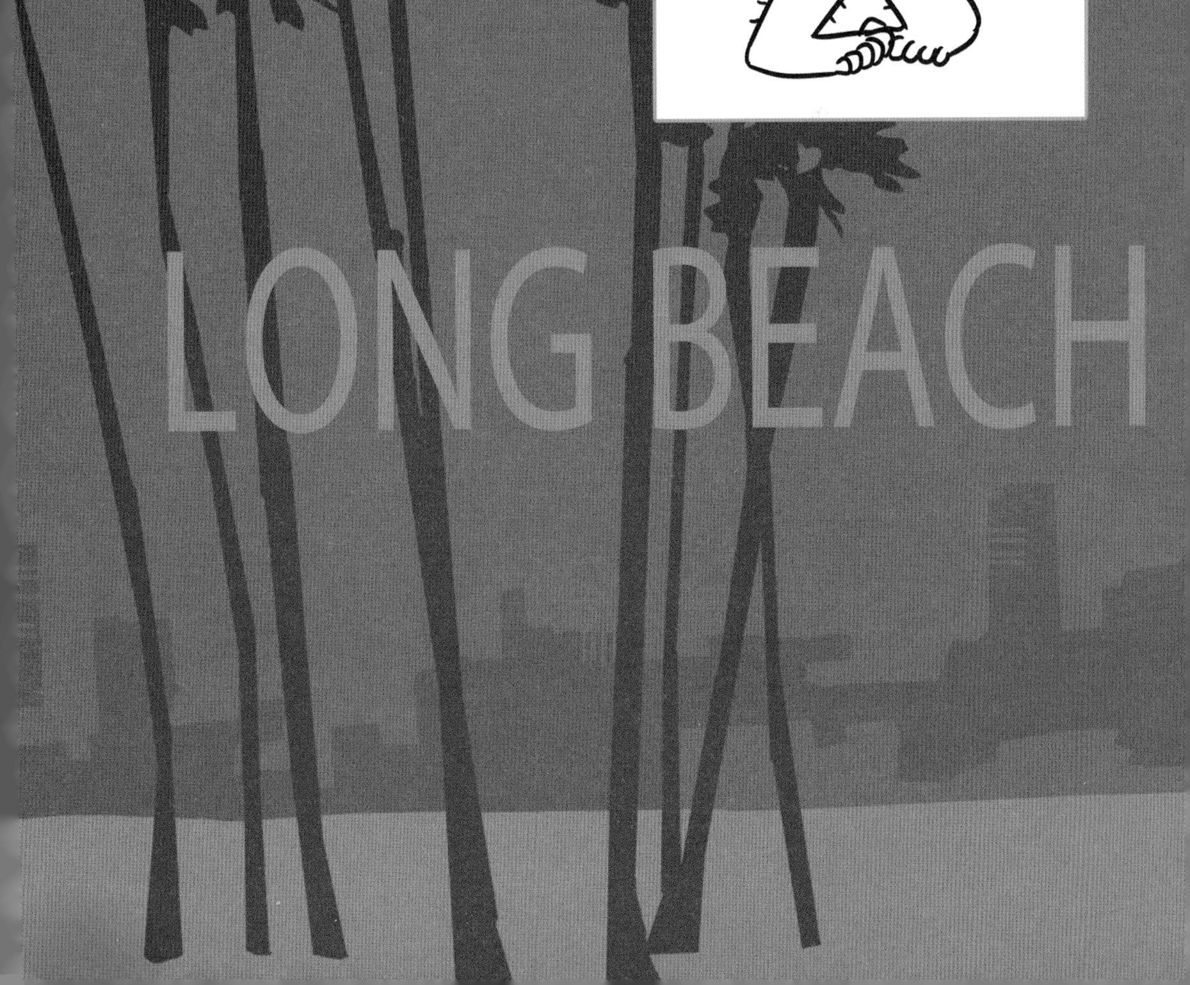
LONG BEACH

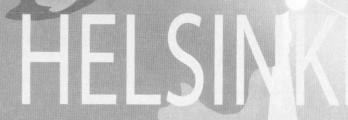

HELSINKI

Aske Rose stems from Hvidovre near Copenhagen.

He enjoys reading things he doesn't understand, cooking things he hasn't cooked, and listening to bands he's heard a billion times.

At the moment, Aske is in rural Canada and it is too cold to draw and write naked. So, the last time he was naked was at his bachelor party where his friends decided that they all had to be naked and he had to draw them.

AskeRose.carbonmade.com
instagram: @aske_rose

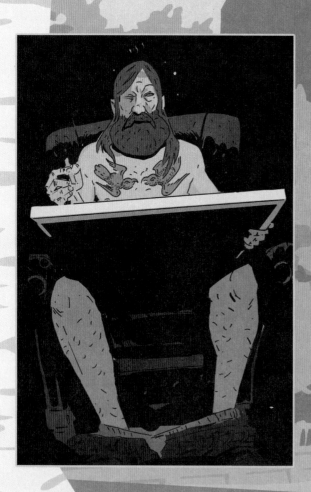

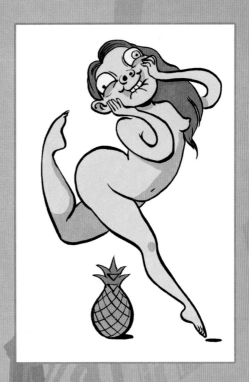

Silja Lin is from Denmark.

Silja enjoys pineapples, mermaids, and
psychological horror.

Silja would like to thank her classmates,
her boyfriend, Mark, and her former
coordinator, Erik Barkman
because they are all awesome.

The last place Silja got naked was in her
curtainless apartment.

www.siljalin.com
tumblr: siljalin.tumblr.com
instagram: siljalin
twitter: siljalin

TALLINN

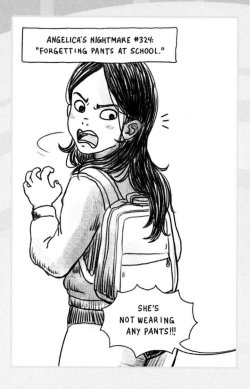

ANGELICA'S NIGHTMARE #324:
"FORGETTING PANTS AT SCHOOL."

SHE'S
NOT WEARING
ANY PANTS!!!

Angelica Inigo Jørgensen is from Vordingborg, Denmark.

Angelica enjoys gathering people for nice cozy dinners,
emotional YouTube videos, and making comics about people.

Angelica would like to thank her boyfriend, Rasmus Schwartz,
for always understanding when she's in her creative mode
by being a good listener and giving feedback while doing the
majority of household chores and massaging sore drawing muscles.

The last place Angelica got naked was at the doctor when she
accepted the offer for preventative examination against cervical
cancer and the doctor assured her that the camera used to record
conversations was off. She still has her doubts.

Her work has appeared in an issue of *Hip Hop Family Tree*
as well as the publishing houses Forlaget Pronto and Forlaget M
ellemgaard in Denmark.

twitter: @angie_inigo
instagram: @angie_inigo
tumblr: artbyangelica.tumblr.com
www.angelicainigo.dk

BALTIC SEA

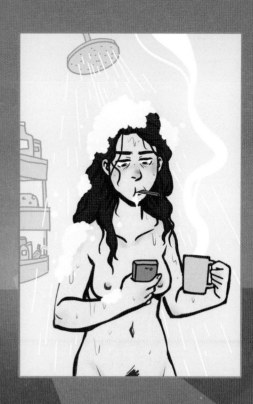

Tina Burholt is from Aalborg, Denmark.

Tina enjoys making food, eating, and chilling in bed.

Tina would like to thank her partner, Mikkel, her family and friends, and the people at TAW.

The last place Tina got **naked** was under the shower one stressful morning while efficiently multitasking.

instagram: artleysart
strikingly: artleysart
facebook: artleysart
artstation: artley
twitter: tinaburholt

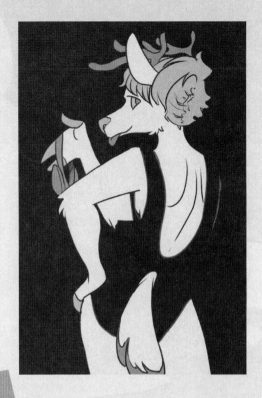

Hope Hjort is from Næstved, Denmark.

Hope enjoys cakes, fat birds, and snowy nights.

Hope would like to thank her parents, her dog,
and all the friends at TAW.

The last place Hope got naked was just before
she nearly drowned herself trying to save a kid's
swimming goggles in the deep end of the pool.

Hope has an ongoing comic on tapastic.

Hopehjort.strikingly.com
Dearhopedeer.tumblr.com
Tapas.io/series/FETCHcomic
twitter: @hopehjort
instagram: @hopehjort

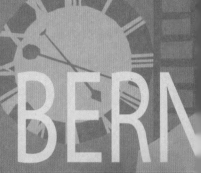

Bob Lundgreen Kristiansen is from Hirtshals, Denmark.

Bob enjoys organic monsters, meat, and mead.

Bob would like to thank his gods, Lilja, and the infinities of the neverending cosmos.

The Last place Bob got naked was years ago in a thunderstorm on top of a mountain in Vermont.

More of Bob's work can be found in Danish anthologies, the next issue of *Standart* and on social media.

www.Blk.gallery
instagram: @bobkristiansen
tumblr: boblk.tumblr.com

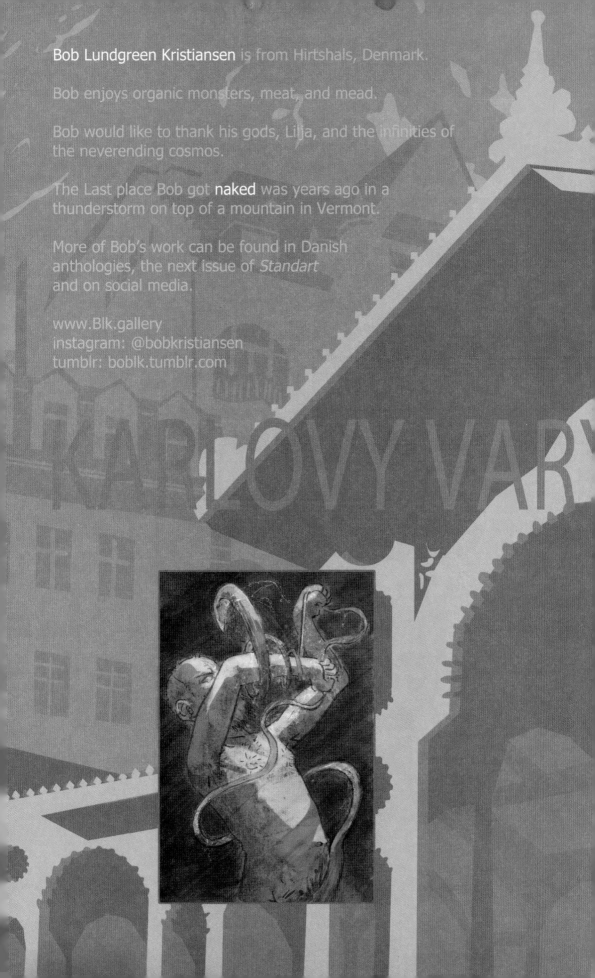

Cecilie "Q" Maintz Thorsen is from
Copenhagen, Denmark.

Q enjoys hugs, singing, and that
one week of Danish summer.

Q would like to thank her whole
family, her really cool classmates,
and the orange cat that left a dead
bird on her doorstep last week.

The last place Q got naked was in
the showers at her local gym,
where she is often reminded that
humans – contrary to popular
media belief – have different shapes
and sizes and all of them are good.

CecilieQ.strikingly.com
tumblr: CecilieQ.tumblr.com
twitter: @QCecilie
instagram: @Q_Cecilie

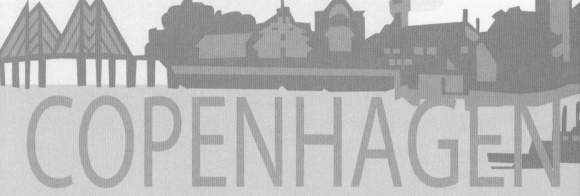

COPENHAGEN

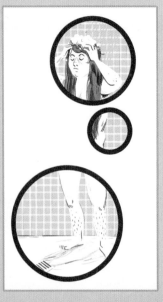

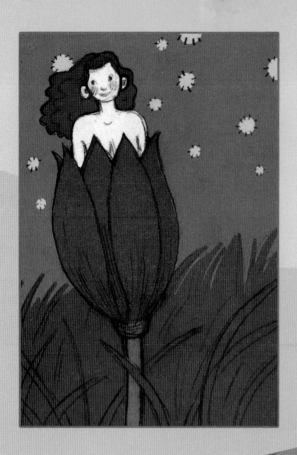

Patricia Amalie Eckerle grew up in a small village in the Black Forest, south Germany.

She enjoys coincidences, putting on newly knitted socks, and biking trough fog.

Patricia would like to thank Pascal for all the love and support.

The last time Patricia got naked was at a little summer house in Sweden close to a lake where there were no people around - just beautiful nature which made her feel like she was a fairy.

Patriciaamalieeckerle.com
tumblr: Patriciaamalie.tumblr.com
twitter:@PatriciaAmalie
instagram:@patricia_amalie

FORWARD

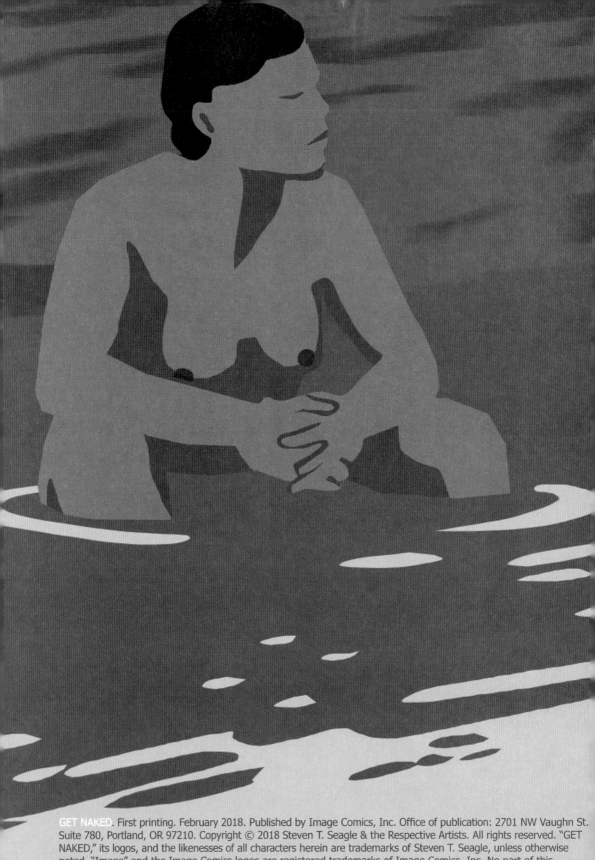

GET NAKED. First printing. February 2018. Published by Image Comics, Inc. Office of publication: 2701 NW Vaughn St. Suite 780, Portland, OR 97210. Copyright © 2018 Steven T. Seagle & the Respective Artists. All rights reserved. "GET NAKED," its logos, and the likenesses of all characters herein are trademarks of Steven T. Seagle, unless otherwise noted. "Image" and the Image Comics logos are registered trademarks of Image Comics, Inc. No part of this publication may be reproduced or transmitted, in any form or by any means (except for short excerpts for journalisti or review purposes), without the express written permission of Steven T. Seagle, or Image Comics, Inc. All names, characters, events, and locales in this publication are entirely fictional. Any resemblance to actual persons (living or dead), events, or places, without satiric intent, is coincidental. Printed in the USA. For information regarding the CPSIA on this printed material call: 203-595-3636 and provide reference #RICH–772939. For international rights, contact: foreignlicensing@imagecomics.com. ISBN: 978-1-5343-0480-2.

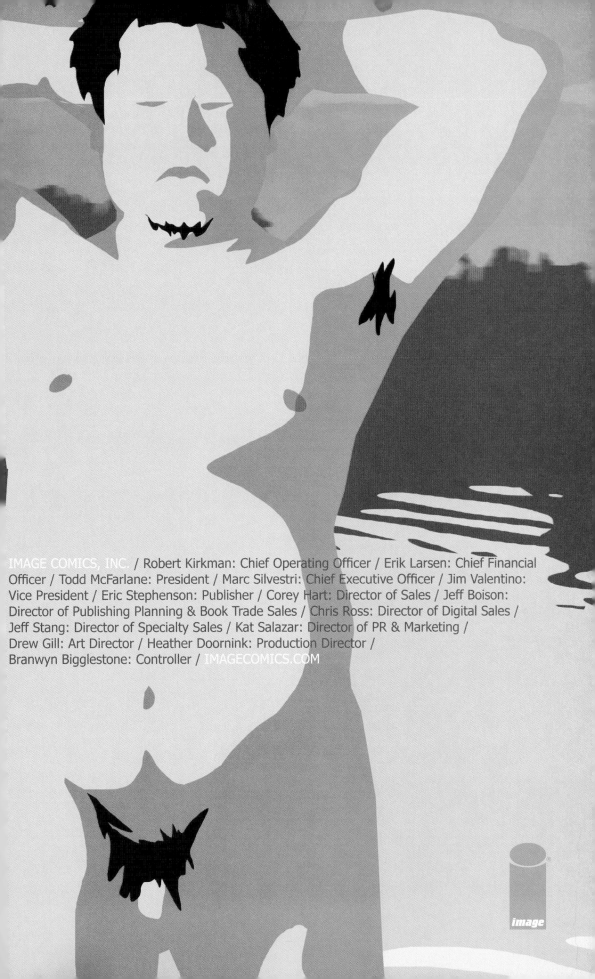

IMAGE COMICS, INC. / Robert Kirkman: Chief Operating Officer / Erik Larsen: Chief Financial Officer / Todd McFarlane: President / Marc Silvestri: Chief Executive Officer / Jim Valentino: Vice President / Eric Stephenson: Publisher / Corey Hart: Director of Sales / Jeff Boison: Director of Publishing Planning & Book Trade Sales / Chris Ross: Director of Digital Sales / Jeff Stang: Director of Specialty Sales / Kat Salazar: Director of PR & Marketing / Drew Gill: Art Director / Heather Doornink: Production Director / Branwyn Bigglestone: Controller / IMAGECOMICS.COM

"In order to swim, one takes off all one's clothes. In order to aspire to the truth, one must undress in a far more inward sense, divest oneself of all one's inward clothes, of thoughts, conceptions, selfishness etc., before one is sufficiently naked."

Søren Kierkegaard

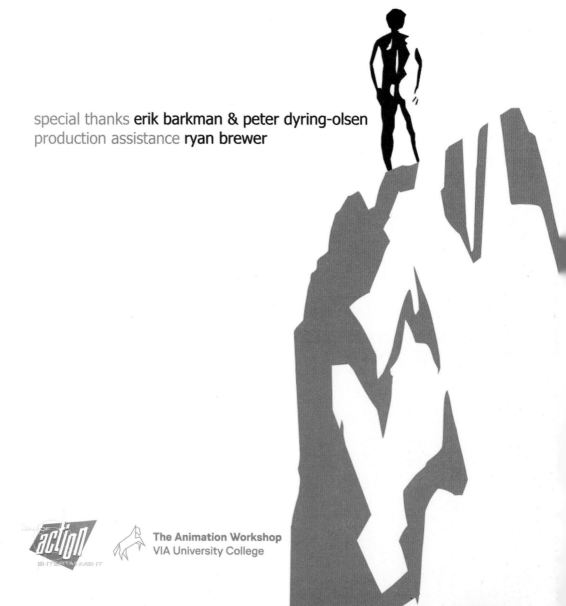

special thanks **erik barkman & peter dyring-olsen**
production assistance **ryan brewer**

The Animation Workshop
VIA University College